Advanced Therapy Medicinal Products for Eye Diseases

Advanced Therapy Medicinal Products for Eye Diseases: Goals and Challenges

Editors

Yolanda Diebold
Laura García-Posadas

MDPI • Basel • Beijing • Wuhan • Barcelona • Belgrade • Manchester • Tokyo • Cluj • Tianjin

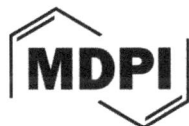

Editors
Yolanda Diebold
Intituto de Oftalmobiología
Aplicada (IOBA)
Universidad de Valladolid
Valladolid
Spain

Laura García-Posadas
Instituto de Oftalmobiología
Aplicada
Universidad de Valladolid
Valladolid
Spain

Editorial Office
MDPI
St. Alban-Anlage 66
4052 Basel, Switzerland

This is a reprint of articles from the Special Issue published online in the open access journal *Pharmaceutics* (ISSN 1999-4923) (available at: www.mdpi.com/journal/pharmaceutics/special_issues/eye_diseases_therapy).

For citation purposes, cite each article independently as indicated on the article page online and as indicated below:

LastName, A.A.; LastName, B.B.; LastName, C.C. Article Title. *Journal Name* **Year**, *Volume Number*, Page Range.

ISBN 978-3-0365-2611-9 (Hbk)
ISBN 978-3-0365-2610-2 (PDF)

© 2021 by the authors. Articles in this book are Open Access and distributed under the Creative Commons Attribution (CC BY) license, which allows users to download, copy and build upon published articles, as long as the author and publisher are properly credited, which ensures maximum dissemination and a wider impact of our publications.

The book as a whole is distributed by MDPI under the terms and conditions of the Creative Commons license CC BY-NC-ND.

Contents

Preface to "Advanced Therapy Medicinal Products for Eye Diseases: Goals and Challenges" . vii

Yolanda Diebold and Laura García-Posadas
Advanced Therapy Medicinal Products for Eye Diseases: Goals and Challenges
Reprinted from: *Pharmaceutics* 2021, *13*, 1819, doi:10.3390/pharmaceutics13111819 1

Marina López-Paniagua, Ana de la Mata, Sara Galindo, Francisco Blázquez, Margarita Calonge and Teresa Nieto-Miguel
Advanced Therapy Medicinal Products for the Eye: Definitions and Regulatory Framework
Reprinted from: *Pharmaceutics* 2021, *13*, 347, doi:10.3390/pharmaceutics13030347 5

Margarita Calonge, Teresa Nieto-Miguel, Ana de la Mata, Sara Galindo, José M. Herreras and Marina López-Paniagua
Goals and Challenges of Stem Cell-Based Therapy for Corneal Blindness Due to Limbal Deficiency
Reprinted from: *Pharmaceutics* 2021, *13*, 1483, doi:10.3390/pharmaceutics13091483 23

Yolanda Diebold and Laura García-Posadas
Is the Conjunctiva a Potential Target for Advanced Therapy Medicinal Products?
Reprinted from: *Pharmaceutics* 2021, *13*, 1140, doi:10.3390/pharmaceutics13081140 57

Rosa M. Coco-Martin, Salvador Pastor-Idoate and Jose Carlos Pastor
Cell Replacement Therapy for Retinal and Optic Nerve Diseases: Cell Sources, Clinical Trials and Challenges
Reprinted from: *Pharmaceutics* 2021, *13*, 865, doi:10.3390/pharmaceutics13060865 71

Promita Bhattacharjee and Mark Ahearne
Significance of Crosslinking Approaches in the Development of Next Generation Hydrogels for Corneal Tissue Engineering
Reprinted from: *Pharmaceutics* 2021, *13*, 319, doi:10.3390/pharmaceutics13030319 97

Noriaki Nagai, Shunsuke Sakurai, Ryotaro Seiriki, Misa Minami, Mizuki Yamaguchi, Saori Deguchi and Eiji Harata
MPC Polymer Promotes Recovery from Dry Eye via Stabilization of the Ocular Surface
Reprinted from: *Pharmaceutics* 2021, *13*, 168, doi:10.3390/pharmaceutics13020168 121

Sandra Ruiz-Alonso, Ilia Villate-Beitia, Idoia Gallego, Markel Lafuente-Merchan, Gustavo Puras, Laura Saenz-del-Burgo and José Luis Pedraz
Current Insights into 3D Bioprinting: An Advanced Approach for Eye Tissue Regeneration
Reprinted from: *Pharmaceutics* 2021, *13*, 308, doi:10.3390/pharmaceutics13030308 133

Lucy A. Bosworth, Kyle G. Doherty, James D. Hsuan, Samuel P. Cray, Raechelle A. D'Sa, Catalina Pineda Molina, Stephen F. Badylak and Rachel L. Williams
Material Characterisation and Stratification of Conjunctival Epithelial Cells on Electrospun Poly(-Caprolactone) Fibres Loaded with Decellularised Tissue Matrices
Reprinted from: *Pharmaceutics* 2021, *13*, 318, doi:10.3390/pharmaceutics13030318 161

Mohammad Mirazul Islam, Dina B. AbuSamra, Alexandru Chivu, Pablo Argüeso, Claes H. Dohlman, Hirak K. Patra, James Chodosh and Miguel González-Andrades
Optimization of Collagen Chemical Crosslinking to Restore Biocompatibility of Tissue-Engineered Scaffolds
Reprinted from: *Pharmaceutics* 2021, *13*, 832, doi:10.3390/pharmaceutics13060832 181

David Sánchez-Porras, Manuel Caro-Magdaleno, Carmen González-Gallardo, Óscar Darío García-García, Ingrid Garzón, Víctor Carriel, Fernando Campos and Miguel Alaminos
Generation of a Biomimetic Substitute of the Corneal Limbus Using Decellularized Scaffolds
Reprinted from: *Pharmaceutics* **2021**, *13*, 1718, doi:10.3390/pharmaceutics13101718 . . . . **197**

Preface to "Advanced Therapy Medicinal Products for Eye Diseases: Goals and Challenges"

The concept of advanced therapy medicinal products (ATMPs) encompasses novel kinds of medicines for human use that are based on genes, cells or tissues. These intend to offer not only regeneration, but complete functional recovery of diseased tissues and organs using different strategies. Gene therapy, cell therapy and tissue engineering are the main areas in which promising advanced therapies are emerging. The eye is a very complex organ whose main structures, the cornea and the retina, play a pivotal role in maintaining normal vision, as severe alterations in these tissues can lead to blindness. Ocular tissues are starting to benefit from ATMPs by fighting against the enormous complexity and devastating potential of many ocular diseases. However, developments arising from this field of work face important challenges related to vectors to deliver drugs and genetic material to target tissues, suitable biomaterials to prepare cell scaffolds and cell stemness, among others—not to mention the complicated legislation around ATMPs, the complexity in production and quality control and the absence of standardized protocols.

The purpose of this Special Issue is to serve as an overview of the current progress in the application of cell and gene therapies, as well as tissue engineering to restore functionality in diseased ocular structures, and the challenges they deal with in order to get to patients.

Yolanda Diebold, Laura García-Posadas
Editors

Editorial

Advanced Therapy Medicinal Products for Eye Diseases: Goals and Challenges

Yolanda Diebold [1,2,*] and Laura García-Posadas [1]

1. Ocular Surface Group, Instituto de Oftalmobiología Aplicada (IOBA), Universidad de Valladolid, 47011 Valladolid, Spain; lgarciap@ioba.med.uva.es
2. Centro de Investigación Biomédica en Red de Bioingeniería, Biomateriales y Nanomedicina (CIBER-BBN), Instituto de Salud Carlos III, 28029 Madrid, Spain
* Correspondence: yol@ioba.med.uva.es

Advanced therapy medicinal products (ATMPs) are a novel class of medicines with enormous potential to improve treatments for a wide range of diseases, including those affecting eye structures. The purpose of ATMPs is to replace or regenerate human cells, tissues, or even organs to restore their normal functions. These complex biological products mainly include gene therapies, somatic cell-based therapies, and tissue-engineered products; the last two are frequently referred to as regenerative medicine. The development of ATMPs is scientifically challenging, but assessment of their clinical success in actual patients is even a more difficult goal to achieve. This fact partly accounts for the low numbers of ATMPs in the market.

The eye is a suitable organ to apply ATMPs for different reasons such as small dimensions, compartmentalized anatomical structure, and good accessibility for treatments, among others; however, there are few examples of ATMPs specific for ocular diseases. Eye structures pose specific challenges which make it difficult for basic and clinical scientists to develop this kind of complex medicines and successfully reach the clinical trial phase.

The aim of this Special Issue is to provide an overview of the current progress in the application of ATMPs to restore functionality in diseased ocular structures. An additional aim is to update the challenges that this novel class of medicines must deal with to effectively reach patients. A series of four research and six review articles is brought together to provide updated information about some of those challenges. Authors who kindly contributed are well-known experts in pre-clinical or clinical research involving the development of ATMPs for the eye, and some of them pioneered their application for specific ocular diseases.

López-Paniagua M. et al. [1] analyze the characteristics that make the eye an ideal organ to receive ATMPs. In their comprehensive review paper, these authors identify all groups of ATMPs according to the European Medicines Agency and deal with the legal framework that regulates their development and classification in the European Union. Regulatory principles associated with this type of innovative medicinal products are revised using specific examples for the treatment of eye diseases.

Cell-based therapy for eye diseases is one of the most successful examples of current regenerative medicine. Two excellent review papers deal with this aspect of ATMPs, one of them focused on cell therapy for diseases leading to corneal blindness [2] and the other one on cell replacement for retinal or optic nerve degeneration [3]. Calonge M. et al. [2] present the goals and challenges of stem cell-based therapy to treat corneal blindness caused by limbal stem cell deficiency, which affects the stem cell niche located at the corneal limbus. This review paper revises the challenges related to the development of cell-based products for the anterior part of the eye and the importance of the close interaction between basic and clinical scientists to succeed. On the other hand, Coco-Martin R. et al. [3] focus their review in the posterior part of the eye, specifically in the potential of cell therapies to restore or replace damaged and/or lost cells in retinal degenerative and optic nerve diseases. The authors describe the available cell sources and the challenges involved in the development of such treatments. They also present those issues that remain to be solved concerning the clinical translation of cell-based therapy for the retina, such as specific retinal subtypes enrichment, cell survival and cell delivery to the target site, and the evaluation of the risk of tumor formation caused by transplanted cells.

The conjunctiva is an underestimated yet incredibly important tissue in maintaining ocular surface homeostasis and contributes to eye protection. Diebold Y. and García-Posadas L. [4] evidence in their review paper how the conjunctiva would benefit from ATMP development because of the relevant pathology that impairs the ocular surface by affecting this tissue. They also provide readers with promising pre-clinical examples mostly oriented to cell therapy and tissue engineering.

Biomaterials are key elements to consider for tissue-engineered products because of their tunable properties. They are used to prepare scaffolds suitable to support cells in 3D tissue equivalents, to deliver active agents, or even to provide tissues with beneficial properties by themselves. Hydrogels are currently being investigated with great interest for ocular tissue-engineering applications. In the eye, the cornea is a good candidate to explore the biocompatibility, mechanical properties, and chemical structure of hydrogels for corneal replacement in different pathologies. Bhattacharjee and Ahearne [5] explore in their review paper different aspects of hydrogel crosslinking for corneal tissue engineering and repair. Issues such as crosslinking techniques, crosslinking chemical additives, and factors influencing crosslinking success including immunogenicity and toxicity are discussed, as well as the limitations and prospects of crosslinking strategies in this field. The research article by Nagai N. et al. [6] present a novel biopolymer (MPCP) with hydrating properties that helps to normalize the tear film in an animal model of the severe immune-based, inflammatory disorder that impairs the homeostasis of the ocular surface known as dry eye disease. Using a specific polymerization procedure, MPCP polymer enhanced tear film volume and prolonged the tear film breakup time in disease animal, indicating promising therapeutic properties.

Another example of advanced therapy is the 3D bioprinting of eye tissues that allows the construction of scaffolds from different biomaterials in which appropriate cell types are incorporated in a custom-fabricated way. Ruiz-Alonso S. et al. [7] update the application of this revolutionary technology to the ocular tissue regeneration field, paying special attention to the manufacture of relevant ocular tissues such as cornea, retina, and conjunctiva in preclinical studies. Issues related to current bioprinting methods and ethical and regulatory aspects are also analyzed.

Other experimental approaches to the design and potential application of biopolymeric scaffolds for ocular tissue regeneration in the context of diverse pathologies are explored in a series of three original research articles. One first approach is the fabrication of fiber scaffolds using the electrospinning technique for conjunctiva regeneration. Bosworth L. A. et al. [8] explored the potential of electrospun scaffolds composed from poly (ε-caprolactone) and decellularized tissue matrices, such as small intestinal submucosa or urinary bladder, to culture human conjunctival epithelial cells and induce their stratification at the air/liquid interface. The bioactive scaffolds created induced an in vitro cell response in terms of changes in cell morphology and stratification. Islam M. M. et al. [9] proposed a double-crosslinking manufacturing approach to fabricate collagen scaffolds with improved mechanical and functional properties, as well as cell biocompatibility. This novel approach would facilitate the use of collagen-based implants in corneal regeneration. Finally, Sánchez-Porras D. et al. [10] evaluated four different protocols to decellularize porcine limbus and further recellularize them with a limbal epithelial cell line and human adipose-derived mesenchymal stem cells. Limbal substitutes generated maintained transparency and other specific limbal characteristics, preliminarily indicating a potential for their use in limbal tissue regeneration.

We would like to thank all the participants in this Special Issue (authors, reviewers, and assistant editors, especially Mr. Albert Yang) for their rigorous work that allowed us to provide the scientific community with an updated collection of research papers and reviews about ATMPs for eye diseases. We hope the readers find their contents useful.

Funding: This research was funded by the Ministerio de Ciencia, Innovación y Universidades (MCIU, Government of Spain), Agencia Estatal de Investigación (AEI, Government of Spain), and the Fondo Europeo de Desarrollo Regional (FEDER), grant number RTI2018–094071-B-C21. L.G.-P. is funded by the Postdoctoral contracts 2017 call (University of Valladolid, Spain).

Conflicts of Interest: The authors declare no conflict of interest.

References

1. López-Paniagua, M.; de la Mata, A.; Galindo, S.; Blázquez, F.; Calonge, M.; Nieto-Miguel, T. Advanced therapy medicinal products for the eye: Definitions and regulatory framework. *Pharmaceutics* **2021**, *13*, 347. [CrossRef] [PubMed]
2. Calonge, M.; Nieto-Miguel, T.; de la Mata, A.; Galindo, S.; Herreras, J.M.; López-Paniagua, M. Goals and challenges of stem cell-based therapy for corneal blindness due to limbal deficiency. *Pharmaceutics* **2021**, *13*, 1483. [CrossRef] [PubMed]
3. Coco-Martin, R.M.; Pastor-Idoate, S.; Pastor, J.C. Cell replacement therapy for retinal and optic nerve diseases: Cell sources, clinical trials and challenges. *Pharmaceutics* **2021**, *13*, 865. [CrossRef] [PubMed]
4. Diebold, Y.; García-Posadas, L. Is the conjunctiva a potential target for advanced therapy medicinal products? *Pharmaceutics* **2021**, *13*, 1140. [CrossRef]
5. Bhattacharjee, P.; Ahearne, M. Significance of crosslinking approaches in the development of next generation hydrogels for corneal tissue engineering. *Pharmaceutics* **2021**, *13*, 319. [CrossRef] [PubMed]
6. Nagai, N.; Sakurai, S.; Seiriki, R.; Minami, M.; Yamaguchi, M.; Deguchi, S.; Harata, E. MPC polymer promotes recovery from dry eye via stabilization of the ocular surface. *Pharmaceutics* **2021**, *13*, 168. [CrossRef] [PubMed]
7. Ruiz-alonso, S.; Villate-beitia, I.; Gallego, I.; Lafuente-merchan, M.; Puras, G.; Saenz-del-burgo, L.; Pedraz, J.L. Current insights into 3D bioprinting: An advanced approach for eye tissue regeneration. *Pharmaceutics* **2021**, *13*, 308. [CrossRef] [PubMed]
8. Bosworth, L.A.; Doherty, K.G.; Hsuan, J.D.; Cray, S.P.; D'sa, R.A.; Molina, C.P.; Badylak, S.F.; Williams, R.L. Material characterisation and stratification of conjunctival epithelial cells on electrospun poly(ε-caprolactone) fibres loaded with decellularised tissue matrices. *Pharmaceutics* **2021**, *13*, 318. [CrossRef] [PubMed]
9. Islam, M.M.; Abusamra, D.B.; Chivu, A.; Argüeso, P.; Dohlman, C.H.; Patra, H.K.; Chodosh, J.; González-Andrades, M. Optimization of collagen chemical crosslinking to restore biocompatibility of tissue-engineered scaffolds. *Pharmaceutics* **2021**, *13*, 832. [CrossRef] [PubMed]
10. Sánchez-Porras, D.; Caro-Magdaleno, M.; González-Gallardo, C.; Garcia-Garcia, Ó.D.; Garzón, I.; Carriel, V.; Campos, F.; Alaminos, M. Generation of a biomimetic substitute of the corneal limbus using decellularized scaffolds. *Pharmaceutics* **2021**, *13*, 1718. [CrossRef] [PubMed]

Review

Advanced Therapy Medicinal Products for the Eye: Definitions and Regulatory Framework

Marina López-Paniagua [1,2,3,†], Ana de la Mata [1,2,3,†], Sara Galindo [1,2,3,†], Francisco Blázquez [4], Margarita Calonge [1,2,3,‡] and Teresa Nieto-Miguel [1,2,3,*,‡]

1. Ocular Surface Group, Instituto de Oftalmobiología Aplicada (IOBA), University of Valladolid, Campus Miguel Delibes, Paseo de Belén 17, 47011 Valladolid, Spain; marina@ioba.med.uva.es (M.L.-P.); adelamatas@ioba.med.uva.es (A.d.l.M.); sgalindor@ioba.med.uva.es (S.G.); calonge@ioba.med.uva.es (M.C.)
2. Centro de Investigación Biomédica en Red de Bioingeniería, Biomateriales y Nanomedicina (CIBER-BBN), Instituto de Salud Carlos III, 28029 Madrid, Spain
3. Centro en Red de Medicina Regenerativa y Terapia Celular de Castilla y León, 47007 Valladolid, Spain
4. Clinical Trials Unit, Instituto de Oftalmobiología Aplicada (IOBA), University of Valladolid, Campus Miguel Delibes, Paseo de Belén 17, 47011 Valladolid, Spain; blazquez@ioba.med.uva.es
* Correspondence: tnietom@ioba.med.uva.es
† These authors contributed equally to this work.
‡ Co-senior authors.

Abstract: Advanced therapy medicinal products (ATMPs) are a group of innovative and complex biological products for human use that comprises somatic cell therapy medicinal products, tissue engineered products, gene therapy medicinal products, and the so-called combined ATMPs that consist of one of the previous three categories combined with one or more medical devices. During the last few years, the development of ATMPs for the treatment of eye diseases has become a fast-growing field as it offers the potential to find novel therapeutic approaches for treating pathologies that today have no cure or are just subjected to symptomatic treatments. Therefore, it is important for all professionals working in this field to be familiar with the regulatory principles associated with these types of innovative products. In this review, we outline the legal framework that regulates the development of ATMPs in the European Union and other international jurisdictions, and the criteria that each type of ATMP must meet to be classified as such. To illustrate each legal definition, ATMPs that have already completed the research and development stages and that are currently used for the treatment of eye diseases are presented as examples.

Keywords: advanced therapy medicinal product; ATMP; cell therapy; tissue engineering; gene therapy; eye; ocular; ophthalmology; regulatory; marketing authorization

1. Introduction

Advanced therapy medicinal products (ATMPs) are a large and diverse group of therapeutic agents for human use. They consist of somatic cell therapy medicinal products (sCTMPs), tissue engineered products (TEPs), gene therapy medicinal products (GTMPs), and the so-called combined ATMPs (cATMPs) that include one of the previous three categories combined with one or more medical devices as an integral part of the product [1].

As with other existing and often less-complex medicinal products, ATMPs must meet the same high standards for scientific, methodological, and regulatory requirements: (1) the safety and efficacy must be demonstrated through both preclinical studies and human clinical trials. Human trials must be designed and conducted following European Union (EU) regulation No. 536/2014 and comply with the principles of good clinical practice (GCP) as stated in Commission Directive 2005/28/EC [2,3]; (2) production must comply with the principles of good manufacturing practices (GMP) [4]; and (3) standard post-authorization and pharmacovigilance requirements must be met [5]. Unlike other more common drugs, ATMPs are medicinal products with a very high degree of complexity that are associated with not only their composition, but also with all of the processes that are necessary for proper development, i.e., manufacturing, characterization, and marketing authorization. Due to the complex nature of ATMPs, they are generating great scientific, clinical, and regulatory challenges for all linked professionals, including researchers, clinicians, developers, and regulators [6].

In the EU, the legal framework for ATMPs is regulated by the European Medicines Agency (EMA), established to guarantee that all products classified as ATMPs were subjected to the proper regulatory assessment prior to clinical and commercial use [1]. A key point in the introduction of ATMP regulation was the establishment of the Committee for Advanced Therapies (CAT) in 2009. The CAT is a multidisciplinary body within the EMA that is responsible for ATMP classification; assessment of quality, safety, and efficacy; performing primary evaluation of marketing authorization applications; and monitoring all of the scientific advancements of the field [7].

The field of ATMPs is currently at the forefront of innovation as it offers novel therapeutic approaches for the treatment of pathologies that, at present, have limited or no effective alternatives. ATMPs hold the potential of curing or preventing the progression of a wide variety of severe and incapacitating diseases, such as some types of cancer, Alzheimer's disease, Parkinson's disease, etc., that today are untreatable or are just subject to palliative treatments [8]. For several reasons, the eye is an ideal organ for application of ATMPs. First, it has small dimensions, thus requiring low amounts of medicinal product for treatment. Second, the anatomical structure is compartmentalized, thus limiting the distribution of medicinal product to non-target tissues. Third, it has good accessibility for applying treatments and examining outcomes. Fourth, it is isolated from the rest of the body due to the blood–retinal barrier. This makes the eyeball an immunologically privileged site, because it restricts the passage of immunoglobulins. These reasons are why ATMPs present a great potential to improve the prognosis and potentially cure ocular diseases that currently have no effective treatment such as age-related macular degeneration, retinitis pigmentosa, Leber's congenital amaurosis, Stargardt's disease, optic nerve pathology, and limbal stem cell deficiency, among others.

During the last few years, the development of ATMPs for the treatment of eye diseases has become a fast-growing field. Therefore, it is important for all professionals working in this field to be familiarized with the regulatory principles associated with these types of innovative products. The aim of this review is to present the legal framework that regulates the development of ATMPs in the EU and the criteria that each type of ATMP must meet to be classified as such. We also identify and describe the ATMPs for the eye that have completed the research and development stages and are currently being used for the treatment of ocular diseases.

2. ATMP Regulatory Framework

2.1. ATMP Regulatory Framework in the EU

In the EU, the legal framework that regulates all medicinal products for human use, among which are ATMPs, is principally established in Directive 2001/83/EC [9]. The EMA is responsible for implementing this framework in cooperation with the national regulatory agencies from each EU member state. Directive 2001/83/EC defines a medicinal product as follows: "(1) any substance or combination of substances presented as having properties for treating or preventing disease in human beings; or (2) any substance or combination of substances which may be used in or administered to human beings, either with a view to restoring, correcting or modifying physiological functions by exerting a pharmacological, immunological, or metabolic action or to making a medical diagnosis".

ATMPs are medicinal products that include engineered cells and/or tissues or recombinant nucleic acids; therefore, they are under the regulatory framework of biological products. The specific legal framework for ATMPs was established by the European Commission in Regulation EC No. 1394/2007, and it provides the regulatory principles for the evaluation, authorization, and post-authorization follow-up for ATMPs that are intended to be commercialized in any EU member state (Table 1).

Table 1. Regulatory framework for cell- and gene-based therapies in the European Union, the United States, and Japan.

Jurisdiction	European Union	United States	Japan
Agency	European Medicines Agency (EMA)	Food and Drug Administration (FDA)	Pharmaceuticals and Medical Devices Agency (PMDA) Ministry of Health, Labour and Welfare (MHLW)
Regulatory framework	Directive 2001/83/EC (related to medical products for human use) European Commission 2007_Regulation EC No. 1394/2007 (related to advanced therapy medicinal products)	Federal Food, Drug, and Cosmetic Act (FDCA) and the Public Health Services Act (PHSA) Regenerative Medicine Advanced Therapy (RMAT) designation: section 3033 of the 21st Century Cures Act.	Act on the Safety of Regenerative Medicine (RM Act) and Pharmaceuticals and Medical Devices Act (PMD Act) 1960 Act No. 145 revised by 2013 Act No. 84
Therapy classification	Somatic cell therapy medicinal products (sCTMPs), tissue engineered products (TEPs), gene therapy medicinal products (GTMPs), and combined ATMPs (cATMPs)	Cell therapy and gene therapy products	Gene-, cell-, and tissue-based therapies

Under the EU regulatory framework, it is compulsory to get a marketing authorization prior to commercializing any medicinal product in any EU member state. As with all medicinal products, to get marketing authorization for an ATMP, it is necessary that the manufacture of the product be performed in compliance with the guidelines for GMPs described in Commission Directive 2003/94/EC [4]. Furthermore, following regulation (EU) No. 536/2014 [2], the product must undergo clinical trials to demonstrate that it is safe and effective in patients. ATMP clinical trial authorization depends on the national competent authorities where the trial will be performed. However, all ATMP marketing authorization applications are evaluated via the EMA's centralized procedure to guarantee that they follow a single evaluation, and get an authorization that is valid throughout the EU [10,11].

EMA's centralized procedure can grant three different types of marketing authorization: standard marketing authorization, conditional marketing authorization, and marketing authorization under exceptional circumstances (Figure 1). The type of marketing authorization requested will depend on whether or not the ATMP meets an unmet medical need and/or on the demonstration of a positive benefit-risk balance provided by enough scientific and medical data obtained during development [12]. Nevertheless, under ATMP Regulation EC No. 1394/2007, the so-called "hospital scheme exemption" opens the possibility for a national authorization of non-industrially manufactured ATMP, i.e., a custom-made product designed and produced for an individual patient. Such an ATMP can be used on a non-routine basis within the same member state in a hospital under the exclusive responsibility of a specific medical practitioner (Figure 1) [1].

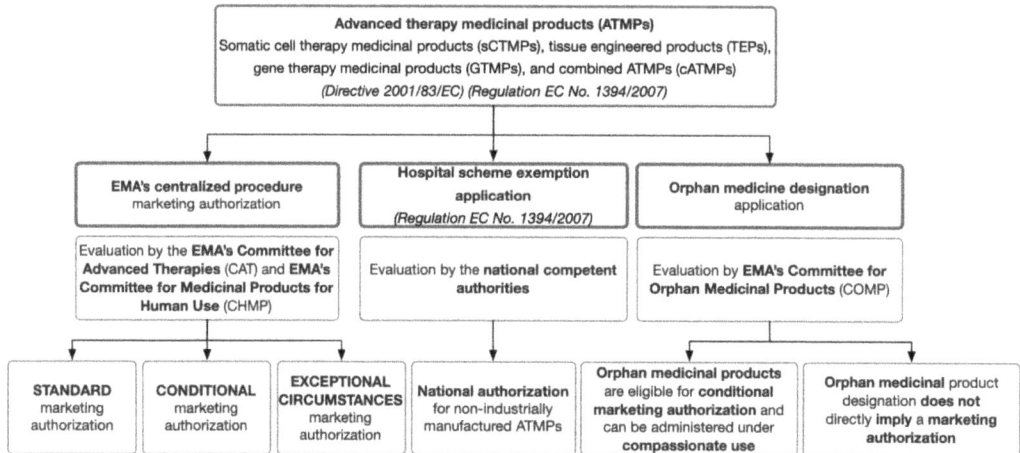

Figure 1. Regulatory pathway for advanced therapy medicinal products (ATMPs) in the European Union (EU). The European Medicines Agency (EMA) is responsible for implementing this regulatory framework in cooperation with the national regulatory agencies from each EU member state.

As described above, the CAT plays a key role in the regulatory oversight of ATMPs. This committee of experts in both the scientific and regulatory aspects of ATMPs is responsible for the primary evaluation of ATMP marketing authorization applications for EMA's Committee for Medicinal Products for Human Use. One of its duties is to provide scientific recommendations for the classification of ATMPs [1,13]. To determine if a putative gene- or cell/tissue-based product fulfills the criteria to be considered as an ATMP, developers can apply for the ATMP classification procedure provided by the CAT. The main purpose of this procedure is to help developers evaluate cases where the classification of a product is not clear. Within 60 days upon receiving the application, the CAT should give its recommendations based on the information supplied by the developer. In this way, the CAT provides assistance regarding the regulatory and development path that should be followed [14]. In the case of cATMPs, the CAT works together with the national regulatory authorities in charge of medical devices of each EU member state with the aim of providing joint recommendations [15].

An ATMP can also be designated as an orphan medicinal product by the Committee for Orphan Medicinal Products (COMP) of the EMA. Orphan designation depends on three criteria: (1) it diagnoses, prevents, or treats a life-threatening or chronically debilitating disease; (2) the disease affects no more than 5 in 10,000 people in the EU or has insufficient returns on investment; and (3) there is a lack of alternative methods of diagnosis, prevention, or treatment [16]. Orphan medicine designation does not directly imply a marketing authorization because demonstration of quality, safety, and efficacy are not preceding requirements. However, designated orphan medicines are eligible for conditional marketing authorization, allowing administration of an unauthorized medicine to patients under compassionate use outside a clinical study. In addition, orphan medicinal products can benefit from incentives such as protection from competition once on the market (Figure 1).

2.2. Regulatory Framework for Cell- and Gene-Based Therapies in Other Jurisdictions

Although the term ATMP is specific for cell- and gene-based therapies developed for commercial use in the EU, other countries such as the United States (US), Japan, Canada, Australia, and Korea also have specific regulatory frameworks for these types of therapies [17]. Despite their differences, the regulatory frameworks of all jurisdictions share the same main goals, i.e., to guarantee the safety and rights of patients and to assure the quality of the results obtained from the preclinical and clinical studies that evaluate the safety and the efficacy of the therapies [17].

Great efforts are being made to achieve international harmonization of the regulatory frameworks for the development of medicinal products. The EU, US, and Japan are the founding members of the International Council for Harmonization of Technical Requirements for Pharmaceuticals for Human Use (ICH). The goal of this international council is to develop and establish worldwide adoption of the scientific, technical, and regulatory requirements for the development of human medicinal products. Therefore, the regulatory frameworks of these jurisdictions have great influence on the international development of specific cell- and gene-based therapies.

In the US, similar to the EU, cell- and gene-based therapies are regulated by the Food and Drug Administration (FDA) as a subset of biological medicinal products known as cellular and gene therapy products (Table 1). Although the inclusion criteria for defining a gene therapy product are similar to the ones in the EU regulatory framework, there is a difference in the criteria for classifying cell and tissue-based products. In both jurisdictions, to classify a cell- or a tissue-based product as an advanced therapy, the processing of the cells must include a manipulation that alters the native biological features; however, in the US, the term "manipulation" distinguishes between structural and non-structural cells and tissues (see Section 3.1) [18–20].

In Japan, the protection of public health safety is the responsibility of the Japanese Ministry of Health, Labour, and Welfare (MHLW) that works with the Pharmaceutical and Medical Devices Agency (PMDA). The PMDA is the regulatory authority responsible for ensuring the safety, efficacy, and quality of medical devices and pharmaceuticals (including biological products). Gene-, cell-, and tissue-based therapies are regulated under a special framework for regenerative medicine products by the Office of Cellular and Tissue-based (Table 1). Under the Japanese Pharmaceuticals and Medical Devices Act, regenerative medicine products are those that consist of processed human/animal cells that are designed to be used for reconstructing, repairing, or substituting human tissues or organs, or for treating or preventing human diseases. Products that contain modified cells with recombinant nucleic acids that are intended to be used for the treatment of human diseases are also considered regenerative medicine products [21,22].

3. Definitions and ATMP Classification Criteria

Legal definitions of ATMPs are essential because they facilitate the classification of a product and therefore determine its whole development plan according to the regulatory framework of each jurisdiction and/or region. Performing a correct classification at an early stage of development is a key step because it determines the itinerary to be followed in research and in preclinical and clinical studies.

In this review, we outline the legal definitions of each type of ATMP according to the EU regulatory framework and the criteria that they should meet to be classified as such. To illustrate each legal definition, we have selected as examples ATMPs that have completed the research and development stages in different jurisdictions and that are currently being used for the treatment of eye diseases.

3.1. Cell-Based Medicinal Products: Somatic Cell Therapy and Tissue-Engineered Medicinal Products

Cell-based or stem cell-based medicinal products encompass two types of therapies, sCTMPs and TEPs. The European Commission, through Regulation EC No. 1394/2007 and Directive 2001/83/EC, has provided precise legal definitions of both. However, due to the complex nature of these medicinal products and the rapid evolution of science in this field, questions about ATMP classification can emerge. This is especially so regarding the classification of an ATMP as sCTMP or TEP because both products include cells. Here, we review the legal definitions for cell-based medicinal products and the main points to be taken into consideration to classify an ATMP as sCTMP or TEP. In addition, we review cell-based therapies already authorized for ocular indication.

The definition of sCTMP is currently included in Directive 2009/120/EC amending Directive 2001/83/EC of the European Parliament and of the Council on the European Community. An sCTMP is "a biological medicinal product whose active substance is made by a living organism" [23]. The product "has the following characteristics: (1) contains or consists of cells or tissues that have been subject to substantial manipulation so that biological characteristics, physiological functions or structural properties relevant for the intended clinical use have been altered, or of cells or tissues that are not intended to be used for the same essential function(s) in the recipient and the donor; (2) is presented as having properties for, or is used in or administered to human beings with a view to treating, preventing or diagnosing a disease through the pharmacological, immunological or metabolic action of its cells or tissues" [11]. For example, in vitro cultivation of cells or genetic modification of cells are considered substantial manipulations [14]. However, the following "shall not be considered as substantial manipulations: cutting, grinding, shaping, centrifugation, soaking in antibiotic or antimicrobial solutions, sterilization, irradiation, cell separation, concentration or purification, filtering, lyophilization, freezing, cryopreservation or vitrification" [1].

The definition of a TEP is provided by Regulation EC No. 1394/2007, where it is defined as "a product that contains or consists of engineered cells or tissues, and is presented as having properties for, or is used in or administered to human beings with a view to regenerate, repair or replace a human tissue" [1]. "Cells or tissues shall be considered 'engineered' if they fulfill at least one of the following conditions: (1) the cells or tissues have been subjected to substantial manipulation or (2) the cells or tissues are not intended to be used for the same essential function or functions in the recipient as in the donor" [1]. "A TEP may contain cells or tissues of human or animal origin, or both. The cells or tissues may be viable or non-viable." [1] However, "products containing or consisting exclusively of non-viable human or animal cells and/or tissues, which do not contain any viable cells or tissues and which do not act principally by pharmacological, immunological or metabolic action, shall be excluded from this definition" [1]. "TEPs may also contain additional substances, such as cellular products, bio-molecules, biomaterials, chemical substances, scaffolds or matrices" [1].

The main difference between sCTMPs and TEPs lies in the therapeutic action of these medicinal products. The sCTMPs are intended for treating, preventing, or diagnosing a disease through its pharmacological, immunological, or metabolic action. In contrast, TEPs are administered for regenerating, repairing, or replacing a human tissue. Therefore, when a researcher or a developer has doubts about whether an ATMP must be classified as a sCTMP or a TEP, the decision-making should be performed based on the mode of action of the ATMP (Figure 2) [14]. It should be considered that when "a product contains viable cells or tissues, the pharmacological, immunological or metabolic action of those cells or tissues shall be considered as the principal mode of action of the product" [1]. In addition, it is necessary to consider that it is possible that a cell-based medicinal product falls within the definition of both sCTMP and TEP. In this case, the medicinal product shall be considered as a TEP [1]. Nevertheless, when developers have doubts in determining if their ATMPs are sCTMPs or TEPs, they can apply for the ATMP classification procedure administered by the CAT and follow its recommendations.

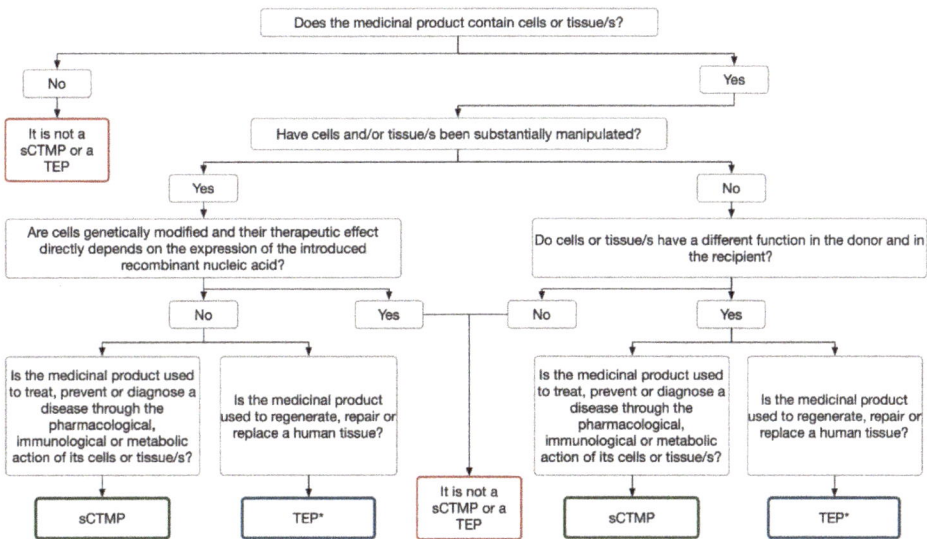

Figure 2. Easy guide to classify a cell-based medicinal product as a sCTMP or a TEP. Abbreviations: sCTMPs, somatic cell therapy medicinal products; TEPs, tissue engineered products. Modified from [14].

Another critical situation related to the classification of the ATMP occurs when cells are modified by adding a mRNA sequence, and the therapeutic effect of the medicinal product depends directly on the protein encoded by the added mRNA. Here, it would be possible to argue the classification of the medicinal product as a GTMP. However, due to the short half-life of mRNA in the modified cells, probably little or no residual mRNA will remain inside the cells administered to the patients. Therefore, the recombinant nucleic acid is not administered to the recipient, and the medicinal therapy is not considered to comply with the definition of a gene therapy (see Section 2.2). This ATMP can be considered to be a sCTMP or TEP, depending on the function of the transplanted cells (with altered phenotype but no altered genotype) to the patient [14]. When an ATMP can fall within the definition of either a GTMP, sCTMP, or TEP, it is considered to be a GTMP [1].

In the US, ATMPs are regulated as biological products by the FDA. Here, cell- and tissue-based products are considered as biological drugs when they are subjected to more than minimal manipulation or non-homologous use. A minimal manipulation, in case of structural tissues, is defined as "processing that does not alter the original relevant characteristics of the tissue relating to the tissue's utility for reconstruction, repair, or replacement", and it is further defined as "processing that does not alter the relevant biological characteristics of cells or tissues" in the case of cells or non-structural tissues [20]. Moreover, there is not a sub-classification for cell-based biological products because all of them are included in the category of cellular therapy products [20]. In Japan, cell-based products are classified as regenerative medicinal products by the PMDA and are defined as processed human cells used to reconstruct, repair, or reform the physical structure of a human, or to treat or prevent disease. In this jurisdiction, "processing" is defined as "the artificial expansion/differentiation of cells, establishment of a cell line, chemical treatment to activate cells or tissues, modification of biological characteristics, combination with non-cell/tissue components, and genetic modification of cells, cells for non-homologous use" [22,24].

Somatic Cell Therapy and Tissue Engineered Medicinal Products for the Eye

Currently, a high percentage of the clinical trials that are being carried out to study the efficacy and/or safety of ATMPs for eye diseases are focused on the analysis of cell-based medicinal products (Figure 3A). Four years ago, this percentage was around 76%, with two-thirds focused on sCTMPs and one-third on TEPs [8]. At the moment, there are several ongoing clinical trials in which efficacy and/or safety of cell-based medicinal products are being tested to treat, regenerate, repair, or replace human ocular tissues in diseases such as limbal stem cell deficiency, presbyopia, cataract, Stargardt's macular dystrophy, acute non-arteritic anterior ischemic optic neuropathy, and retinitis pigmentosa [25]. In a recent search for the terms "cell therapy or tissue engineering" and "eye diseases" in the US National Library of Medicine (ClinicalTrials.gov, accessed on 4 February 2021), there were 607 clinical trials, but actually only 93 of them were performed to evaluate cell-based therapies. Of these 93 clinical trials, 22.5% (21 out of 93) had already been completed. Most of them (74.2%; 69 out of 93) were associated with retinal or optic nerve diseases, while another important proportion (22.5%; 21 out of 93) were associated with ocular surface pathologies. Only one out of 93 (1.1%) clinical trials was associated with glaucoma, and two were associated with uveal melanoma (2.2%) (Figure 3B).

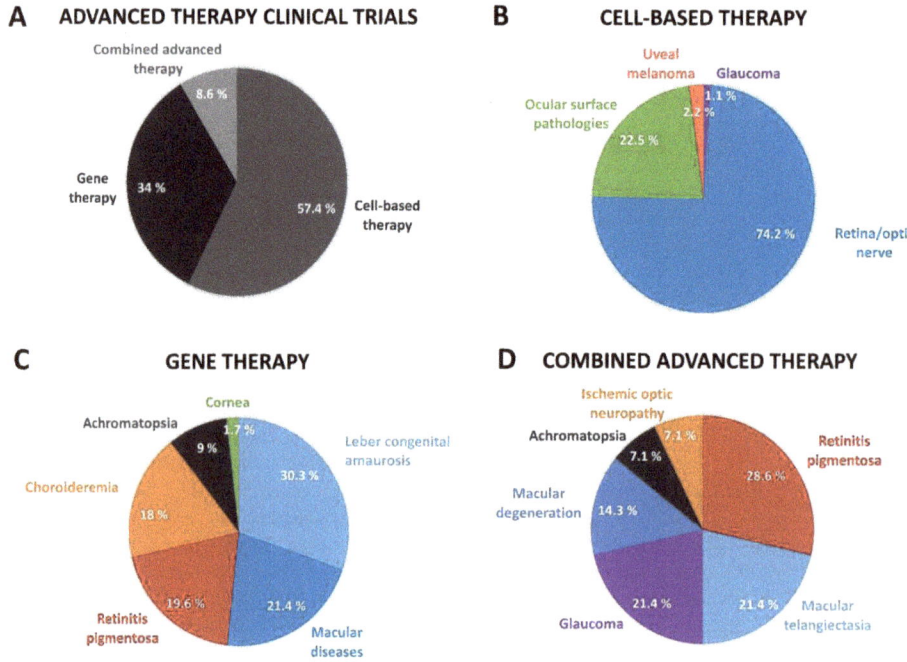

Figure 3. Clinical trials in which the safety and/or efficacy of advanced therapies for eye diseases are evaluated: (**A**) Advanced therapy clinical trials; (**B**) Cell-based therapy clinical trials; (**C**) Gene therapy clinical trials; (**D**) Combined advanced therapy clinical trials.

The number of authorized sCMTPs or TEPs is not very large (Table 2), probably due to the technical difficulty and the high costs involved in developing a cell-based therapy and proving its safety and efficacy.

Table 2. Somatic cell therapy and tissue engineering medicinal products for the eye.

Product (Commercial Name or Number Designated by EMA [1])	sCTMP [2] or TEP [3]	Manufacturer	Active Substance	Administration Route	Indication	Regulatory Status
EU/3/11/874	sCTMP, as implanted cells are expected to help retinal function	Astellas Pharma Europe B.V. (Leiden, The Netherlands)	Human embryonic stem-cell-derived retinal pigment epithelial cells	Intravitreal injection	Stargardt's disease	Orphan medicinal product designation by the EMA in 2011. Orphan medicinal product designation by the FDA [4] for the treatment of Stargardt's macular dystrophy
EU/3/13/1168	TEP, as implanted cells expected to help corneal regeneration	University of Newcastle. (Newcastle upon Tyne, United Kingdom)	Ex Vivo expanded autologous human corneal epithelium containing stem cells	Transplantation of a cell sheet	Limbal stem cell deficiency	Orphan medicinal product designation by the EMA in 2013
EU/3/14/1340	TEP, as implanted cells, expected to help corneal regeneration	NHS National Services Scotland, trading as Scottish National Blood Transfusion Service. (Edinburgh, United Kingdom)	Culture allogeneic corneal limbal stem cells	Transplantation of a cell sheet	Limbal stem cell deficiency	Orphan medicinal product designation by the EMA in 2014
OraNera (EMEA/H/C/002443)	TEP, as OraNera, expected to replace damaged corneal cells	CellSeed Europe Ltd.. (London, United Kingdom)	Autologous oral mucosal epithelial cells	Transplantation of a cell sheet	Limbal stem cell deficiency	Application for a marketing authorization withdrawn from the EMA in 2013
Holoclar (EU/3/08/579)	TEP (EMA classification)	Holostem Terapie Avanzate S.R.L. (Modena, Italy)	Ex vivo expanded autologous human corneal epithelium containing stem cells	Transplantation of a cell sheet	Moderate-severe limbal stem cell deficiency, unilateral or bilateral, due to chemical or physical burns	Orphan medicinal product designation by the EMA in 2008. Conditional marketing authorization by the EMA in 2015. The orphan medicinal product designation was maintained
Nepic	Human somatic stem cell-processed products (Japanese PMDA [5] classification)	Japan Tissue Engineering Co., Ltd. (Gamagori, Japan)	Human autologous corneal limbus-derived corneal epithelial cell sheet	Transplantation of a cell sheet	Limbal stem cell deficiency	Orphan regenerative medical product designation by the Japanese PMDA in 2020

[1] EMA, European Medicines Agency. [2] sCTMPs, somatic cell therapy medicinal products. [3] TEPs, tissue engineered products. [4] FDA, Food and Drug Administration. [5] PMDA, Pharmaceutical and Medical Devices Agency.

Nevertheless, several cell-based therapies have been authorized in the EU under the orphan medicinal product designation (Table 2). In June 2011, orphan medicinal product designation (EU/3/11/874) was approved by the EMA to a company in the United Kingdom (TMC Pharma Services Ltd., Hampshire, United Kingdom) for "human embryonic stem-cell-derived retinal pigment epithelial cells for the treatment of Stargardt's disease", a genetic disorder that affects retinal pigment epithelial cells and that leads to gradual loss of vision [26]. The human embryonic stem-cell-derived retinal pigment epithelial cells are administered to the patient by injection directly into the eye, under the retina, and are expected to help its function. Before its authorization in the EU, this medicinal product was granted approval in the US for the treatment of Stargardt's macular dystrophy [27]. In December 2016, the sponsorship for this cell-based therapy was transferred to Astellas Pharma Europe B.V., The Netherlands.

In July 2013, orphan medicinal product designation (EU/3/13/1168) was approved by the European Commission to the University of Newcastle, United Kingdom, for "ex vivo expanded autologous human corneolimbal epithelium, containing stem cells, for the treatment of limbal stem cell deficiency". Limbal stem cell deficiency is a pathology resulting from a critical reduction and/or dysfunction of the limbal epithelial stem cells that are responsible for the continuous renewal of the corneal epithelium. This pathology often results in corneal opacity, loss of vision, and/or chronic pain [28]. In this case, autologous human corneolimbal epithelial cells are cultured in vitro using a culture system that includes cells derived from the human placenta. Finally, with the expectation that the implanted stem cells will help the cornea to regenerate, the cultured corneolimbal epithelial cells are implanted on the damaged ocular surface [29]. In October 2014, orphan medicinal product designation (EU/3/14/1340) was awarded by the European Commission to NHS National Services Scotland (trading as Scottish National Blood Transfusion Service, United Kingdom), for "cultured allogeneic corneolimbal stem cells" to be used in the treatment of the same disease. Here, limbal stem cells are obtained from a donor eye and cultivated on a membrane. The membrane with the cultured cells is implanted onto the ocular surface of the patient, with the expectation that it will help corneal regeneration [30].

Another cell-based therapy, OraNera (CellSeed Europe Ltd.), to treat limbal stem cell deficiency in adults, was evaluated by the EMA (Table 2). In this case, the active substance was composed of autologous oral mucosal epithelial cells. In March 2013, after an application for a pediatric investigation plan, the company CellSeed Europe Ltd. informed the EMA that it wished to remove its application for a marketing authorization for OraNera. The basis for the removal request was the negative benefit–risk balance established by the CAT to use this medicinal product in patients with limbal stem cell deficiency [31].

The first ATMP approved, with marketing authorization, for ocular treatment in the EU was Holoclar, a cell-based therapy, specifically a TEP, to replace damaged ocular surface epithelium in patients suffering limbal stem cell deficiency. In 1997, Pellegrini et al. reported the first successful clinical trial, in which autologous epithelium from a limbal biopsy was cultured in vitro on petrolatum gauze or on a soft contact lens. It was then transplanted into two patients with limbal stem cell deficiency. After several studies that showed the presence of limbal epithelial stem cells in these types of cultures [32,33], and the selection of fibrin as a more suitable substratum for limbal epithelial cell cultivation [34], the product became a "routine treatment" in Italy in 2004 and was accepted in India some years after. However, this treatment was not established in the US because the regulatory requirements were not achieved [35]. In November 2008, orphan designation was approved by the European Commission to the Chiesi Farmaceutici S.P.A. (Italy), for "ex vitro expanded autologous human corneal epithelium containing stem cells for the treatment of corneal lesions, with associated corneal (limbal) stem cell deficiency, due to ocular burns" [36]. Finally, in February 2015, Holoclar, while the orphan designation, became the first stem cell-based ATMP to be approved with marketing authorization by the EMA [37], and given a conditional marketing authorization. This means that more clinical evidence on the safety and efficacy of this cell-based medicinal product must be collected and reported to the EMA to get the standard marketing authorization [38]. Currently, Holoclar is manufactured by Holostem Terapie Avanzate S.R.L. (Italy), which received the ownership of this product from Chiesi Farmaceutici S.P.A. in June 2020 [36].

Currently there are no FDA-authorized cellular therapy products for ophthalmic indications in the US [19]. In Japan, the PMDA has so far approved only one cell-based regenerative medicinal product to treat ocular diseases. In March 2020, the human somatic cell-processed orphan product Nepic (Japan Tissue Engineering Co., Ltd., Gamagori, Japan) was authorized. The active substance is a human autologous corneal-derived epithelial cell sheet to treat limbal stem cell deficiency (Table 2) [39].

3.2. Gene Therapy Medicinal Products

According to the EU, part IV of Annex I to Directive 2001/83/EC and the update of Directive 2009/120/EC, "a GTMP is defined as a biological medicinal product that presents the following two characteristics: (1) it contains and active substance that contains or consist of a recombinant nucleic acid used in or administered to human beings with a view to regulating, repairing, adding or deleting a genetic sequence; (2) its therapeutic, prophylactic or diagnostic effect relates directly to the recombinant nucleic acid sequence it contains, or to the product of genetic expression of this sequence. Moreover, GTMPs shall not include vaccines against infectious diseases" [1,9].

The obtention of these products involves the generation and amplification of genetic constructs in cell lines. The most commonly used technology for gene transfer is based on viral vectors, although non-viral vectors are also used, as they can be assembled synthetically. Further, the constructs are either purified for direct administration (non-cell-based), in vivo gene therapies, or used for the transduction of therapeutic cells (cell-based, or ex vivo, gene therapies) [12].

The goal of GTMPs is to deliver a gene with the intention to obtain, through its expression, a therapeutic effect in a patient. This gene should encode a protein that replaces the dysfunctional or absent protein in the patient, or a protein that inhibits the function related to the respective pathology [6]. A GTMP usually consists of a vector including the inserted sequence and the target cells that are modified by the vector, which finally encodes a protein and is expressed if the gene transfer is successful.

Considering part IV of Annex I to Directive 2001/83/EC, there are some specific requirements for GTMPs: "(1) GTMP containing recombinant nucleic acid sequences or genetically modified microorganisms or virus, should contain an active substance consist of nucleic acid sequences or genetically modified microorganisms or viruses in its carrier for medical use. The product could also be combined with medical devices. (2) Regarding GTMP containing genetically modified cells, the finished medicinal product shall comprise genetically modified cells formulated in the final container for the proposed medical application. The final product could be also combined with a medical device" [9,11].

One important challenge of these products is to achieve a stable gene expression. The duration of the product depends on the promoter used to drive the transgene, the cell survival, the persistence of the transgene, and the immune response against the vector or the genetically modified cells. Another challenge of GTMPs is related to the clinical efficacy and safety. These depend on the gene transfer efficiency, the capacity of directing the vector to the target cells, and the expression level of the gene of interest. In parallel, the target cell type, the type of vector, and the administration are also important factors to be considered [40].

Gene Therapy Medicinal Products for the Eye

At present, a large number of gene therapy clinical trials, around 2700 performed in 38 different countries, have been approved since 1989. Most of them have addressed cancer (66.6%), while only 1.3% have been directed towards ocular diseases [41]. Nevertheless, among the organs targeted by gene therapy, the eye is at the vanguard of translational gene therapy largely due to appropriate disease targets and its suitable anatomic features: it presents a well-defined anatomy, it is relatively immune-privileged, it is easy to access and examine, and it is possible to use one eye as an experimental target and the other one as a control in the same subject [42].

Gene therapy could offer an improvement in the treatment of several ocular diseases like glaucoma, X-linked retinoschisis, Stargardt's disease, choroideremia, retinitis pigmentosa, age-related macular degeneration (AMD), and Leber's congenital amaurosis [42], among others. Some corneal diseases are also potentially open to gene therapy, including the monogenic lysosomal storage disorders like mucopolysaccharidosis type IV and VII, corneal scarring, corneal neovascularization, anterior and stromal dystrophies linked to genetic mutations, corneal graft rejection, and the maintenance of corneal endothelial cell density [43].

Currently, 56 clinical trials related to gene therapy for eye diseases are reported (ClinicalTrials.gov, accessed on 4 February 2021) to be approved, in progress, or completed. Among all of the studies, 16 have already been completed. Interestingly, most of them (41) are associated with hereditary diseases, mostly retinal diseases (29 out of 56 trials). More precisely, 30.3% (17 out of 56) are related to Leber's congenital amaurosis, 21.4% (12 of 56) to macular diseases, 19.6% (11 out of 56) to retinitis pigmentosa, 18.0% (10 out of 56) to choroideremia, 9% (5 out of 56) to achromatopsia, and just 1.7% (1 out of 56) are related to corneal diseases (Figure 3C). Considering the types of vectors that are used, adeno-associated virus (AAV) is the most common, confirming that gene replacement therapy is the most widely applied modality in the clinical approach.

Concerning GTMPs for ocular diseases (Table 3), Vitravene (fomivirsen) was the first GTMP approved by the FDA in 1998, and later by the EMA in 1999. This product, administered by intravitreal injection, was indicated for the treatment of cytomegalovirus (CMV) retinitis in patients with acquired immune deficiency syndrome (AIDS), as these patients are not capable of fighting these infections. The fomivirsen is an antisense phosphorothioate oligodeoxynucleotide complementary to mRNA of the region 2 of human CMV. Hybridization of this antisense molecule to CMV mRNA prevents RNA transcription of the region 2 gene. This inhibits viral replication, a potent antiviral property, and delays the progression of CMV-associated retinitis. Due to commercial motivations, Novartis stopped the US marketing in 2006 and the EU marketing in 2020. However, it is still commercialized in Switzerland. The second authorized GTMP was Macugen (pegaptanib), a product indicated for the wet form of the AMD. It consists of a RNA aptamer that binds to the 165 isoform of vascular endothelial growth factor, producing an anti-angiogenic effect that prevents both the excessive growth of blood vessels and the formation of defective ones [44]. This product was approved by the FDA and EMA in 2006. However, the application was withdrawn in 2011 by Pfizer to include it in the treatment of diabetic macular oedema (Table 3).

Finally, the FDA in 2017 and EMA in 2018 approved Luxturna (voretigene neparvovec), the only GTMP for eye disease currently commercially authorized. This product was designated as orphan medicine by the EMA for the treatment of Leber´s congenital amaurosis in 2012, and for retinitis pigmentosa in 2015, where the RPE65 gene is mutated, producing retinal dystrophy [45]. This product consists of a recombinant AAV vector that delivers a functional RPE65 gene, and it is administered by subretinal injection. Since 2018, this GTMP has been commercialized by Novartis Europharm Limited (Table 3).

Table 3. Gene therapy medicinal products for the eye.

Product (Commercial Name or Number Designated by EMA [1])	Manufacturer	Active Substance	Administration Route	Indication	REGULATORY STATUS
Vitravene EMA/H/C/000244	Novartis (Basel, Switzerland)	Fomivirsen (antisense PODN [2])	Intravitreal injection	CMV [3] retinitis in HIV [4] infection	Marketing authorization by the FDA [5] 1998 and by the EMA 1999. Withdrawn in 2002 in the EU [6] and in 2006 in the US [7] Currently authorized in Switzerland
Macugen EMA/671614/2010	Pfizer (New York, USA)	Pegaptanib (RNA aptamer)	Intravitreal injection	Wet form of AMD [8]/Diabetic macular edema	Marketing authorization by the EMA and by the FDA in 2006/ Withdrawn in 2011 to include a new application (diabetic macular edema)
Luxturna EU/3/15/1518; EU/3/12/981	Novartis	Voretigene neparvovec (AAV [9]-RPE65)	Subretinal injection	Retinitis pigmentosa/Leber´s congenital amaurosis	Marketing authorization by the EMA in 2018 and by the FDA in 2017

[1] EMA, European Medicines Agency. [2] PODN, phosphorothioate oligodeoxynucleotide. [3] CMV, cytomegalovirus. [4] HIV, human immunodeficiency virus. [5] FDA, Food and Drug Administration. [6] EU, European Union. [7] US, United States. [8] AMD, age-related macular degeneration. [9] AAV, adeno-associated virus.

3.3. Combined ATMPs

As described above and in accordance with Regulation EC No. 1394/2007, cATMPs are composed of a GTMP, sCTMP, or TEP in combination with one or more medical devices or one or more active implantable medical devices as an integral part of the product [1]. Additionally, the biological components of the cATMP must fulfill one of two conditions: "(1) its cellular or tissue part must contain viable cells or tissues, or (2) its cellular or tissue part containing non-viable cells or tissues must be liable to act upon the human body with action that can be considered as primary to that of the devices referred to".

To clarify those descriptions, it will be helpful to understand the differences between "medical devices" and "active implantable medical devices". According to Directive 93/42/EEC, a "medical device" is "any instrument, apparatus, appliance, material or other article whether used alone or in combination, including the software necessary for its proper application intended by the manufacturer, to be used for human beings for the purpose of diagnosis, prevention, monitoring, treatment or alleviation of disease, diagnosis, monitoring, treatment, alleviation of or compensation for an injury or handicap, investigation, replacement or modification of the anatomy or of a physiological process or control of conception, and which does not achieve its principal intended action in or on the human body by pharmacological, immunological or metabolic means" [46]. In contradistinction to a "medical device", an "active implantable medical device" is "any active medical device (i.e., "any medical device relying for its functioning on a source of electrical energy or any source of power other than that directly generated by the human body or gravity") which is intended to be totally or partially introduced, surgically or medically, into the human body or by medical intervention into a natural orifice, and which is intended to remain after the procedure" [47]. Both medical device directives are currently under revision to keep up with advances in science and technology, and it is estimated that they will be replaced by new regulations before 2022.

Following these regulations (Directive 93/42/EEC and Directive 90/385/EEC) and the MEDical DEVices guidance document (MEDDEV), a medical device must be approved with the CE marking, an abbreviation in French of "Conformité Européenne" (European Conformity), for it to be commercially available in the EU [46–48]. The notified bodies are organizations designated by an EU country to assess the conformity of certain products such as medical devices before being placed on the market. To obtain the CE marking, the manufacturer or marketing company must demonstrate to the notified bodies that their medical device has benefits and an absence of risk. In this regard, any medical device that includes a cATMP must be previously approved with the CE marking by the notified bodies for its commercialization in the EU.

The CAT is the committee responsible for the adoption of scientific recommendations on ATMP classification. Also, for the marketing authorization of a cATMP, the CAT can request the assistance of the notified bodies. Importantly, to qualify as a cATMP, the medicinal product containing a medical device or active implantable medical device must be used in the authorized combination as an integral part of the ATMP. Thus, it must be used for the same purpose as was intended and without additional components [1]. Thus, if the medical device or active implantable medical device is not used, or is no longer used, with the same function as the CE marked medical device, it should be considered as an "excipient" in the final formulation of the drug and not as an integral part. In that case, the ATMP is a non-combined ATMP.

Combined ATMPs for the Eye

cATMPs represent only 1% of the ATMPs that are under development in the EU [8,49]. In 2013, the only cATMP approved in the EU was for the repair of knee cartilage defects. However, it was withdrawn in 2014 for commercial reasons due to the closure of the EU manufacturing site [8,50,51]. To date, 14 clinical trials have been developed (ClinicalTrials.gov, accessed on 4 February 2021) to study ophthalmic applications of a cATMP, NT-501 (Neurotech Pharmaceuticals Inc. (Cumberland, RI, USA) / Enpharma Ltd., Oxford, United Kingdom), to treat retinitis pigmentosa (28.6%; 4 out of 14 trials), macular telangiectasia (21.4%; 3 out of 14 trials), glaucoma (21.4%; 3 out of 14 trials), macular degeneration (14.3%; 2 out of 14 trials), achromatopsia (7.1%; 1 out of 14 trials), and ischemic optic neuropathy (7.1%; 1 out of 14 trials) [51] (Figure 3D). NT-501 consists of encapsulated human retinal pigment epithelial cells genetically modified to secrete therapeutic doses of ciliary neurotrophic factor (CNTF) into the back of the eye (Table 4). The cells are encapsulated by the so-called Encapsulated Cell Technology® (ECT), an intravitreal implant (medical device) that consists of a semi-permeable exterior capsule and an internal scaffolding that allows controlled cell growth [52,53]. The NT-501 implant has demonstrated controlled and continuous release of CNTF at effective doses, with no CNTF or antibodies against CNTF or the cell line in the systemic circulation [51,54–59]. This cATMP was designated as orphan drug by the FDA for the treatment of retinitis pigmentosa in 2004 and for treatment of macular telangiectasia type 2 in 2012. Subsequently, the EMA classified NT-501 implant as orphan medicinal product for the treatment of macular telangiectasia type 2 in 2012 and for the treatment of retinitis pigmentosa in 2013 (Table 4) [60,61].

Table 4. Combined advanced therapy medicinal product for the eye.

Product (Commercial Name or Number Designated by EMA [1])	Manufacturer	Active Substance	Administration Route	Indication	Regulatory Status
NT-501 (EMA/COMP/808529/2012) (EMA/COMP/682942/2012)	Neurotech Pharmaceuticals Inc. (Cumberland, RI, USA) / Enpharma Ltd. (Oxford, United Kingdom)	Encapsulated human retinal pigment epithelial cell line transfected with plasmid vector expressing human CNTF [3]	Intravitreal implant	Retinitis pigmentosa/Macular telangiectasia type 2	Orphan designation by the FDA [2] in 2004 and by the EMA in 2013/Orphan designation by the EMA and the FDA in 2012

[1] EMA, European Medicines Agency. [2] FDA, Food and Drug Administration. [3] CNTF, ciliary neurotrophic factor.

4. Conclusions

ATMPs provide novel therapeutic approaches to a large variety of diseases and therefore hold the potential to improve the prognosis and even cure certain eye diseases that currently have no effective treatment. However, because of the complexity and novelty of these innovative products, the regulatory procedures have the potential to be excessively rigid and complex, creating new challenges to both developers and regulators. These challenges can be especially significant for small ATMP developers that often have limited budgets and regulatory expertise and for whom a deep understanding and compliance with ATMP regulations can be difficult. It should be noted that, in the EU, most of the ATMP developers are universities, hospitals, charities, and small- and medium-sized enterprises. Therefore, developers normally feel overwhelmed with the regulatory requirements, because they increase both the financial and administrative burden and consequently hamper the market access of ATMP products.

Recently, the development of ATMPs for eye diseases has grown at a very fast and active pace, with many clinical trials conducted worldwide. However, the number of ATMPs that have been approved and that currently have a Marketing Authorization is rather small, as some of them showed poor results and market performance that finally led to their withdrawal. Because the pathway to get the regulatory approval of an ATMP involves a significant amount of expertise, time, and investment, the ATMP classification procedure provided by the CAT is a very helpful tool for developers. The CAT can be consulted to verify whether or not a product based on genes, cells, or tissues is an ATMP, to determine what type of ATMP product it is, and therefore to clarify the development and regulatory path that should be followed.

In recent years, regulatory agencies from the EU, US, and Japan have implemented schemes such as PRIME (PRIority MEdicines) designation, Breakthrough Therapy designation, and Sakigake designation, respectively, that are accelerating the development of priority cell- and gene-based therapies. To expedite and optimize the approval of ATMPs in these jurisdictions in the near future, a regulatory convergence among these regulatory agencies should be strongly promoted.

Currently, there are many ongoing clinical trials taking place worldwide for testing the safety and efficacy of new medicinal products based on gene, cells, and tissues for treating ocular conditions. Therefore, if these products provide good results, the number of authorized ATMPs for eye diseases is expected to significantly increase in the coming years. The number of ATMPs under development is growing not only in the regions participating in the International Council for Harmonization of Technical Requirements for Pharmaceuticals for Human Use, but also in all global jurisdictions. As compliance with national and international regulations is of paramount importance in the development of these types of products, stronger efforts should be made to set an international harmonization of the regulatory frameworks that control the development of ATMPs for commercial use. Regulators should be flexible and responsive to the unique and evolving challenges created by ATMPs. Accordingly, scientists and developers must work together with the regulators and act within the requirements of the regulatory system to improve the chances of successfully reaching the market. This will enable patients to have faster access to safe products and get the benefits from them as soon as possible.

Author Contributions: Conceptualization, T.N.-M.; investigation, M.L.-P., A.d.l.M. and S.G.; writing—original draft preparation, M.L.-P., A.d.l.M., S.G. and T.N.-M.; writing—review and editing, F.B. and M.C.; funding acquisition, M.C. and T.N.-M. All authors have read and agreed to the published version of the manuscript.

Funding: This work was funded by the Department of Education, Castilla y León Regional Government (Grant VA168P18 FEDER, EU) Spain; Ministry of Science and Innovation (Grant PID2019-105525RB-100, MICINN/FEDER, EU), Spain; Institute of Health Carlos III, CIBER-BBN (CB06/01/003 MICINN/FEDER, EU), Spain; and the Regional Center for Regenerative Medicine and Cell Therapy of Castilla y León, Spain.

Institutional Review Board Statement: Not applicable.

Informed Consent Statement: Not applicable.

Data Availability Statement: Publicly available datasets were analyzed in this review. This data can be found here: https://www.clinicaltrials.gov/ (accessed on 4 February 2021).

Acknowledgments: We thank B. Bromberg (Certified Editor in Life Sciences, Xenofile Editing, www.xenofileediting.com (accessed on 4 February 2021).) for his assistance in the final editing and preparation of this manuscript.

Conflicts of Interest: The authors declare no conflict of interest. The funders had no role in the design of the study; in the collection, analyses, or interpretation of data; in the writing of the manuscript, or in the decision to publish the results.

References

1. Regulation (EC) No. 1394/2007 of the European Parliament and of the Council of 13 November 2007 on Advanced Therapy Medicinal Products and Amending Directive 2001/83/EC and Regulation /EC) N0 726/2004. Available online: https://eur-lex.europa.eu/LexUriServ/LexUriServ.do?uri=OJ:L:2007:324:0121:0137:en:PDF (accessed on 4 February 2021).
2. Regulation (EU) No. 536/2014 of the European Parliament and of the Council of 16 April 2014 on Clinical Trials on Medicinal Products for Human Use, and Repealing Directive 2001/20/EC. Available online: https://ec.europa.eu/health/sites/health/files/files/eudralex/vol-1/reg_2014_536/reg_2014_536_en.pdf (accessed on 4 February 2021).
3. Commission Directive 2005/28/EC of 8 April 2005 Laying down Principles and Detailed Guidelines for Good Clinical Practice as Regards Investigational Medicinal Products for Human Use, as well as the Requirements for Authorisation of the Manufacturing or Importation of Such Products. Available online: https://eur-lex.europa.eu/LexUriServ/LexUriServ.do?uri=OJ:L:2005:091:0013:0019:en:PDF (accessed on 4 February 2021).
4. Commission Directive 2003/94/EC of 8 October 2003 Laying down the Principles and Guidelines of Good Manufacturing Practice in Respect of Medicinal Products for Human Use and Investigational Medicinal Products for Human Use. Available online: https://eur-lex.europa.eu/LexUriServ/LexUriServ.do?uri=OJ:L:2003:262:0022:0026:en:PDF (accessed on 4 February 2021).
5. Salmikangas, P.; Schuessler-Lenz, M.; Ruiz, S.; Celis, P.; Reischl, I.; Menezes-Ferreira, M.; Flory, E.; Renner, M.; Ferry, N. Marketing Regulatory Oversight of Advanced Therapy Medicinal Products (ATMPs) in Europe: The EMA/CAT Perspective. *Adv. Exp. Med. Biol.* **2015**, *871*, 103–130. [CrossRef] [PubMed]
6. Committee for Advanced Therapies (CAT); CAT Scientific Secretariat; Schneider, C.; Salmikangas, P.; Jilma, B.; Flamion, B.; Todorova, L.; Paphitou, A.; Haunerova, I.; Maimets, T.; et al. Challenges with advanced therapy medicinal products and how to meet them. *Nat. Rev. Drug Discov.* **2010**, *9*, 195–201. [CrossRef] [PubMed]
7. European Medicines Agency. Procedural Advice on the Evaluation of Advanced Therapy Medicinal Product in Accordance with Article 8 of Regulation (EC) No. 1394/2007. Available online: https://www.ema.europa.eu/en/documents/regulatory-procedural-guideline/procedural-advice-evaluation-advanced-therapy-medicinal-product-accordance-article-8-regulation-ec/2007_en.pdf (accessed on 4 February 2021).
8. Hanna, E.; Rémuzat, C.; Auquier, P.; Toumi, M. Advanced therapy medicinal products: Current and future perspectives. *J. Mark. Access Health Policy* **2016**, *4*. [CrossRef] [PubMed]
9. Directive 2001/83/EC of the European Parliament and of the Council of 6 November 2001 on the Community Code Relating to Medicinal Products for Human Use. Available online: https://ec.europa.eu/health/sites/health/files/files/eudralex/vol-1/dir_2001_83_consol_2012/dir_2001_83_cons_2012_en.pdf (accessed on 4 February 2021).
10. Regulation (EC) No. 726/2004 of the European Parliament and of the Council of 31 March 2004 Laying down Community Procedures for the Authorisation and Supervision of Medicinal Products for Human and Veterinary Use and Establishing a European Medicines Agency. Available online: https://ec.europa.eu/health/sites/health/files/files/eudralex/vol-1/reg_2004_726/reg_2004_726_en.pdf (accessed on 4 February 2021).
11. Commission Directive 2009/120/EC of 14 September 2009 Amending Directive 2001/83/EC of the European Parliament and of the Council on the Community Code Relating to Medicinal Products for Human Use as Regards Advanced Therapy Medicinal Products. Available online: https://ec.europa.eu/health//sites/health/files/files/eudralex/vol-1/dir_2009_120/dir_2009_120_en.pdf (accessed on 4 February 2021).
12. Detela, G.; Lodge, A. EU Regulatory Pathways for ATMPs: Standard, Accelerated and Adaptive Pathways to Marketing Authorisation. *Mol. Ther. Methods Clin. Dev.* **2019**, *13*, 205–232. [CrossRef]
13. European Medicines Agency, Committee for Advanced Therapies (CAT). Available online: https://www.ema.europa.eu/en/committees/committee-advanced-therapies-cat (accessed on 4 February 2021).
14. European Medicines Agency. Reflection Paper on Classification of Advanced Therapy Medicinal Products. Available online: https://www.ema.europa.eu/en/documents/scientific-guideline/reflection-paper-classification-advanced-therapy-medicinal-products_en-0.pdf (accessed on 4 February 2021).

15. European Medicines Agency. Procedural Advice on the Evaluation of Combined Advanced Therapy Medicinal Products and the Consultation of Notified Bodies in Accordance with Article 9 of Regulation (EC) No. 1394/2007. Available online: https://www.ema.europa.eu/en/documents/regulatory-procedural-guideline/procedural-advice-consultation-notified-bodies-accordance-article-9-regulation-ec-no-1394/2007_en.pdf (accessed on 4 February 2021).
16. Regulation (EC) No. 141/2000 of the European Parliament and of the Council of 16 December 1999 on Orphan Medicinal Products. Available online: https://ec.europa.eu/health/sites/health/files/files/eudralex/vol-1/reg_2000_141_cons-2009-07/reg_2000_141_cons-2009-07_en.pdf (accessed on 4 February 2021).
17. Galli, M.C.; Serabian, M. *Regulatory Aspects of Gene Therapy and Cell Therapy Products*; Springer International Publishing: Cham, Switzerland, 2015; Volume 871, ISBN 978-3-319-18617-7.
18. U.S. Food and Drug Administration. Framework for the Regulation of Regenerative Medicine Products. Available online: https://www.fda.gov/vaccines-blood-biologics/cellular-gene-therapy-products/framework-regulation-regenerative-medicine-products (accessed on 4 February 2021).
19. U.S. Food and Drug Administration. Cellular & Gene Therapy Products. Available online: https://www.fda.gov/vaccines-blood-biologics/cellular-gene-therapy-products (accessed on 4 February 2021).
20. Iglesias-Lopez, C.; Agustí, A.; Obach, M.; Vallano, A. Regulatory Framework for Advanced Therapy Medicinal Products in Europe and United States. *Front. Pharmacol.* **2019**, *10*, 921. [CrossRef]
21. Azuma, K. Regulatory Landscape of Regenerative Medicine in Japan. *Curr. Stem Cell Rep.* **2015**, *1*, 118–128. [CrossRef]
22. Jokura, Y.; Yano, K.; Yamato, M. Comparison of the new Japanese legislation for expedited approval of regenerative medicine products with the existing systems in the USA and European Union. *J. Tissue Eng. Regen. Med.* **2018**, *12*, 1056–1062. [CrossRef] [PubMed]
23. European Medicines Agency. Biological Medicine. Available online: https://www.ema.europa.eu/en/glossary/biological-medicine (accessed on 4 February 2021).
24. Okada, K.; Koike, K.; Sawa, Y. Consideration of and Expectations for the Pharmaceuticals, Medical Devices and Other Therapeutic Products Act in Japan. *Regen. Ther.* **2015**, *1*, 80–83. [CrossRef] [PubMed]
25. Bobba, S.; Di Girolamo, N.; Munsie, M.; Chen, F.; Pébay, A.; Harkin, D.; Hewitt, A.W.; O'Connor, M.; McLenachan, S.; Shadforth, A.M.A.; et al. The current state of stem cell therapy for ocular disease. *Exp. Eye Res.* **2018**, *177*, 65–75. [CrossRef] [PubMed]
26. Tsang, S.H.; Sharma, T. Stargardt Disease. *Adv. Exp. Med. Biol.* **2018**, *1085*, 139–151. [CrossRef]
27. European Medicines Agency. EU/3/11/874. Available online: https://www.ema.europa.eu/en/medicines/human/orphan-designations/eu311874 (accessed on 4 February 2021).
28. Dua, H.S.; Azuara-Blanco, A. Limbal Stem Cells of the Corneal Epithelium. *Surv. Ophthalmol.* **2000**, *44*, 415–425. [CrossRef]
29. European Medicines Agency. EU/3/13/1168. Available online: https://www.ema.europa.eu/en/medicines/human/orphan-designations/eu3131168 (accessed on 4 February 2021).
30. European Medicines Agency. EU/3/14/1340. Available online: https://www.ema.europa.eu/en/medicines/human/orphan-designations/eu3141340 (accessed on 4 February 2021).
31. European Medicines Agency. OraNera. Available online: https://www.ema.europa.eu/en/medicines/human/withdrawn-applications/oranera (accessed on 4 February 2021).
32. Pellegrini, G.; Golisano, O.; Paterna, P.; Lambiase, A.; Bonini, S.; Rama, P.; De Luca, M. Location and Clonal Analysis of Stem Cells and Their Differentiated Progeny in the Human Ocular Surface. *J. Cell Biol.* **1999**, *145*, 769–782. [CrossRef] [PubMed]
33. Pellegrini, G.; Dellambra, E.; Golisano, O.; Martinelli, E.; Fantozzi, I.; Bondanza, S.; Ponzin, D.; McKeon, F.; De Luca, M. p63 identifies keratinocyte stem cells. *Proc. Natl. Acad. Sci. USA* **2001**, *98*, 3156–3161. [CrossRef] [PubMed]
34. Pellegrini, G.; Ranno, R.; Stracuzzi, G.; Bondanza, S.; Guerra, L.; Zambruno, G.; Micali, G.; De Luca, M. The control of epidermal stem cells (holoclones) in the treatment of massive full-thickness burns with autologous keratinocytes cultured on fibrin1. *Transplantation* **1999**, *68*, 868–879. [CrossRef]
35. Pellegrini, G.; Lambiase, A.; Macaluso, C.; Pocobelli, A.; Deng, S.; Cavallini, G.M.; Esteki, R.; Rama, P. From discovery to approval of an advanced therapy medicinal product-containing stem cells, in the EU. *Regen. Med.* **2016**, *11*, 407–420. [CrossRef] [PubMed]
36. European Medicines Agency. EU/3/08/579. Available online: https://www.ema.europa.eu/en/medicines/human/orphan-designations/eu308579 (accessed on 4 February 2021).
37. Pellegrini, G.; Ardigò, D.; Milazzo, G.; Iotti, G.; Guatelli, P.; Pelosi, D.; De Luca, M. Navigating Market Authorization: The Path Holoclar Took to Become the First Stem Cell Product Approved in the European Union. *Stem Cells Transl. Med.* **2018**, *7*, 146–154. [CrossRef]
38. European Medicines Agency. Holoclar. Available online: https://www.ema.europa.eu/en/medicines/human/EPAR/holoclar (accessed on 4 February 2021).
39. Pharmaceuticals and Medical Devices Agency. New Regenerative Medical Products. Available online: https://www.pmda.go.jp/english/review-services/reviews/approved-information/0002.html (accessed on 4 February 2021).
40. Somia, N.; Verma, I.M. Gene therapy: Trials and tribulations. *Nat. Rev. Genet.* **2000**, *1*, 91–99. [CrossRef]
41. del Pozo-Rodríguez, A.; Rodríguez-Gascón, A.; Rodríguez-Castejón, J.; Vicente-Pascual, M.; Gómez-Aguado, I.; Battaglia, L.S.; Solinís, M.Á. Gene Therapy. *Adv. Biochem. Eng. Biotechnol.* **2020**, *171*, 321–368. [CrossRef]
42. Solinís, M.Á.; del Pozo-Rodríguez, A.; Apaolaza, P.S.; Rodríguez-Gascón, A. Treatment of ocular disorders by gene therapy. *Eur. J. Pharm. Biopharm.* **2015**, *95*, 331–342. [CrossRef] [PubMed]

43. Williams, K.A.; Coster, D.J. Gene therapy for diseases of the cornea a review. *Clin. Exp. Ophthalmol.* **2009**, *38*, 93–103. [CrossRef]
44. Parashar, A. Aptamers in Therapeutics. *J. Clin. Diagn. Res.* **2016**, *10*. [CrossRef]
45. Russell, S.; Bennett, J.; Wellman, J.A.; Chung, D.C.; Yu, Z.-F.; Tillman, A.; Wittes, J.; Pappas, J.; Elci, O.; McCague, S.; et al. Efficacy and safety of voretigene neparvovec (AAV2-hRPE65v2) in patients with RPE65-mediated inherited retinal dystrophy: A randomised, controlled, open-label, phase 3 trial. *Lancet* **2017**, *390*, 849–860. [CrossRef]
46. Council Directive 93/42/EEC of 14 June 1993 Concerning Medical Devices. Available online: https://eur-lex.europa.eu/LexUriServ/LexUriServ.do?uri=CONSLEG:1993L0042:20071011:en:PDF (accessed on 4 February 2021).
47. Council Directive of 20 June 1990 on the Approximation of the Laws of the Member States Relating to Active Implantable Medical Devices (90/385/EEC). Available online: https://eur-lex.europa.eu/LexUriServ/LexUriServ.do?uri=CONSLEG:1990L0385:20071011:EN:PDF (accessed on 4 February 2021).
48. European Commission. Guidelines on Medical Devices. Available online: http://ec.europa.eu/DocsRoom/documents/17522/attachments/1/translations/ (accessed on 4 February 2021).
49. ten Ham, R.M.T.; Hoekman, J.; Hövels, A.M.; Broekmans, A.W.; Leufkens, H.G.M.; Klungel, O.H. Challenges in Advanced Therapy Medicinal Product Development: A Survey among Companies in Europe. *Mol. Ther. Methods Clin. Dev.* **2018**, *11*, 121–130. [CrossRef] [PubMed]
50. European Medicines Agency. Closure of EU Manufacturing Site for MACI. Available online: https://www.ema.europa.eu/en/documents/referral/maci-article-20-procedure-closure-eu-manufacturing-site-maci_en.pdf (accessed on 4 February 2021).
51. Eldem, T.; Eldem, B. Ocular Drug, Gene and Cellular Delivery Systems and Advanced Therapy Medicinal Products. *Türk Oftalmol. Derg.* **2018**, *48*, 132–141. [CrossRef]
52. Emerich, D.F.; Thanos, C.G. NT-501: An ophthalmic implant of polymer-encapsulated ciliary neurotrophic factor-producing cells. *Curr. Opin. Mol. Ther.* **2008**, *10*, 506–515. [PubMed]
53. European Medicines Agency. Scientific Recommendation on Classification of Advanced Therapy Medicinal Products. Available online: https://www.ema.europa.eu/en/documents/report/scientific-recommendation-classification-advanced-therapy-medicinal-products-human-ciliary_en.pdf (accessed on 4 February 2021).
54. Kauper, K.; McGovern, C.; Sherman, S.; Heatherton, P.; Rapoza, R.; Stabila, P.; Dean, B.; Lee, A.; Borges, S.; Bouchard, B.; et al. Two-Year Intraocular Delivery of Ciliary Neurotrophic Factor by Encapsulated Cell Technology Implants in Patients with Chronic Retinal Degenerative Diseases. *Investig. Opthalmol. Vis. Sci.* **2012**, *53*, 7484–7491. [CrossRef] [PubMed]
55. Zhang, K.; Hopkins, J.J.; Heier, J.S.; Birch, D.G.; Halperin, L.S.; Albini, T.A.; Brown, D.M.; Jaffe, G.J.; Tao, W.; Williams, G.A. Ciliary neurotrophic factor delivered by encapsulated cell intraocular implants for treatment of geographic atrophy in age-related macular degeneration. *Proc. Natl. Acad. Sci. USA* **2011**, *108*, 6241–6245. [CrossRef]
56. Birch, D.G.; Weleber, R.G.; Duncan, J.L.; Jaffe, G.J.; Tao, W. Randomized Trial of Ciliary Neurotrophic Factor Delivered by Encapsulated Cell Intraocular Implants for Retinitis Pigmentosa. *Am. J. Ophthalmol.* **2013**, *156*, 283–292. [CrossRef] [PubMed]
57. Talcott, K.E.; Ratnam, K.; Sundquist, S.M.; Lucero, A.S.; Lujan, B.J.; Tao, W.; Porco, T.C.; Roorda, A.; Duncan, J.L. Longitudinal Study of Cone Photoreceptors during Retinal Degeneration and in Response to Ciliary Neurotrophic Factor Treatment. *Investig. Opthalmol. Vis. Sci.* **2011**, *52*, 2219–2226. [CrossRef]
58. Pilli, S.; Zawadzki, R.J.; Telander, D.G. The dose-dependent macular thickness changes assessed by fd-oct in patients with retinitis pigmentosa treated with ciliary neurotrophic factor. *Retina* **2014**, *34*, 1384–1390. [CrossRef]
59. Birch, D.G.; Bennett, L.D.; Duncan, J.L.; Weleber, R.G.; Pennesi, M.E. Long-term Follow-up of Patients With Retinitis Pigmentosa Receiving Intraocular Ciliary Neurotrophic Factor Implants. *Am. J. Ophthalmol.* **2016**, *170*, 10–14. [CrossRef] [PubMed]
60. European Medicines Agency. Public Summary of Opinion on Orphan Designation. Available online: https://www.ema.europa.eu/en/documents/orphan-designation/eu/3/12/1072-public-summary-opinion-orphan-designation-encapsulated-human-retinal-pigment-epithelial-cell_en.pdf (accessed on 4 February 2021).
61. European Medicines Agency. Public Summary of Opinion on Orphan Designation. Available online: https://www.ema.europa.eu/en/documents/orphan-designation/eu/3/12/1098-public-summary-opinion-orphan-designation-encapsulated-human-retinal-pigment-epithelial-cell_en.pdf (accessed on 4 February 2021).

Review

Goals and Challenges of Stem Cell-Based Therapy for Corneal Blindness Due to Limbal Deficiency

Margarita Calonge [1,2,3,*], Teresa Nieto-Miguel [1,2,3], Ana de la Mata [1,2,3], Sara Galindo [1,2,3], José M. Herreras [1,2,3,4] and Marina López-Paniagua [1,2,3,*]

1. IOBA (Institute of Applied Ophthalmobiology), University of Valladolid, 47011 Valladolid, Spain; tnietom@ioba.med.uva.es (T.N.-M.); adelamatas@ioba.med.uva.es (A.d.l.M.); sgalindor@ioba.med.uva.es (S.G.); herreras@ioba.med.uva.es (J.M.H.)
2. CIBER-BBN (Biomedical Research Networking Center in Bioengineering, Biomaterials and Nanomedicine), Carlos III National Institute of Health, 47002 Valladolid, Spain
3. Castile and Leon Networking Center for Regenerative Medicine and Cell Therapy, 47008 Valladolid, Spain
4. Ophthalmology Service, University Clinic Hospital, 47003 Valladolid, Spain
* Correspondence: calonge@ioba.med.uva.es (M.C.); marina@ioba.med.uva.es (M.L.-P.)

Abstract: Corneal failure is a highly prevalent cause of blindness. One special cause of corneal failure occurs due to malfunction or destruction of the limbal stem cell niche, upon which the superficial cornea depends for homeostatic maintenance and wound healing. Failure of the limbal niche is referred to as limbal stem cell deficiency. As the corneal epithelial stem cell niche is easily accessible, limbal stem cell-based therapy and regenerative medicine applied to the ocular surface are among the most highly advanced forms of this novel approach to disease therapy. However, the challenges are still great, including the development of cell-based products and understanding how they work in the patient's eye. Advances are being made at the molecular, cellular, and tissue levels to alter disease processes and to reduce or eliminate blindness. Efforts must be coordinated from the most basic research to the most clinically oriented projects so that cell-based therapies can become an integrated part of the therapeutic armamentarium to fight corneal blindness. We undoubtedly are progressing along the right path because cell-based therapy for eye diseases is one of the most successful examples of global regenerative medicine.

Keywords: blindness; cell therapy; CLET; cornea; limbal niche; limbal stem cell; LSCD; mesenchymal stem cell transplantation; MSCT; ocular surface

1. Introduction

Ophthalmology is among the first medical science branches that have benefited from stem cell-based therapy and regenerative medicine. Many facts can account for this success, such as easy accessibility to the stem cell niches (especially those located in the anterior segment of the eye); a relatively easy follow-up of the applied therapies; the fact that the eyes are paired, non-vital organs; and the immune-privileged nature of the intraocular tissues and cornea [1].

Of all of the potential stem cell niches in the visual system [1], those located at the ocular surface are the most accessible for study and extraction of the stem cells, and they can be repaired if they fail and produce disease. Consequently, second only to hematopoietic stem cell transplantation, regenerative medicine of the ocular surface is the most well developed. In fact, epithelial stem cell transplantation to repair the corneal surface is the most widely used stem cell-based therapy in clinical medicine.

The anterior segment of the eye is composed of the ocular surface, the anterior sclera, the corneal stroma and endothelium, the anterior and posterior chambers containing the aqueous humor, the anterior uvea composed of the iris and ciliary body, and the crystalline lens. The posterior segment of the eye consists of the posterior uvea containing the choroid, the retina, the optic nerve head, the vitreous body, and the posterior sclera. The concept of the ocular surface includes those structures and tissues directly exposed to the environment. Thus, the ocular surface is comprised of the overlying tear film, superficial cornea (the epithelium; Bowman's layer; and for some eyes, the superficial stroma), conjunctiva, and the corneoscleral limbus. The main tissue at the ocular surface is the epithelium because, in general, only epithelial tissues have direct contact with the environment through either the skin or diverse mucosal sites, including the ocular surface.

Several potential stem cell niches are present in the ocular surface. Some are still under investigation, and in the future, these sites may enable the isolation of human adult stem cells from the conjunctiva, corneal stroma, and/or the meibomian glands [2]. The procedures for isolating the stem cells and the knowledge learned from them could provide fundamental insights and new regenerative therapies for many diseases, such as cicatricial conjunctivitis (i.e., Stevens–Johnson syndrome and the associated spectrum), conjunctival trauma, and meibomian gland disease, for which there are currently no effective, long-term treatments.

In the ocular surface, the most well-known and documented stem cell niche is located at the limbus, where the transparent cornea transitions to the opaque sclera and is overlain by the conjunctiva. Stem cells in that location have been identified, extracted, and used therapeutically in attempts to repair the severe corneal pathology when these cells and/or their niche are damaged. The goals and challenges that this therapy constitute are the topic of this review.

2. The Past: The Beginnings of Stem Cell-Based Therapy for Corneal Failure

Much of the knowledge regarding the location of corneal epithelial stem cells in the limbal area came from clinical observations and subsequent experimentation in the field of corneal epithelial wound healing, coupled with the research in the field of skin stem cells. At the beginning of the 20th century, ophthalmologists and scientists began studying the first phenomenon in the process of corneal epithelium wound healing: sliding or migration of the surrounding epithelial cells (reviewed in Schwab, 1999 [3]), and the subsequent cell replication and proliferation to generate replacement cells. In 1944, Ida Mann demonstrated pigment movement from the limbus in a rabbit model of corneal injury [4], which matched the observations by clinicians that epithelial lines seemed to move from the peripheral cornea to the wound site in the central cornea. Friedenwald and Buschke, also in 1944, demonstrated that the mitotic index of corneal epithelium tended to be higher towards the periphery of the cornea [5]. Maumenee, in 1964, was the first to suggest that the corneal epithelium could be regenerated efficiently from the limbal epithelium and, to a lesser extent, from the conjunctival epithelium [6]. In 1971, Davanger and Evenson described the rapid movement of peripheral cells in response to an acute central defect [7]. They referred to the source of the migrating cells as the "pericorneal papillary structure", which today, is called the palisade of Vogt, located at the limbus. They proposed that the essential role of the migrating cells was the renewal of the corneal epithelium and suspected that, to maintain corneal transparency, the source of these cells had to be in the nearest vascular stroma, i.e., the limbus. In 1983, Richard Thoft and Julie Friend published their famous X, Y, Z hypothesis [8], where they established that there are three different phenomena that kept the corneal epithelial cell mass more or less constant under physiological conditions: The X component of this hypothesis is the proliferation of basal epithelial cells and migration toward the surface. The Y component is the contribution to the corneal epithelial cell mass by the centripetal movement of peripheral cells. The Z component is the loss of epithelial cells through normal desquamation. When the hypothesis was proposed, the Y component was not proven, though there was evidence of it. For instance, following corneal transplantation, the centripetal movement of cells from the host peripheral cornea replaced the loss of the corneal epithelial cells from the donor transplant [9]. This elegant hypothesis was validated later as the Y component was proven to be the mass of limbal stem cells. The simplicity of Thoft's statement that "corneal epithelial maintenance, essential to avoid pathology, could be defined by the equation 'X + Y = Z'" could not be truer to this day [8] (Figure 1).

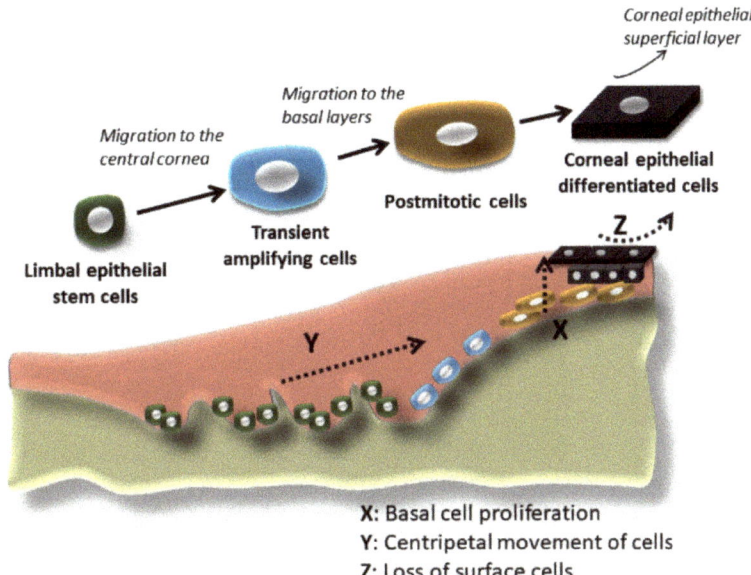

Figure 1. Graphical representation of the limbal stem cell niche with all of the cell states implicated in the corneal epithelium regeneration (limbal epithelial stem cells, transient amplifying cells, postmitotic cells, and corneal epithelial differentiated cells). The X, Y, Z hypothesis published by Thoft and Friend in 1983 [8] is also represented, presenting the three different phenomena that allow the corneal epithelial cell mass to remain constant. X: proliferation of basal epithelial cells; Y: contribution to the cell mass by centripetal movement of peripheral cells; Z: epithelial cell loss or constant desquamation from the surface.

In 1986, Schermer et al. offered strong evidence that the location of the corneal epithelial stem cells was at the limbus [10]. By studying keratin expression patterns, they demonstrated that limbal basal cells were less differentiated than corneal epithelial basal cells. This supported the clinical observation of the centripetal migration of corneal epithelial cells. They concluded that corneal epithelial stem cells were likely located in the limbus and, furthermore, that the basal corneal epithelial cells corresponded to cells then known as "transient amplifying cells" because the more apically located epithelial cells were terminally differentiated [10].

Based on those early studies, multiple researchers have contributed to better defining the limbal epithelial stem cells along with other cells located in the limbal niche and the niche itself. Additionally, a wide range of markers have been identified to define each of the different cell types in that niche [11].

Clinically, ophthalmologists have now defined the term "limbal stem cell deficiency" (LSCD) to describe what had previously been called "conjunctivalization" or "neovascular pannus" before the presence of stem cells was even suspected. LSCD describes certain severe conditions in which cells of the damaged ocular surface epithelium are not replaced with centripetally migrating cells derived from the limbal niche. Consequently, the conjunctiva encroaches upon the cornea, replacing the injured corneal epithelium and preventing further irreversible structural damage such as infection, stromal necrosis, or even perforation. While conjunctival overgrowth results in the loss of functionality, i.e., visual loss due to corneal opacification, it prevents the loss of corneal anatomical integrity that could ensue otherwise (Figure 2).

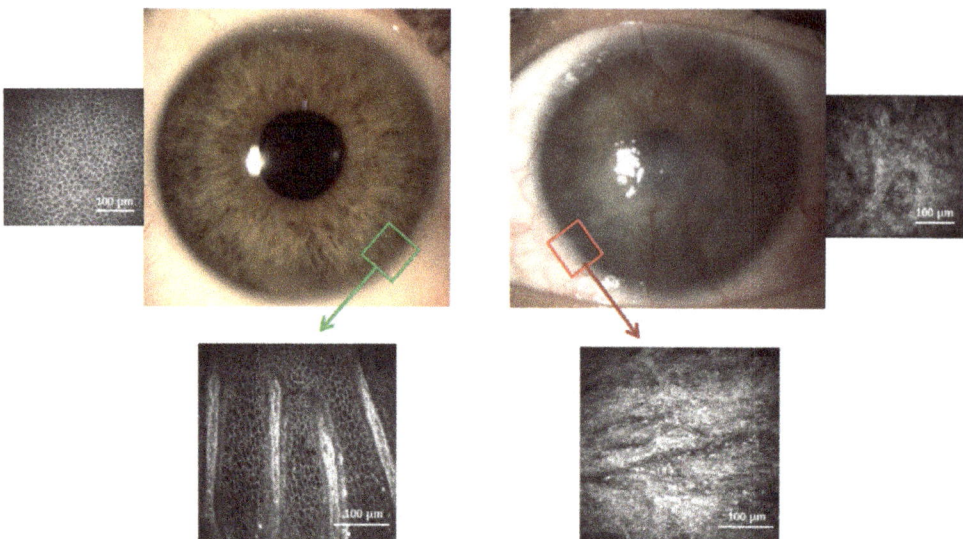

Figure 2. (**Top Left**) Location of the limbal niche (**green box**) in the normal eye of a 26-year-old man. (**Lower Left**) Confocal image of the limbal niche that is responsible for maintaining the corneal epithelial phenotype. (**Top Right**) The left eye of the man suffered a chemical injury 2 years before. The injury destroyed his limbal niche (**red box**). Consequently, the corneal epithelium has a conjunctival phenotype derived from the adjacent conjunctiva. (**Lower Right**) Confocal image of the damaged limbal niche.

Primary LSCD is currently defined as an end-stage pathology resulting from multiple diseases that destroy the corneal niche located at the corneoscleral limbus. Secondary LSCD refers to the loss of the resident corneal epithelium stem cells even though the limbal niche remains intact. LSCD can be hereditary, e.g., congenital aniridia, or acquired, e.g., immune-mediated diseases such as Stevens–Johnson/toxic epidermal necrolysis, atopic keratoconjunctivitis, rosacea-related pathology, and non-immune mediated pathologies such as chemical injuries [12].

LSCD results in recurrent corneal epithelial ulceration, conjunctivalization (pannus with superficial neovascularization), and opacification because of the inability of the limbal niche to renew the corneal epithelium. It is well established that LSCD, when extended and/or severe, usually leads to corneal opacity and subsequent blindness with accompanying symptomatology. Diseases leading to LSCD and LSCD itself are extremely difficult to manage, and in most instances, they need proper, aggressive medical therapy before proceeding with surgical treatment [12].

Understanding the functionality of the limbal niche and the consequences of its pathology explain why corneal transplants in patients with ocular surfaces diseases in which LSCD is concomitantly present are doomed to fail. Failure of the initial transplant and of subsequent ones is due to the incapacity of the host limbus with LSCD to replace the epithelium of the transplanted corneas as the cells are lost through desquamation during the post-transplant period. At present, ophthalmologists have now agreed that corneal transplantation is not a viable primary solution if extensive LSCD is present because transplantation does not replace the damaged corneal epithelial stem cells [13]. Repair of the limbal stem cell niche must be achieved first. Consequently, ophthalmologists began to design strategies to remove limbal tissue from the fellow healthy or the less affected eye of the patient or, alternatively, from allogenic sources such as cadaveric eyes or healthy living relatives, to transplant into the LSCD-affected eye.

Kenyon and Tseng pioneered the transplantation of limbal tissue in 1989. They reported good results at 6 months after surgery for 21 of 26 LSCD cases subjected to limbal autograft transplantation in which the limbal tissue was removed from the less injured eye [14]. Following that report, large auto- and allo-limbal grafts were performed for LSCD, but soon, two problems became evident: the risk of limbal failure in the donor eye in case of autografts, and the need for potent and protracted immunosuppression for allografts.

Since the initial years of limbal tissue transplantation, the methodology has evolved and is now performed as keratolimbal autografts, keratolimbal allografts, conjunctival limbal autografts, or conjunctival limbal allografts. Allografts must be chosen for cases of bilateral disease, and the donor source is from a cadaver or from a living related or non-related donor. For all of the transplantation methods, keratoplasty can be performed either concomitantly or following a delay, though in both cases the outcomes are highly variable, ranging from very poor to good.

One important problem with transplantation of allogeneic limbal tissue is the need for long-term systemic immunosuppression, even in HLA-matched donors, without which long-term survival of the transplanted niche tissue is unlikely [15]. Furthermore, two limbal grafts measuring approximately 6 mm at the limbus (3 h clock quadrants) and extending 5–8 mm posterior to the limbus are removed from the healthy donor eye. This extensive extirpation could lead to pathology in the donor eye [16]. In any case, these procedures are still in current clinical practice [17].

Tissue-based transplantations require a significant amount of tissue that is derived from the fellow eye for transplantation into the damaged eye. An alternative approach is to harvest small amounts of healthy limbal niche tissue from the donor eye and then to generate more autologous stem cells through tissue culture (see below). However, this approach requires the use of good manufacturing practice (GMP) cell culture facilities, which are expensive to maintain and may not be generally available to all ophthalmologists and patients who need them. Based on these limitations, in 2012, Virender Sangwan and his group in India pioneered another tissue-based technique of tissue transplantation known as simple limbal epithelial transplantation (SLET) [18]. It uses a smaller limbal tissue biopsy (3–4 mm) from the contralateral healthy eye (autologous). The tissue is then cut into 8–10 tiny pieces and placed on top of an amniotic membrane that was previously glued by fibrin to the scraped, diseased corneal bed of the recipient eye. The more than 30 reports published so far suggest good mid-term results as long as autologous tissue is used [19]. A modification of this technique uses a double layer of cryopreserved amniotic membrane to sandwich the limbal cells [20] and has been approved by the US Food and Drug Administration (FDA). As an alternative for bilateral cases in which healthy autograft donor tissue is not available, the alloSLET, using allogeneic tissue, was recently introduced by Shanbhag et al. with apparent good results [21]. It is important to understand that no matter how small the allogeneic tissue is, systemic immunosuppression is still needed. With alloSLET, Shanbhag et al. used a pulsed intravenous immunosuppression regimen for long term, i.e., more than 2 years, or the usual oral protocols used for cultivated limbal cells (see below) for an amount of time not yet specified [21].

To reduce the high rate of immune rejection of tissue-based transplants, Pellegrini et al. described for the first time, in 1997, stem cell-based therapies (as distinct from tissue-based therapies) that transplanted cultivated, autologous limbal epithelial cells that were extracted from small biopsies of the contralateral donor eye [22]. Although it was described for just two patients and did not follow GMP techniques, this cultured cell approach represented a significant breakthrough in regenerative medicine.

3. The Present: Available Stem Cell-Based Therapies

At the beginning of the 21st century, bilateral cases of LSCD continued to be a challenge because allogenic limbal tissue transplantation was generally unsuccessful without long-term immunosuppression. Furthermore, the availability of stem cell-based transplantation was becoming more limited due to the implementation of new regulatory guidelines that guaranteed safety but restricted the conditions under which auto- and allograft treatments could be used. This section describes the stem cell-based therapies currently available for both unilateral and bilateral LSCD.

3.1. Cultivated Limbal Epithelial Transplantation

Limbal epithelial stem cells, the adult stem cells of the corneal epithelium, have been widely used in both preclinical and clinical studies for LSCD therapy, as described in this review. The transplantation of limbal epithelial cells facilitates ocular surface regeneration, and consequently, it improves the prognosis of a subsequent corneal graft [23–31]. Molecular and functional characterization of these cells and their use for LSCD therapy are also being vigorously investigated in preclinical and clinical ophthalmological research.

Although the fate of transplanted limbal stem cells on the ocular surface is still not certain, some potential mechanisms of action have been identified: (1) donor cell migration to the host niche and subsequent regeneration of the niche before corneal epithelial repair, (2) donor cell creation of a new pseudo-niche before regeneration of the corneal epithelium, (3) donor-cell stimulated regeneration of the corneal epithelium through paracrine or direct interaction, and (4) donor transit-amplifying cells acting as the principal cells responsible for regeneration of the host epithelium [32–34].

After the first publication by Pellegrini et al. in 1997 of two patients treated with cultivated limbal cells extracted from a small (approximately 2 × 2 mm) biopsy of limbal tissue from the contralateral healthy eye [22], other authors began developing similar techniques and published different reports on autologous cultivated limbal epithelial transplantation (CLET). In 2008, the European Medicines Agency (EMA) granted orphan drug status for a product that provided "ex vivo expanded autologous human corneal epithelium containing stem cells for the treatment of corneal lesions, with associated corneal (limbal) stem cell deficiency, due to ocular burns" [35]. In 2010, Rama et al. reported a 76.6% success rate in the 2–3 years of follow-up of 112 cases treated with a stem cell-derived product that was similar to the one used in 1997 by the same group [36]. In 2015, that product received the trade name of Holoclar and it became the first stem cell-based therapy to be approved by the EMA with a conditional marketing authorization pending on further clinical evidence of safety and efficacy [37,38]. Holoclar has not yet achieved approval for standard commercialization; however, if and when it is, it will only be authorized for treatment of chemical injuries with stem cells derived from an autologous source.

The great advancement of Pellegrini and Rama's group [22,36,37] prompted many other groups to start developing similar protocols with some modifications in culture, evaluation procedures, and surgical techniques. There are consequently some published reports, especially in Asia and Europe [39], on autologous CLET with success rates varying from 60% to 100% [40,41].

Soon after starting treatments with autologous CLET, ophthalmologists realized that there were many cases of bilateral LSCD where this therapy was not an option, usually because the disease or trauma caused bilateral LSCD, leaving no healthy limbal tissue available for biopsy. Then, encouraged by the good results of autologous transplants, ophthalmologists began investigating allogeneic CLET. The first attempts of allogeneic CLET in patients with LSCD were by Schwab in 1999 [3], who published two partially successful allogeneic cases that utilized stem cells derived from living relatives of the patients, and by Koizumi et al. (Kinoshita's group) in 2001 [42]. The latter publication was a retrospective case series, reporting success in 10 of 13 eyes followed for 11.2 months. Cells were obtained from cadaveric limbal explants, cultured on a carrier composed of denuded amniotic membrane coated with a layer of 3T3 fibroblasts to assist epithelial cell growth. The cultivated epithelium consisted of four to five stratified cell layers and was positive for corneal specific keratins (K3/12). None of the patients were immunosuppressed, but only three eyes suffered epithelial rejection.

In the following years, other authors began using allogeneic limbal tissue from cadaveric sources. These were used mainly for cultivation and extraction of limbal epithelial cells. Initially this was conducted in regular tissue culture laboratories; however, stem cell-based therapies are considered to be medicinal products. Therefore, it was necessary to move production into GMP-based cell culture facilities to comply with the same regulatory principles as conventional drugs [43,44].

The techniques for the cultivation of allogeneic stem cells and surgeries are diverse but are the same as those for autologous cells. The main difference is that the patients receiving allogeneic cell-based transplants need to be systemically immunosuppressed but require only one drug and endure a shorter period of immunosuppression (12 months maximum) [40] than required for high risk corneal transplants or for allogeneic limbal tissue transplantation (full segments or SLET). The best culture, surgical, medical, and evaluation protocols, however, have not yet been defined for either autologous or allogeneic CLET.

In 2015, Zhao et al. published a systematic review and meta-analysis of ex vivo CLET using amniotic membranes as a substratum in LSCD [45]. In 18 publications involving 572 eyes (562 patients), the success rate was about 67% for both autografts and allografts, provided that the allografts receive systemic immunosuppression, which were less intense than required for the transplantation of non-cultured allografts [45]. These results were consistent with previous reviews by Baylis et al. [28] and Shortt et al. [46] of 28 reports and 17 reports, respectively, that compared autografts and allografts. Another more recent meta-analysis by Mishan et al. of autologous versus allogeneic CLET included 30 studies, with sample sizes ranging from 6 to 200 and follow-up periods of 0.6–156 months [41]. Of the 1306 eyes, 982 (75.2%) received autografts and 324 (24.8%) received allografts from living or deceased donors. The meta-analysis revealed that the odds of success were similar for both CLET procedures.

One prospective comparative study stated that allogeneic CLET yields far worse results than autologous CLET [47]. However, the authors of this study failed to give the necessary immunosuppressive treatment to their allogeneic transplantation patients, and this most likely explains why these patients had unsuccessful transplantations.

Another recent meta-analysis of 40 studies (2202 eyes) concluded that autologous grafts had a higher rate of ocular surface restoration and a lower rate of complications than allogeneic grafts [40]. In their analysis, the authors combined the outcomes for cases treated with allo-CLET and allo-limbal tissue transplantation. However, these two approaches are fundamentally independent and incompatible with one another for the purpose of being combined in a meta-analysis. Thus, their finding of differences in the rate of ocular surface restoration and in the rate of complications for autologous and allogeneic treatments was flawed.

In conclusion, CLET results seem to be similar whether the cell source is autologous or allogeneic (Figure 3). Even though the objective assessment of outcome is difficult because the cases are extremely variable in every possible aspect, the success rates range between 60% and 100%. Additionally, following LSCD treatment, eyes with significant stromal and/or endothelial damage require subsequent corneal transplantation. In these cases, visual acuity is not a good indicator of success [24], something that it is very difficult for patients, relatives, and even referring clinicians to understand.

However, without a doubt, significant clinical improvements have been achieved in the treatment of ocular surface pathology due to LSCD. These improvements are based on the evolution of our understanding of the disease origin and advances in treatment methodology, all of which have improved the prognosis, with or without the need for subsequent corneal transplants. Consequently, patient quality of life has vastly improved [34].

In terms of safety, xenobiotic-free conditions are now broadly used to minimize the risk of diseases or immune reaction [45,48]. For instance, in the case of allogeneic grafts, CLET reduces the exposure of the host to non-self-antigens. With the in vitro expansion of cells from a small biopsy, most antigen-presenting Langerhans cells and other cells found in the normal limbal stem cell niche are lost [49]. Importantly, tumorigenic events have not been reported in either preclinical studies or in clinical practice.

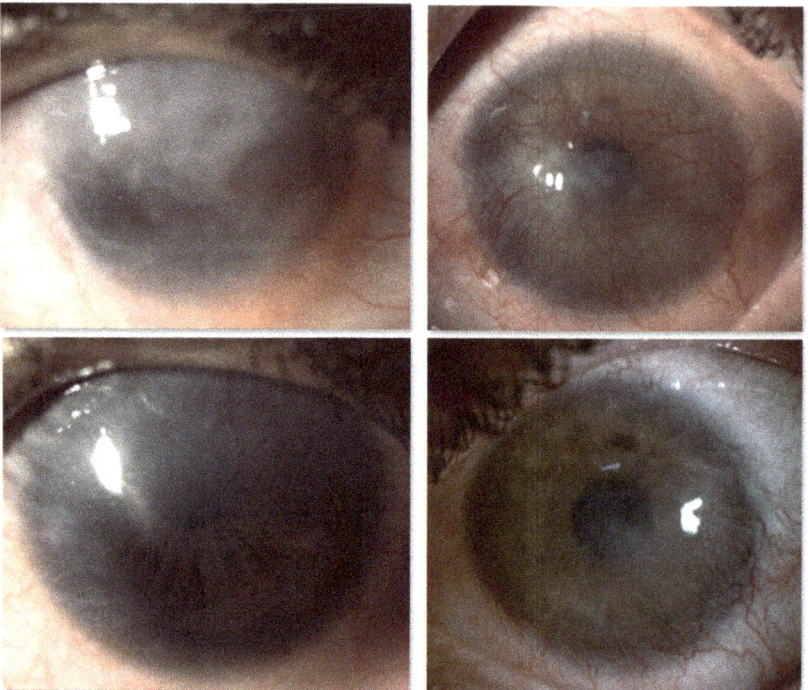

Figure 3. Chemical injury in two different patients, before (**upper panel**) and 12 months after (**lower panel**) successful cultivated limbal epithelial transplantation (CLET). The source of the limbal epithelial cultivated stem cells was autologous, from the fellow healthy eye (**left panel**) or allogeneic from cadaveric limbal ring (**right panel**).

3.2. Autologous Non-Limbal Epithelial Cell Transplantation

Another potential solution for bilateral cases of LSCD, where autologous limbal tissue is not available, is the transplantation of cultured cells from autologous non-limbal tissues. Different preclinical studies have demonstrated that cultivated oral mucosal epithelial cell transplantation (COMET) in the treatment of the ocular surface in experimental models of LSCD in rabbits reduces corneal epithelial defects, corneal opacity, and vascularization [50–53]. However, some corneas had irregular epithelial surfaces associated with peripheral neovascularization after COMET [50,51]. In 2004, Nakamura et al. published the first clinical studies that used autologous COMET [54]. In a recent review of 24 publications between 2004 and 2019 [55], the authors concluded that COMET is the most frequently used non-limbal autologous cell procedure in the treatment of bilateral LSCD, possibly because it eliminates the risk of graft rejection and thus avoids the need for immunosuppression. The COMET approach has been preferentially performed in Japan, and based on published cases from the last 15 years, they offer promising mid-term results with a stable ocular surface reported in 70.8% of LSCD eyes [55]. However, neo-angiogenesis following transplantation is a drawback associated with this procedure, but solutions for this problem have been proposed. For example, the mucosal epithelial cells can be co-cultured with limbal mesenchymal niche cells instead of the usual 3T3 cells [56]. The oral mucosal cells obtained from this alternative culture system seem to be less likely to induce postsurgical neovascularization and therefore improve postsurgical outcomes.

Although the molecular mechanisms of COMET are still unknown, the transplanted cells remain in the cornea for at least 24 weeks in rabbits [51] and up to 22 months in humans [57]. In addition, the expression of corneal epithelial marker K3 [52,57] and the limbal epithelial marker p63 [51,57] were found in rabbit and human corneas after COMET. In contrast, the corneal epithelial marker K12 showed variable expression, being absent from many corneas but present in others after COMET [51,57].

It is extremely difficult to make comparisons among techniques. Nevertheless, Wang et al. compared the success rate of COMET to allogeneic CLET [58]. The success rate of COMET, 52.9% (18 of 34 eyes), was lower than that for allogeneic CLET, 71.4% (30 of 42 eyes). The difference was attributed mainly to a higher incidence of postoperative complications with COMET due mostly to persistent epithelial defects. The authors attributed the different results to the unique morphology, function, and microenvironment of oral mucosal epithelium compared to the limbal epithelium despite the expression of similar gene markers.

Another more recent review by Samoila et al. in 2020 [59] compared the clinical outcomes of allogeneic CLET (18 publications between 2005 and 2019) and COMET (11 publications between 2004 and 2019) for total bilateral LSCD. They identified the advantages of COMET, including the lack of graft rejection (as it is autologous), the achievement of cell culture in a shorter period of time, and the absence of keratinization over a prolonged time span. In addition, tumorigenic events have not been reported. However, they also reiterated the previously identified shortcomings such as the lower success rate of the oral mucosal epithelial cells due to the higher incidence of post-operative persistent epithelial defects and subsequent graft failure, and lower cell proliferation and differentiation activities. They concluded that allogenic limbal epithelial stem cells may have a better ability to form a stable and integrated corneal epithelium.

In summary, there is no current agreement regarding the preferred use of COMET or allogeneic CLET for total LSCD patients. Most publications agree that allogeneic CLET should be prioritized over COMET because the limbal epithelial cells may have a better capacity to maintain ocular surface stability, provided that immunosuppression is used, which is not necessary with COMET.

3.3. Allogeneic Non-Limbal Stem Cell-Based Transplantation

The only non-limbal allogenic stem cells that have been used clinically are mesenchymal stem cells (MSCs). As recently documented, MSCs were the most commonly used stem cell type for cellular and tissue-engineering therapies in Europe between 2016 and 2017 [39]. This is mainly due to the capacity of MSCs to produce growth factors, to modulate immune and inflammatory properties, and to differentiate into multiple cell lineages depending on the environmental signals [60]. MSCs secrete epithelial growth factor, which increases corneal epithelial cell proliferation [61,62]. Other growth factors secreted by MSCs include hepatocyte growth factor, fibroblast growth factor, and nerve growth factor [63,64]. To modulate the inflammatory response, MSCs secrete anti-inflammatory molecules, such as transforming growth factor β, thrombospondin 1, and tumor necrosis factor-stimulated gene-6 [61,65]. Other secreted molecules have either pro- or anti-inflammatory effects depending on the microenvironment. These include interleukin 6, which is increased in the presence of damaged corneal epithelial cells [63]. In addition, MSCs can produce antioxidant enzymes such as dioxygenase-2,3-indolamine and cyclooxygenase 2 in the oxidative stress environment associated with damaged corneas [66]. MSCs can also reduce T lymphocyte proliferation and can inhibit differentiation of immature macrophages to mature (active) macrophages [67–69], thus regulating the immune response by reducing rejection and inflammatory reactions [70].

When applied to the ocular surface in preclinical animal models of LSCD, MSCs exerted potent reductions of inflammation, corneal opacity, and neovascularization, all while promoting re-epithelialization [66,71–78]. Other important preclinical studies showed that MSCs can migrate specifically to the damaged corneolimbal tissues [73,78–80] and can improve the therapeutic response of the ocular surface affected by LSCD.

Regarding safety-related issues in preclinical studies, the transplantation of MSCs to treat LSCD does not induce adverse events, and no toxicologic effects have been reported [73–76,78,81]. Nevertheless, several preclinical works to analyze the tumorigenic potential of MSCs have been reported, confirming that the transplantation of this type of cell does not induce tumorigenesis in either healthy vital organs or in damaged target organs [82–86].

MSCs also have potential advantages over limbal epithelial cells because they can be easily obtained from many tissue types without the dependence of deceased donors. Additionally, they can be cultured in vitro, achieving clinical scales in a short period of time by less expensive procedures than those required for limbal epithelial stem cells. Importantly, 100% of the MSCs in a transplant are stem cells, while only a variable proportion of the cells cultured for CLET are indeed stem cells, as they are extracted from limbal tissue, and the limbal epithelium consists of only about 5–10% of stem cells [87]. Finally, the MSCs can be cryopreserved without loss of potency and allogeneic MSCs can be transplanted without the need of host immunosuppression [88].

The first and only published clinical use of MSCs for LSCD was by Calonge et al. in 2019 [89]. These authors designed a 12-month proof-of-concept double-masked clinical trial in which 22 patients with severe and total LSCD were randomized to either allogeneic bone marrow-derived mesenchymal stem cell transplantation (MSCT) or allogeneic CLET. All patients had immunosuppression with one drug for one year to maintain investigator masking, even though MSCT did not require it. Both cell types produced similar results and were equally safe. MSCT was successful in 85.7%, and CLET was successful in 77.8%. The central corneal epithelial phenotype evaluated by in vivo confocal microscopy improved in 71.4% and 66.7% of MSCT and CLET cases, respectively (Figure 4). There were no adverse events related to MSCT or CLET [89]. Therefore, the tumorigenic potential of MSCs has been discounted. If these good results are corroborated in a large series of patients, MSC therapy is deemed a safe, efficacious alternative for both unilateral and bilateral LSCD cases.

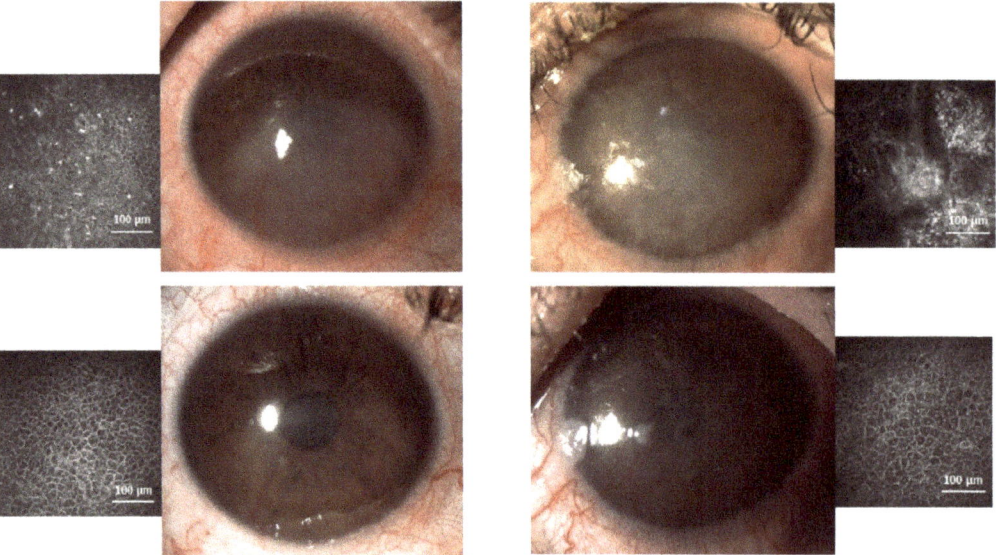

Figure 4. Bilateral limbal stem cell deficiency due to Stevens–Johnson syndrome. The right eye (**left panel**) was randomized to receive allogeneic limbal stem cell transplantation (CLET), and the left eye (**right panel**) received a mesenchymal stem cell transplantation (MSCT). The upper panels show that both corneas have a mixed epithelial phenotype as imaged by in vivo confocal microscopy. The lower panels show the same eyes after 12 months. Both corneas have an epithelial phenotype in the central cornea. Both transplants were successful.

Finally, Table 1 summarizes the distinctive characteristics and success rates of different published stem cell-based therapies that report comparative studies among different sources of cells.

Table 1. Published studies using stem cell-based transplants compared with other techniques (in at least five eyes) in the management of severe limbal stem cell deficiency (LSCD).

Publication's First Author, Year (Reference No.) Country	Type of Clinical Study/No. Surgeries or Eyes/Mean Time to Final Evaluation (months)	Type of Transplant (n), GMP [1] Followed for Product Preparation	Systemic Immunosuppressants in Allogeneic Transplants	Anatomical Success (Method of Evaluation)/Statistically Significant (s), Non-Significant (ns) or Not Mentioned (nm)
Shimazaki et al., 2007 [90] Japan	Retrospective, observational case series/27/31.6	Auto [2]-CLET [3] (7) Allo [5]-CLET (20) No	CsA [4] for 6 months	Global: 59.3% (clinical) Auto-CLET 85.7% Allo-CLET: 50.0%/ns
Shortt et al., 2008 [91] UK	Prospective, noncomparative, interventional case series/10/6 or 13	Auto-CLET (3) Allo-CLET (7) Yes	CsA for 6 months	Global: 60% (clinical, ccp-IVCM [6], impression cytology) Auto-CLET: 33% Allo-CLET: 71%/nm [7]
Pauklin et al., 2010 [92] Germany	Prospective noncomparative interventional case series/44/28.5	Auto-CLET (30) Allo-CLET (14) No	CsA for 12–15 months (one case had none)	Global: 68% (clinical) Auto-CLET: 76.7% Allo-CLET: 50%/s
Prabhasawat et al., 2012 [93] Thailand	Prospective, noncomparative case series/19/26.1	Auto-CLET (12) Allo-CLET (7) No	CsA for 6–12 months	Global: 73.7% (clinical) Auto-CLET: 66.7% Allo-CLET: 85.7%/ns
Zakaria et al., 2014 [94] Belgium	Phase I-II non-randomized clinical trial/18/22	Auto-CLET (15) Allo-CLET (3) No	CsA for 12 months	Global: 66.7% (clinical) Auto-CLET: 66.7% Allo-CLET: 66.7%/ns
Ramírez et al., 2015 [24] Spain	Prospective noncomparative interventional case series/20/12, 24, 36	Auto-CLET (11) Allo-CLET (9) Yes	Mycophenolate CsA or azathioprine for 12 months	Global (clinical, ccp-IVCM): 80% at 1–2 years; 75% at 3 years Auto-CLET: 90.9% Allo-CLET: 66.7%/ns
Ganger et al., 2015 [95] (India)	Retrospective case series/62 (38 children, 24 adults)/12	Auto-CLET (54) Allo-CLET (8) No	No	Global: nm Auto-CLET: 87.8% children, 99.9% adults/ns Allo-CLET: 62.5%/ns
Parihar et al., 2017 [96] India	Prospective interventional/50/12	Allo-CLET (25) Allo-LTT [8] (25) No	CsA for 12 months	Global (clinical): nm Both groups had significant improvement/ns
Sharma et al., 2018 [97] India, USA, Australia	Prospective comparative/40/12	Auto-CLET (20) AMT [9] (20) No	Na [10]	Global (clinical): nm Similar results in both groups
Calonge et al., 2019 [89] Spain	Phase I-II, randomized, controlled, double-masked clinical trial/28/12	Allo-MSCT [11] (17) Allo-CLET (11) Yes	Yes	Global (clinical ccp-IVCM): Allo-MSCT: 85.7% Allo-CLET: 77.8%/ns MSCT was as safe as CLET

Table 1. Cont.

Publication's First Author, Year (Reference No.) Country	Type of Clinical Study/No. Surgeries or Eyes/Mean Time to Final Evaluation (months)	Type of Transplant (n), GMP [1] Followed for Product Preparation	Systemic Immunosuppressants in Allogeneic Transplants	Anatomical Success (Method of Evaluation)/Statistically Significant (s), Non-Significant (ns) or Not Mentioned (nm)
Campbell et al., 2019 [98] UK	Randomized, controlled, single-masked, multicenter clinical trial/16	Allo-CLE (11) AMT (5) Yes	Prednisolone plus CsA or mycophenolate for 12 months	Global (clinical): nm sustained significant improvement in allo-CLET but not in AMT
Borderie et al., 2019 [47] France	Phase II, noncomparative clinical trial: CLET vs. retrospective control: LTT/30 /72 vs. 132	Auto-CLET (7) Allo-CLET (7) Auto-LTT (8) Allo-LTT (8) No	Allo-CLET: NO Allo-LTT: CsA, steroids or chloraminophen for 12 months	Global survival (clinical) at 5 years/nm Auto-CLET: 71% Allo-CLET: 0% Auto-LTT: 75% Allo-LTT: 33%
Wang et al., 2019 [58] China	Retrospective cohort study/76/23.3 vs. 16.1	Allo-CLET (42) Auto-COMET [12] (34) No	No (only oral corticosteroids for 2–3 months)	Global (clinical): nm Allo-CLET: 71.4% (Immune rejections: 9.5%) COMET: 52.9%)
Behaegel et al., 2019 [99] Belgium	Prospective, noncomparative case series (first 2 years); Later follow-up or retrospective review/13/2.1 (short-term) vs. 6.7 (long-term)	Auto-CLET (9) Allo-CLET (4) Yes	Not specified	Global short-term: 46.1% Auto-CLET: 77.8% Allo-CLET: 75% Global long-term: 23.1%/ns Auto-CLET: 55% Allo-CLET: 0% Success decreased over time
Shimazaki et al. [100] 2020 Japan	Retrospective analysis/246/89.3	Auto-CLET + auto-COMET (171) Allo-CLET (75) No	CsA for unknown period	Global (clinical): 65.1% Auto-CLET + COMET: 65.6% Allo-CLET: 63.0%/ns

[1] GMP, good manufacturing practice. [2] Auto, autologous. [3] CLET, cultivated limbal epithelial transplantation. [4] CsA, cyclosporin A. [5] Allo, allogeneic. [6] ccp-IVCM, central corneal phenotype by in vivo confocal microscopy. [7] nm, not mentioned. [8] LTT, limbal tissue transplantation. [9] AMT, amniotic membrane transplantation. [10] na, non-applicable. [11] MSCT, mesenchymal stem cell transplantation. [12] COMET, cultivated oral mucosal epithelial cell transplantation.

3.4. Regulatory Status of Stem Cell-Based Therapy for Treatment of LSCD in Different Countries

Autologous and allogeneic CLET are now performed in several European centers. The procedures require permission from national or European regulatory agencies and must be conducted within GMP guidelines. In the European Union (EU), the specific legal framework for advanced therapy medicinal products (ATMPs) was established by the European Commission in Regulation EC No. 1394/2007 and is regulated by EMA [43,101]. Currently, only Holoclar, the first and only stem cell-based therapy for autologous LSCD, has a conditional marketing authorization with orphan designation in the EU. Moreover, although the UK has recently left the EU, the UK Medicines and Healthcare products Regulatory Agency (MHRA) continues regulating ATMPs following the European regulations. In this regard, Holoclar is still authorized in the UK. In other European countries outside the EU, the regulation of stem cell therapy is at the national level. In Turkey, where autologous CLET has been conducted, the stem cell therapy must follow the guidelines entitled "The Guide to Non-embryonic Cell Studies for Clinical Purposes", prepared by

The Scientific Advisory Board of Stem Cell Transplantations [102]. In the US, stem cell-based therapies are regulated by the FDA and, similar to the EU, cell-based products are considered as biological drugs when they are subjected to more than minimal manipulation or non-homologous use. Currently, in the US, there are no FDA-authorized cellular therapy products for ophthalmic indications [20,103]. Nevertheless, the SLET, not considered as a cell-based therapy, was approved by the FDA for clinical use in 2014 [20]. In addition, autologous or allogeneic limbal epithelial stem cells expanded ex vivo on human amniotic membrane were designated in 2005 as orphan drugs by the FDA to treat LSCD. Allogeneic ABCB5-positive limbal epithelial stem cells were similarly designated in 2019. In Japan, stem cell-based therapy products are regulated by the Pharmaceuticals and Medical Devices Agency (PMDA), Ministry of Health, Labour, and Welfare. These medicines are classified as regenerative medicinal products [104,105]. Autologous CLET, allogeneic CLET, and autologous COMET clinical trials have been developed under Japanese legislation. In 2020, commercial use of a stem cell-based regenerative medicinal product, Nepic, was authorized by the PMDA to treat LSCD, and it is currently manufactured by the Japan Tissue Engineering Co., Ltd. (Gamagori, Japan). In India, the National Stem Cell Guidelines regulate stem cell therapies. They were jointly written in 2007 by the Indian Council of Medical Research and the Indian Department of Biotechnology. The guidelines were revised in 2013 and 2017, and since then, stem-cell-based products derived from substantial, or more than minimal, manipulation have been considered as drugs. However, these amendments exclude minimally manipulated stem cells from the category of drugs [106,107]. At present, in India, there are no approved indications for stem cell-based therapy apart from hematopoietic stem cell transplantation. Therefore, any other stem cell-based therapy must be treated as investigational and conducted only in the form of a clinical trial after obtaining regulatory authorization. Finally, in Australia, cell-derived products are regulated under the Therapeutic Goods Administration regulatory framework for biologicals and must comply with the Therapeutic Goods Order No. 88 [108] and the Australian Code of Good Manufacturing Practice [109].

4. The Future: Challenges to Overcome in Stem Cell-Based Therapies

The ideal goal in the management of corneal blindness due to LSCD is to restore the architecture of the limbal niche so that new stem cells, coming from internal and/or external sources, can repopulate the niche and can replicate in a successful way such that the corneal epithelium can be regenerated with its original properties: transparency, uniformity, and self-renewing capacity.

We have made enormous progress since our preceding colleagues began tissue-based techniques and then stem cell-based techniques (Figure 5). The farthest we have achieved at present is to transplant stem cell-containing tissues or cultivated stem cells extracted from those tissues.

Selection of the best techniques by comparisons among the different therapeutic approaches available at present can hardly be made. Variations in LSCD diagnosis and grading, cell culture protocols, transplantation techniques, postoperative management, evaluation of success vs. failure, etc. are so great that comparative analyses would be inaccurate and unfair. Additionally, there are still no clear answers as to how these therapies work when the stem cells or tissues are transplanted into the human eye. Thus, we have a long way to go as to be able to anatomically and functionally repair a destroyed limbal niche and the stem cells that normally reside there. With no intention of being comprehensive, we selected and described some examples of the relevant clinical and pre-clinical challenges that must be faced and overcome below.

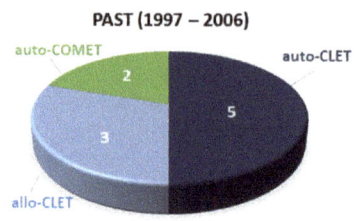
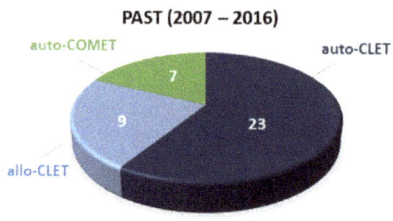
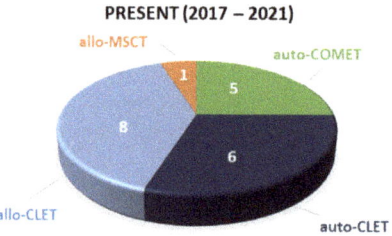

Figure 5. Evolution of stem cell-based therapies to treat corneal failure due to limbal stem cell deficiency from 1997 until the present. The data are for only published clinical trials. CLET, cultivated limbal epithelial transplantation; COMET, cultivated oral mucosal epithelial cell transplantation; MSCT, mesenchymal stem cell transplantation; auto, autologous; allo, allogeneic.

4.1. Clinical Challenges

At present, autologous and allogeneic CLET are performed in several specialized centers around the world, and COMET techniques are being redesigned to offer better results. MSC-based therapies are showing promising results while waiting for larger confirmatory clinical trials [89].

Clinicians have not yet reached full agreement about the clinical stages and gradations of LSCD or even about how to diagnose LSCD [12,110], although efforts are being made [12]. For example, some defend that clinical slit-lamp biomicroscopy findings as observed by experienced ophthalmologists, e.g., loss of limbal normal features, whorl-like epitheliopathy, superficial opacification, neovascularization, persistent epithelial defects, and fluorescein late staining, are sufficient evidence to support a diagnosis of LSCD; however, others feel that more proof is necessary. It is possible that the slit-lamp biomicroscopy findings are sufficient for everyday clinical practice but that more evidence should be considered in the context of clinical trials. The presence of conjunctival or mixed epithelial phenotypes in the central cornea is proof of conjunctivalization or, in other words, LSCD (Figures 2 and 4). Undoubtedly, demonstration of the corneal epithelial phenotype in at least the central cornea following treatment by a stem cell-dependent method can be considered as objective proof of restoration and validation of the LSCD diagnosis. Whether to prove the presence of LSCD by in vivo confocal microscopy or impression cytology is debatable, and each clinical center uses their available resources. However, it is also clear that the epithelium that develops after the transplantation should not be jeopardized by removing the 2–3 layers that corneal impression cytology requires. Anterior segment optical coherence tomography (OCT) is also a good tool to provide high resolution images of the limbal niche [111] and corneal abnormalities pre-, intra- and post-operatively [112,113]. OCT can be especially helpful in showing more clearly how deep the opacification of the cornea is in cases where a clinical inspection at the slit-lamp is unreliable. This allows the clinician to make a therapy plan and to apprise patients and referring physicians whether a further corneal transplantation is probably needed for visual recovery purposes after cell transplantation. The presence of corneal opacification deeper than the anterior stroma due to the etiology of the LSCD, e.g., chemical burn, is an obvious reason for which visual acuity alone is not an adequate parameter to judge the potential efficacy of stem cell-based techniques [37].

Among the many clinical considerations with these challenging patients is the importance of maximizing medical therapy before planning any surgical approaches. The ocular surface must be as quiet as possible for the delicate transplanted stem cells to survive and have a chance to be effective. Thus pre-, peri-, and post-transplant medications need to effectively reduce or eliminate, if possible, ocular surface inflammation. Thus, any eyedrop applied to the eye must be gentle, i.e., unpreserved, and, ideally, applied with a clearly planned protocol that is tailored to each specific case [34]. The issue of systemic immunosuppression for 6–12 months when transplanting allogeneic cells has been addressed above, although this is not a concern for allogeneic MSCs.

A particular aspect of medical treatment and how to best prepare the ocular surface for a future cell transplant is whether corneal neovascularization can be diminished before cell transplant. A related issue is when and how to deal with the remaining neovessels after transplantation. The currently used protocols for treating neovessels are rarely successful [114] and could affect stem cell viability; thus, there is uncertainty about the most adequate timing of treatments. However, the encouraging protocol developed by Yin and Jacobs using the Prosthetic Replacement of Ocular Surface Ecosystem (PROSE) as a delivery system for topical bevacizumab has shown spectacular long-term results [115], and it may be applied to LSCD cases before cell transplantation or even after.

An important strategic consideration prior to stem cell transplantation is to avoid concomitant surgeries that cause additional inflammation and place the transplanted stem cells at risk. For example, the repair of adnexal abnormalities associated with the health and function of the eyelids, conjunctival fornices, symblephara, etc., must be assessed and improved prior to cell transplantation to ensure the best chance of stem cell survival and epithelial healing. Cataract surgery, if needed, must be performed before if possible. Corneal transplantation must not be performed at the same time as stem cell transplantation, and all ocular procedures must wait until cell transplantation is considered finished, between 6 and 12 months [24].

Although the most common practice is to excise any conjunctival tissue encroaching upon the cornea just prior to placing the stem cells on the ocular surface, there is a debate about the best technique to prepare the recipient bed. Another concern is the level of aggressiveness that the ocular surgeon should take in certain etiologies, such as in Stevens–Johnson's syndrome and its spectrum, where the response to surgical aggression can be enormous.

An important consideration, though rarely mentioned, is how to treat limbal scar tissue. Surgically removing it could stimulate neovessel encroachment upon the cornea; therefore, uncertainty exists regarding the best option, i.e., leave it in place or totally or partially removing it.

Clinicians also do not know with certainty if it is better to place the stem cell-based products with cells facing down, i.e., in close contact with tissues, or with cells facing up, i.e., with the carrier in contact with the tissues. There is no agreement or data supporting one way over the other, and each medical team fervently defends its position.

At this stage of clinical development, there are many questions that remain to be asked and answered. For instance, what is the best way to protect the transplant during the immediate post-operative period? Several approaches have been tried, e.g., scleral contact lens, partial tarsorrhaphy, and botulin toxin injection to promote ptosis. However, no protocols have been systematically designed and investigated.

In summary, better-designed randomized and parallel-controlled clinical trials at multiple centers are needed to address the clinical challenges presented here and others as well. Extensive follow-up is necessary to ascertain which technique is best for each specific clinical scenario, how long each type of transplant lasts, and how often each can be repeated. In addition, to help clinicians arrive at a consensus for each of the challenges described here, they need answers from scientists focused on the cellular and molecular aspects of treatments that show promising clinical results.

4.2. Preclinical Challenges

Despite the large number of clinical studies that have shown quite high success rates in different stem cell-based LSCD therapies, there are still many preclinical challenges to overcome and many questions to answer that could further improve the current and yet to come available techniques.

Among the remaining challenges, there is the fact that we still do not fully understand the mechanism by which the transplanted stem cells help repair the damaged ocular surface. Additionally, it is clear that transplantation of just a sheet of stem cells is not enough for reconstructing a damaged limbal stem cell niche. Therefore, alternative routes of cell administration and tissue-engineering techniques must be developed and investigated. Additionally, there is an ongoing research effort to find alternative sources of non-limbal stem cells that have not achieved clinical application but which have promising preclinical results with different degree of success that are also summarized in this section (Figure 6).

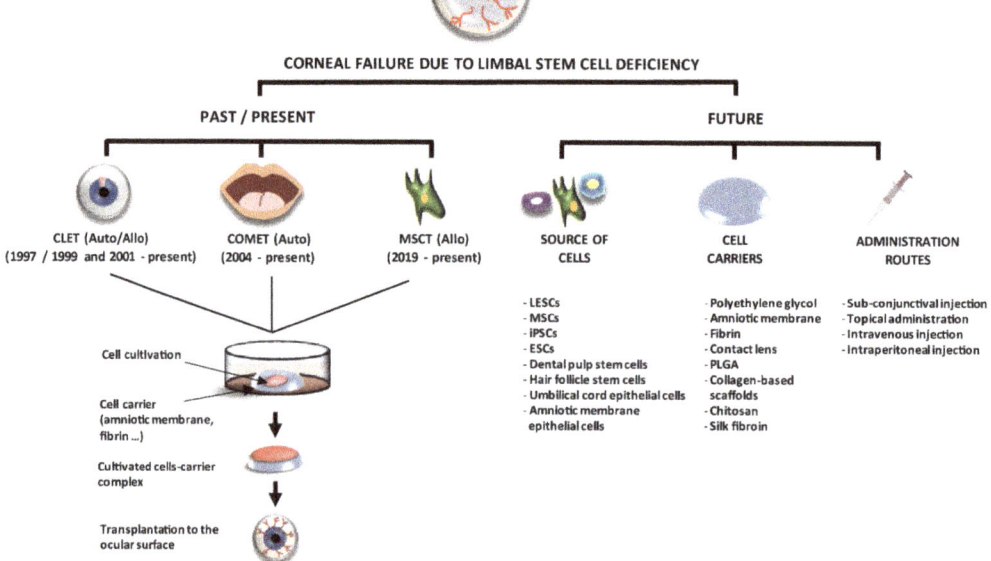

Figure 6. Representation of the different stem cell-based therapy techniques, sources of cells, cell carriers, and alternative administration routes that were used in the past, are being used at present, or will likely be used in the future. Auto: autologous; Allo: allogeneic; CLET: cultivated limbal epithelial transplantation; COMET: cultivated oral mucosa epithelial cells; ESCs: embryonic stem cells; iPSCs: induced pluripotent stem cells; LESCs: limbal epithelial stem cells; LSCD: limbal stem cell deficiency; MSCs: mesenchymal stem cells; MSCT: mesenchymal stem cell transplantation; PLGA: poly lactide-co-glycolic acid.

4.2.1. Analysis of the Corneal Epithelium after Stem Cell-Based Transplantation

At present, the mechanism of action and the fate of the administered stem-cells are still uncertain. The possible cell fates include (1) being metabolized and degraded after application, (2) remaining embedded in the administration place, (3) migration to damaged tissues, or (4) other unknown fates. The mechanism(s) by which transplanted stem cells act could include replicating as stem cells, hopefully after they settle in their niche, and/or by delivering soluble factors into their milieu [34,116].

Although many of these questions are difficult to solve in humans, different techniques have been used in patients to identify the phenotype of cells at the ocular surface after a stem cell transplantation. For instance, the histologic characteristics of the corneal epithelium can be analyzed after the host corneal tissue has been replaced by a corneal transplantation performed in the months following stem cell transplantation [22].

For example, Sangwan et al. showed a normal stratified corneal epithelium in 15 corneal buttons from penetrating keratoplasties where limbal and conjunctival epithelial cells had been grafted in 125 patients with LSCD [117].

Corneal impression cytology has also been used to analyze the phenotype of ocular surface epithelium after a stem cell transplantation. In these specimens, the presence of corneal epithelial markers keratin K3 or K12, conjunctival epithelial goblet cells, and conjunctival epithelial markers K19 and MuC5AC can be identified to determine if the transplanted stem cells achieved a corneal, conjunctival, or mixed phenotype [33,91,118,119].

Currently, corneal in vivo confocal microscopy has mostly replaced corneal impression cytology to study the quality of the new epithelium after stem cell transplantation. This technology is currently used not only to recognize the epithelium phenotype in the central corneal but also to analyze the limbal niche (Figures 2 and 4). When performed on the cornea, the basal epithelium phenotype can be defined as corneal, conjunctival, or mixed. Additionally, inflammatory cells, such as dendritic cells and leucocytes, can be imaged as well as some other structures such as corneal nerves, limbal palisades of Vogt, blood vessels, etc. [33,120–122]. Several authors showed that the confocal microscopy results are correlated with the data obtained by impression cytology [91] with a concordance of 77% (10/13 eyes) [33]. However, the histological study of the ocular tissues obtained from a clinically necessary penetrating keratoplasty should not be replaced by in vivo confocal microscopy, as both techniques are complementary and both have been performed in parallel in recent years [22,24,33,47,89,94,117,122,123].

It is important to know the correlation between the characteristics of stem cell-based grafts and the success of the treatment. Rama et al. showed that 78% of the eyes with stem cell transplants were successful when more than 3% of the transplanted cells were positive for the limbal epithelial stem cell marker p63 [36]. The estimate of p63-positive cells was based on cells in primary culture, but the transplanted cells were harvested from secondary cultures that were derived from the primary cultures [36]. Later, the same authors confirmed that the number of clonogenicity cells, colony size, growth rate, and presence of conjunctival cells in grafts is not directly correlated with clinical outcomes [124].

Several groups have also analyzed the cell phenotype of cultured stem cells before developing a clinical transplantation protocol with the harvested cells [42,93,94,97,117,119,125]. For example, Zakaria et al. reported the expression of ABCG2, ΔNp63, and K14 markers in more than 50% of the amniotic membrane–limbal epithelial cell grafts [94].

Other researchers have used "replicated grafts" to analyze the expression of different markers [89,98]. Replicated grafts are cultures obtained in parallel to the graft to be transplanted; thus, they are composed of cells taken at the same culture passage and grown under the same GMP conditions as the actual graft cells. Replicated grafts, as surrogates for grafts that were actually used in clinical transplants, were analyzed for cell markers in cultured allogeneic limbal cells and allogeneic MSCs cultured on amniotic membrane [89]. The authors showed that 80% of the cells in both cell type cultures expressed the limbal cell markers K15 and p63alpha and corneal marker K3.

In summary, although there are many studies in which the markers and quality of the transplanted stem cells have been studied, there are inherent limitations to the investigation of the mechanism(s) of action and fate(s) of transplanted stem cell-based medicines in humans. As moral and ethical considerations restrict the in vivo use of humans as research models, other approaches must be developed to ask and answer the important questions about the use of stem cells for treating human diseases. Preclinical research tries to answer all of these questions to help clinicians offer patients better cell therapy products.

4.2.2. The Need to Reconstruct the Limbal Stem Cell Niche

The well-known importance of the limbal niche in stem cell regulation, maintenance, proliferation, and differentiation has prompted researchers to seek the best substrata for the culture and transplantation of stem cells, trying to mimic the limbal natural niche. Several types of materials, both natural, such as human amniotic membrane or fibrin, and synthetic, such as poly lactide-co-glycolic acid (PLGA) or siloxane, have been developed over the years to facilitate the cell culture, handling, and corneal regeneration as well as to protect the graft itself (Figure 6).

Currently, the most frequently used substratefor stem cell culture and transplantation of cultured cells into patients with LSCD is human amniotic membrane. This tissue has unique characteristics, including anti-angiogenic, anti-inflammatory, and anti-bacterial properties, which help in the corneal regeneration process [126,127]. Moreover, the culture of limbal epithelial stem cells on amniotic membrane promotes the expression of stem cell markers such as p63α and ABCG2 and reduces some corneal differentiated markers such as K3, K12, and Cx43 [128]. Thus, the amniotic membrane has been successfully used in multitude of clinical studies [24,28,45,46,89,91,93,128–135].

Another natural carrier used in corneal regeneration is fibrin, previously isolated from human plasma [136]. This material has been widely used in ophthalmology as a surgical adhesive and as a biodegradable carrier for tissue engineering [137–139]. In fact, the first CLET was performed using fibrin as a carrier [22], and subsequently, many other studies have used it as a scaffold [36,124,140,141]. Additionally, the EMA-approved product Holoclar also uses fibrin in its composition [37,38].

Apart from natural products, some synthetic materials have also been developed for clinical use since 2007. One of these is a contact lens, Lotrafilcon A siloxane hydrogels, which serves as a cell carrier that supports limbal cell culture and expansion [48,142]. Contact lenses have some benefits compared with natural carriers, as they are transparent and easy to use in ophthalmology, the production is standardized, and some of these materials are commercially approved. However, these substrata are not biodegradable, and the use of contact lenses has not become widely accepted.

Additionally, synthetic biodegradable PLA polymers have been recently used for the treatment of LSCD by serving as a substratum for freshly excised limbal tissue [143]. The use of PLGA membranes as substitute for amniotic membranes or fibrin for limbal epithelial transplantation is a novel technique that will potentially benefit patients, reduce costs, and avoid the risk of disease transmission. A clinical trial completed by Sangwan et al. in 2018 (ClinicalTrials.gov: NCT02568527), evaluated the safety and efficacy of PLGA scaffolds to regenerate limbal epithelial stem cells for autologous limbal grafts in five patients with total unilateral LSCD. No results concerning this study have yet been published.

Several preclinical studies have been developed by using different biomaterials as carrier substrata for limbal cells. Among them are collagen-based scaffolds composed of type I or type IV collagen. They are nontoxic and support corneal epithelial cell culture in animal models. However, they have not yet been implemented in vivo in humans [144–147]. A variation of these materials is plastic compressed collagen, which has been used for co-cultures of limbal epithelial cells and fibroblasts [148–150]. This substratum simulates an artificial stroma and increases the capacity of limbal epithelial cell expansion.

Chitosan, a polysaccharide obtained from natural chitin, is a biocompatible, non-toxic, and bioresorbable polymer with antibacterial properties. It has been widely used as a carrier for limbal epithelial cells in preclinical studies [151–153]. De la Mata et al. demonstrated that glutaraldehyde-crosslinked chitosan, functionalized with gelatin, was suitable for the expansion and maintenance of human stem cells derived from the limbal niche, cultivated with non-xenogeneic supplements [151].

Silk fibroin has also demonstrated the potential to support the culture of both human and rabbit limbal epithelial cells [154]. Moreover, silk fibroin modified with polyethylene glycol was recently established as a potential carrier for limbal cell transplantation in rabbits [155]. Other synthetic polymers such as polyethylene glycol and some temperature-responsive substratum, such as poly(N-isopropylacrylamide), which facilitates cell adhesion, spreading, and growth, have been successfully used in preclinical studies to analyze their potential as carriers for further cell transplantation [156].

All of these potential carriers can be considered opportunities to improve the currently available LSCD therapies. The use of a substratum serves not only to facilitate the process of cell transplantation but also to simulate the limbal niche, providing cells with an ideal environment to grow, proliferate, and maintain their phenotype. Additionally, combining different sources of cells, such as MSCs and others, together with appropriate biological scaffolds, appears to be a promising strategy for long-term revitalization of the limbal niche [157].

In summary, although many different substrata have been investigated with the initial idea of providing an environment similar to the limbal niche, a realistic approach has not yet been achieved in the reconstruction of the architecture of the human healthy limbal niche.

4.2.3. Alternative Routes of Delivering Stem Cell-Therapy

The most commonly used route of stem cell administration to treat LSCD is by affixing with sutures or biological glues the cultivated cells onto the top of the damaged cornea and limbal areas. However, other routes of administration have been studied, some of them with promising results (Figure 6). Topical administration of cells is one of the easiest ways to apply them to the ocular surface. It avoids the need of carriers, surgical sutures, or glues. Indeed, it avoids the whole surgical procedure. However, there are some drawbacks to topical application of the stem cells, such as low retention time, high washing off rate, and low penetration of the corneal epithelium.

The topical administration of MSCs provides therapeutic and anti-inflammatory effects in different experimental models of corneal epithelial damage [79,158]. A clinical trial performed by Boto et al. (ClinicalTrials.gov: NCT01808378) administered adipose tissue-derived MSCs (AT-MSCs) topically in combination with subconjunctival injection of AT-MSCs; however, the results of this study have not yet been published. A clinical trial by Auffarth et al. (ClinicalTrials.gov: NCT03549299), active since 2018 but not yet recruiting, proposes topical application of four different doses of allogeneic ABCB5-positive limbal stem cells. The results from these and future clinical trials are needed to determine if topical administration of cells can be a fully effective route of administration for ocular surface treatment.

The subconjunctival injection of cells is another local route of administration that has been extensively studied. This technique has numerous advantages: (1) It is minimally invasive and does not require a surgical facility. (2) The cell product can be prepared easily, and carriers are not needed. (3) It allows for the administration of high cell doses in a small volume. (4) The cell dose administered can be effectively controlled. (5) It can be used in severe cases of LSCD [159]. However, a large volume of solution cannot be injected into the subconjunctiva, and there are yet no consensus on the best vehicle solution, the number and location of injections, and the dose of cells to be administered. In spite of this, there are several works showing that the subconjunctival injection of MSCs reduces inflammation of the ocular surface in different experimental models of corneal epithelial damage [80,160,161]. It also reduces clinical signs such as corneal neovascularization, opacity, and epithelial defects [162–164]. The most frequently injected cell type is MSCs, but oral mucosal epithelial cells have also been subconjunctivally injected in a rat experimental LSCD model [165].

After the transplantation of expanded cells on a human amniotic membrane or fibrin, the subconjunctival injection of AT-MSCs or bone marrow-derived MSCs (BM-MSCs) for the treatment of corneal epithelial damage is the most studied technique in humans. To date, three clinical trials have been completed (ClinicalTrials.gov: NCT01808378, NCT04484402, and NCT02325843) but not yet published. Additionally, there are two other clinical trials registered in which umbilical cord MSCs or allogeneic BM-MSCs will be injected subconjunctivally (ClinicalTrials.gov: NCT03237442 and NCT03967275). Although more clinical evidence is needed to determine if subconjunctival injection is an effective route of cell administration for the treatment of LSCD, the advantages and preclinical evidence makes it one of the most promising techniques.

Another option in preclinical study phases for the treatment of ocular surface pathology is the systemic injection of stem cells. The ability of MSCs to migrate into damaged or inflamed tissues [166] makes MSCs the most suitable cell type for systemic administration in the treatment of LSCD. However, systemic administration presents a high risk of side effects, and the number of cells that reach the target tissue is low [65,167]. Moreover, as with all cell administration by injection, there is still no consensus regarding the best vehicle solution. However, in contrast with subconjunctival injection, systemic administration allows for large volumes to be administered and much higher cell doses can be achieved [159].

Both intraperitoneal and intravenous administration of BM-MSCs have reduced corneal opacity [64,65,74,168,169] and ocular surface inflammation [65,75,169] in different experimental models of corneal epithelial damage. However, to the best of our knowledge, these routes of administration have not been used in humans yet for the treatment of corneal failure due to LSCD.

In summary, interesting new alternative routes and doses could undergo further preclinical investigations before finally being translated into clinical use.

4.2.4. Other Potential Sources of Non-Limbal Cells

As described above, limbal epithelial cells have limitations with respect to providing a sufficient number of stem cells to ensure successful treatment of LSCD. For that reason, other cell sources have been sought. Up to now, oral mucosa epithelial cells and MSCs are the only non-limbal epithelial cells that have been proven to be safe and effective for treating patients with ocular surface failure due LSCD [55,89]. Nevertheless, during the last few years, other alternative sources of non-limbal cells have also been investigated in experimental studies with different degrees of success [34,170–172] (Figure 6).

Embryonic Stem Cells

Human embryonic stem cells (hESCs) are pluripotent stem cells derived from the inner cell mass of human blastocysts, and they can differentiate into derivatives of all three germ layers [173]. Therefore, the differentiation of hESCs into corneal or limbal epithelial cells offers the potential of an unlimited source of cells to treat patients suffering from LSCD.

The significance of reproducing the corneal stem cell environment to induce hESCs to differentiate towards a corneal or limbal epithelial-like cell phenotype has been supported by several studies [174–177]. By mimicking the microenvironment of the corneal epithelial stem cell niche in vitro, Ahmad et al. successfully induced hESC differentiation into corneal epithelial-like cells. To that end, they cultured hESCs on type IV collagen, a component of the corneal epithelial basement membrane, using media conditioned by limbal fibroblasts [177]. Other authors differentiated hESCs into corneal epithelial-like cells by seeding them onto a partially de-epithelialized or de-cellularized human corneal buttons [174]. Others coaxed the hESCs to develop into limbal epithelial stem cell-like cells by using a culture medium conditioned by limbal epithelial stem cells [175]. However, all of these differentiation techniques depend on corneal tissue donors to either culture the hESCs on them or to prepare the conditioned media. With the potential biological variations among tissues from different donors, this greatly limits the potential of these differentiation techniques.

To overcome these limitations, Zhang et al. developed a protocol to differentiate hESCs into corneal epithelial progenitor cells using a defined serum-free medium [178]. They demonstrated the functionality of the progenitor cells grown on an acellular porcine corneal matrix and transplanted onto rabbit eyes [179]. Very recently, He et al. have also demonstrated that clinical-grade hESC-derived corneal epithelial cell sheets successfully helped repair the damaged ocular surface of a rabbit LSCD model [180].

Despite being a potential limitless source of cells, the future clinical use of hESCs for treating patients with LSCD might be hampered due to some drawbacks, such as the ethical controversy regarding their embryonic origin, their immunogenicity, and their potential tumorigenicity [181].

Induced Pluripotent Stem Cells

Human-induced pluripotent stem cells (hiPSCs), which have characteristics that are similar to hESCs, are generated by manipulation of differentiated adult cells [182]. Since the reprogramming technique was described, great efforts have been made to generate corneal and limbal epithelial cells from hiPSCs. This technology could provide an unlimited supply of limbal and corneal epithelial cells without any ethical issue for treating patients with LSCD (reviewed in [183–185]).

Hayashi et al. reported the first method to generate corneal epithelial cells from hiPSCs derived from both adult corneal limbal epithelial cells and human dermal fibroblasts [186]. Later, these same authors described a strategy to generate corneal stem and progenitor cells from hiPSCs by reproducing in vitro the whole eye development. Using this approach, they generated an epithelial cell sheet that successfully restored corneal function in a rabbit model of LSCD [187,188]. Using small molecules, Mikhailova et al. developed a directed two-stage differentiation protocol to generate corneal epithelial-like progenitor cells with the capacity to terminally differentiate towards mature corneal epithelial-like cells [189]. This same research group later published another reproducible and clinical compatible differentiation method using xeno-free conditions to generate limbal epithelial stem cells from hiPSCs [190]. Apart from the ones already mentioned, several other methods have been published with the aim to generate functional corneal and limbal epithelial cells from hiPSCs (reviewed in [183–185]). However, before translating these methodologies to clinical applications, further improvements must be made on the derivation protocols because they are extremely expensive. They also require a considerable amount of time, first, for hiPSC generation and, later, for corneal and limbal cell induction. The creation of HLA-typed hiPSC banks has been proposed as a potential solution to partially overcome these two limitations and to also reduce the potential problems of immunogenicity [191,192]. Furthermore, given that hiPSC generation could induce mutagenicity, extensive genetic analyses must be performed on the hiPSCs intended for transplantation into patients to ensure genetic fidelity and stability [193]. Among these, reprogramming vector analysis and karyotype analysis are considered mandatory, while performing single nucleotide polymorphism arrays, whole genome analysis, and other genetic and disease marker analyses are considered to be for informational purposes only [193]. Considering that the tumorigenic potential of hiPSC-derived corneal epithelial cells has not been fully tested [194], the likelihood of it cannot be conclusively ruled out due to the possible presence of undifferentiated or partially differentiated iPSCs in the cell population intended to be transplanted [194]. Consequently, the development of protocols to directly reprogram adult cells towards a designated phenotype, thus avoiding the pluripotent state, could help to diminish the tumorigenicity of the transplanted cells [195]. In this context, a direct transdifferentiation protocol to generate corneal/limbal epithelial cells from human dermal fibroblasts has already been published [196]. Therefore, this new methodology that bypasses the hiPSC stage might provide a safer source of corneal epithelial cells devoid of tumorigenic potential.

Dental Pulp Stem Cells

Human immature dental pulp stem cells isolated from exfoliated teeth express both MSC, ESC, and limbal epithelial stem cell markers such as p63 and ABCG2. The transplantation of these stem cells into a LSCD rabbit model reduced corneal neovascularization and conjunctivalization, and reconstructed the damaged ocular surface by developing a well-formed corneal epithelium that expressed limbal epithelial stem cell and corneal epithelial cell markers [197,198]. These and other authors further developed the capacity of dental pulp stem cells to acquire corneal and limbal epithelial features using different cell culture techniques [199,200] and cell carriers [201,202]. However, although these cells seem to represent a valid alternative source of cells for treating patients with LSCD, more preclinical evidence should be gathered, especially related to their tumorigenicity, before translating this technology into clinical practice.

Hair Follicle Bulge-Derived Epithelial Stem Cells

Hair follicle bulge-derived stem cells are a population of epithelial stem cells involved in forming hair follicles and in regenerating the epidermis during wound healing [203,204]. Blazejewska et al. demonstrated that these cells were also able to differentiate into corneal epithelial-like cells. They reported that, by mimicking the limbal microenvironment, hair follicle bulge-derived stem cells cultivated on laminin-5 in a culture medium conditioned by limbal fibroblast showed the structural, morphological, and molecular features of corneal epithelial cells [205]. Later, the functionality and therapeutic potential of these stem cells was further confirmed in a mouse model of LSCD [206]. Mainly because of their easy accessibility, hair follicle bulge-derived epithelial stem cells might be an interesting alternative source of stem cells for treating LSCD. However, apart from these initial studies, not much further work has been performed.

Amniotic Membrane Epithelial Cells

The inner surface of the human amniotic membrane is covered by a continuous single layer of ectodermal cells, the amniotic membrane epithelial cells. These cells not only express hESC markers and pluripotent stem cell-like characteristics but also have a MSC-like phenotype. As a consequence, they also have both low immunogenicity and high immunomodulatory properties [207,208]. Studies have reported the potential of human amniotic membrane epithelial cells to differentiate into corneal epithelial cells and to reconstruct the damaged ocular surface of rabbit LSCD models [209–212]. Therefore, this type of cell represents another alternative source of stem cells for treating LSCD, and similar to other potential sources of stem cells other than hESCs, their use does not provoke any ethical issues. It is important to highlight that these cells are also genetically stable because they do not form tumors upon transplantation into immunodeficient mice [207]. However, the data regarding the mechanism by which these cells exert their immunomodulatory properties is still not fully known. That is why further studies to elucidate the mechanism underlying this effect are required before they are used for clinical purposes [208].

Umbilical Cord Lining Epithelial Cells

Human umbilical cord lining epithelial cells are a population of pluripotent stem cells that express a cytokeratin pattern similar to human epidermal cells [213] and are capable of forming stratified epithelial sheets [214,215]. Reza et al. investigated the effectiveness of a mucin-expressing cell line derived from the cord lining for treating LSCD in a rabbit model using denuded human amniotic membrane as a cell carrier [216]. The mucin-expressing cord lining epithelial cells regenerated the damaged ocular surface with minimal neovascularization and opacification and formed a stratified epithelium that expressed the corneal epithelial markers K3/12. These cells showed no tumorigenicity, and there was no immune rejection, indicating low immunogenicity. Nevertheless, additional studies must be performed to verify those results before using this source of cells for treating patients.

Besides the cell-based therapies that are currently used in clinical practice, an increasing range of alternative sources of stem cells is being investigated. Many highly varied inducing protocols have been published to culture and later differentiate all of these types of human stem cells into corneal and limbal epithelial cells. However, there are no studies that compare the outcomes obtained among the different methodologies, and as a consequence, there are no standardized differentiation protocols. Therefore, efforts should be made to elaborate standard and reproducible differentiation protocols for each of the different types of stem cells [185]. There is also a need to develop cell culture techniques with chemically defined xeno-free culture media that meet the clinical grade requirements. This will increase the reproducibility, the quality, and the safety of the final stem cell-based product. Although any of these alternative stem cell sources could become a successful therapy for treating ocular surface failure due to LSCD, there are still some other challenges, such as tumorigenicity and immunogenicity that need to be overcome.

4.3. Regulatory Challenges

Stem cell-based therapies for corneal blindness due to ocular surface failure must meet the same regulatory requirements as other cell-based products for any other indication. Under most of the regulatory frameworks, this means that, among other requirements, the production of the cell-based product must comply with the principles of GMP. Furthermore, human clinical trials must be designed and conducted in compliance with the principles of good clinical practice. As the regulatory procedure to obtain approval of a cell-based therapy requires a lot of expertise, time, and investment, the process of bringing a new stem cell-based product to the clinic is very challenging. This is especially significant for small developers, such as universities, hospitals, and small- to medium-sized enterprises for which compliance with the regulations of cell-based products can be difficult and unaffordable. To this end, several agencies from different jurisdictions, such as the ones from the EU, Japan, and the US, have implemented mechanisms to accelerate and optimize the development of this type of medicinal product. The compliance with national and international regulations is vital for the development and commercialization of these therapies. Therefore, one of the greatest regulatory challenges for the coming years will be to establish an international harmonization of the regulatory frameworks that control the development of stem cell-based medicinal products throughout the globe [30].

5. Conclusions

The application of surgical therapies to treat corneal pathology due stem cell destruction, just a decade after the discovery of stem cells at the ocular surface, has made an extraordinary progress over the last three decades. A new name, LSCD, was given to the corneal failure caused by a wide variety of pathologies that can destroy the corneoscleral limbus. Transplantation of limbal tissues (either whole or minced limbal segments) began and was followed some years later by stem cell-based transplants in an effort to repair these severe clinical entities.

At present, to avoid the need for immunosuppression, only unilateral cases of LSCD are eligible for autologous transplantations, either tissue-based or cultivated stem cell-derived. Bilateral severe cases can benefit from autologous transplants only when extraocular stem cells can be used. For that purpose, only COMET has been translated into clinical practice. Another alternative in bilateral LSCD cases is to use allografts. In the case of whole or minced limbal tissue tissue-based allografts, long-term immunosuppression is needed to avoid immune rejection. Short-term immunosuppression is needed if cultivated stem cell-based therapies, such as allogeneic CLET, are planned. However, to avoid host immunosuppression, immune-privileged stem cells such as allogeneic MSCs, the most often used stem cell type in regenerative medicine, has just entered the ophthalmic armamentarium. As only allogeneic therapies are of interest for commercialization purposes at affordable prices, more efforts must be made by both research and clinical scientists to develop medicinal products based on allogeneic sources. Even with all of the progress made thus far, we must be aware that, while current therapies are delivering stem cells or stem cell-rich products onto the cornea and limbal area, the limbal niche itself has not yet been reconstructed.

In summary, only the close collaboration between preclinical and clinical scientists, international regulatory agencies, governmental and non-governmental financial sources, and the pharmaceutical industry make meaningful achievements that can effectively reach patients affected by LSCD pathologies, making the statement "from the bench to the bedside" truer than ever.

Author Contributions: Conceptualization, M.C.; investigation, M.C., T.N.-M., A.d.l.M., S.G. and M.L.-P.; writing—original draft preparation, M.C., T.N.-M., A.d.l.M., S.G. and M.L.-P.; writing—review and editing, J.M.H. and M.C.; funding acquisition, M.C. and T.N.-M. All authors have read and agreed to the published version of the manuscript.

Funding: This work was funded by the Department of Education, Castilla y León Regional Government (grant VA268P18 FEDER, EU) Spain; Ministry of Science and Innovation (grant PID2019-105525RB-100, MICINN/FEDER, EU), Spain; Institute of Health Carlos III, CIBER-BBN (CB06/01/003 MICINN/FEDER, EU), Spain; and the Regional Center for Regenerative Medicine and Cell Therapy of Castilla y León, Spain.

Institutional Review Board Statement: Not applicable.

Informed Consent Statement: Not applicable.

Data Availability Statement: Publicly available datasets were analyzed in this review. This data can be found here: https://www.clinicaltrials.gov/ (accessed on 12 July 2021).

Acknowledgments: We thank B. Bromberg for his assistance in the final editing and preparation of this manuscript.

Conflicts of Interest: The authors declare no conflict of interest. The funders had no role in the design of the study; in the collection, analyses, or interpretation of data; in the writing of the manuscript; or in the decision to publish the results.

References

1. Dhamodaran, K.; Subramani, M.; Ponnalagu, M.; Shetty, R.; Das, D. Ocular stem cells: A status update! *Stem Cell Res. Ther.* **2014**, *5*, 56. [CrossRef]
2. Ramos, T.; Scott, D.; Ahmad, S. An Update on Ocular Surface Epithelial Stem Cells: Cornea and Conjunctiva. *Stem Cells Int.* **2015**, *2015*, 601731. [CrossRef]
3. Schwab, I.R. Cultured corneal epithelia for ocular surface disease. *Trans. Am. Ophthalmol. Soc.* **1999**, *97*, 891–986.
4. Mann, I. A Study of Epithelial Regeneration in the Living Eye. *Br. J. Ophthalmol.* **1944**, *28*, 26–40. [CrossRef] [PubMed]
5. Friedenwald, J.S.; Buschke, W. Some Factors Concerned in the Mitotic and Wound-Healing Activities of the Corneal Epithelium. *Trans. Am. Ophthalmol. Soc.* **1944**, *42*, 371–383.
6. Maumenee, A. Repair in cornea. *Adv. Biol. Ski.* **1964**, *5*, 208–215.
7. Davanger, M.; Evensen, A. Role of the pericorneal papillary structure in renewal of corneal epithelium. *Nature* **1971**, *229*, 560–561. [CrossRef]
8. Thoft, R.A.; Friend, J. The X, Y, Z hypothesis of corneal epithelial maintenance. *Investig. Ophthalmol. Vis. Sci.* **1983**, *24*, 1442–1443.
9. Kinoshita, S.; Friend, J.; Thoft, R.A. Sex chromatin of donor corneal epithelium in rabbits. *Investig. Ophthalmol. Vis. Sci.* **1981**, *21*, 434–441.
10. Schermer, A.; Galvin, S.; Sun, T.T. Differentiation-related expression of a major 64K corneal keratin in vivo and in culture suggests limbal location of corneal epithelial stem cells. *J. Cell Biol.* **1986**, *103*, 49–62. [CrossRef]
11. Guo, P.; Sun, H.; Zhang, Y.; Tighe, S.; Chen, S.; Su, C.W.; Liu, Y.; Zhao, H.; Hu, M.; Zhu, Y. Limbal niche cells are a potent resource of adult mesenchymal progenitors. *J. Cell. Mol. Med.* **2018**, *22*, 3315–3322. [CrossRef] [PubMed]
12. Deng, S.X.; Borderie, V.; Chan, C.C.; Dana, R.; Figueiredo, F.C.; Gomes, J.A.; Pellegrini, G.; Shimmura, S.; Kruse, F.E. Global consensus on definition, classification, diagnosis, and staging of limbal stem cell deficiency. *Cornea* **2019**, *38*, 364–375. [CrossRef]
13. Nakamura, T.; Inatomi, T.; Sotozono, C.; Koizumi, N.; Kinoshita, S. Ocular surface reconstruction using stem cell and tissue engineering. *Prog. Retin. Eye Res.* **2016**, *51*, 187–207. [CrossRef] [PubMed]
14. Kenyon, K.R.; Tseng, S.C. Limbal Autograft Transplantation for Ocular Surface Disorders. *Ophthalmology* **1989**, *96*, 709–722. [CrossRef]

15. Ballios, B.G.; Weisbrod, M.; Chan, C.C.; Borovik, A.; Schiff, J.R.; Tinckam, K.J.; Humar, A.; Kim, S.J.; Cole, E.H.; Slomovic, A.R. Systemic immunosuppression in limbal stem cell transplantation: Best practices and future challenges. *Can. J. Ophthalmol.* **2018**, *53*, 314–323. [CrossRef]
16. Ozer, M.D.; Altinkurt, E.; Yilmaz, Y.C.; Gedik, A.C.; Alparslan, N. The surgical outcomes of limbal allograft transplantation in eyes having limbal stem cell deficiency. *J. Curr. Ophthalmol.* **2020**, *32*, 132–141. [CrossRef]
17. Cheung, A.Y.; Eslani, M.; Kurji, K.H.; Wright, E.; Sarnicola, E.; Govil, A.; Holland, E.J. Long-term outcomes of living-related conjunctival limbal allograft compared with keratolimbal allograft in patients with limbal stem cell deficiency. *Cornea* **2020**, *39*, 980–985. [CrossRef]
18. Sangwan, V.S.; Basu, S.; MacNeil, S.; Balasubramanian, D. Simple limbal epithelial transplantation (SLET): A novel surgical technique for the treatment of unilateral limbal stem cell deficiency. *Br. J. Ophthalmol.* **2012**, *96*, 931–934. [CrossRef] [PubMed]
19. Jackson, C.J.; Myklebust Ernø, I.T.; Ringstad, H.; Tønseth, K.A.; Dartt, D.A.; Utheim, T.P. Simple limbal epithelial transplantation: Current status and future perspectives. *Stem Cells Transl. Med.* **2020**, *9*, 316–327. [CrossRef]
20. Amescua, G.; Atallah, M.; Nikpoor, N.; Galor, A.; Perez, V.L. Modified simple limbal epithelial transplantation using cryopreserved amniotic membrane for unilateral limbal stem cell deficiency. *Am. J. Ophthalmol.* **2014**, *158*, 469–475.e2. [CrossRef] [PubMed]
21. Shanbhag, S.; Patel, C.; Goyal, R.; Donthineni, P.; Singh, V.; Basu, S. Simple limbal epithelial transplantation (SLET): Review of indications, surgical technique, mechanism, outcomes, limitations, and impact. *Indian J. Ophthalmol.* **2019**, *67*, 1265–1277. [CrossRef]
22. Pellegrini, G.; Traverso, C.E.; Franzi, A.T.; Zingirian, M.; Cancedda, R.; De Luca, M. Long-term restoration of damaged corneal surfaces with autologous cultivated corneal epithelium. *Lancet* **1997**, *349*, 990–993. [CrossRef]
23. Notara, M.; Alatza, A.; Gilfillan, J.; Harris, A.R.; Levis, H.J.; Schrader, S.; Vernon, A.; Daniels, J.T. In sickness and in health: Corneal epithelial stem cell biology, pathology and therapy. *Exp. Eye Res.* **2010**, *90*, 188–195. [CrossRef]
24. Ramírez, B.E.; Sánchez, A.; Herreras, J.M.; Fernández, I.; García-Sancho, J.; Nieto-Miguel, T.; Calonge, M. Stem Cell Therapy for Corneal Epithelium Regeneration following Good Manufacturing and Clinical Procedures. *Biomed Res. Int.* **2015**, *2015*, 408495. [CrossRef]
25. Angunawela, R.I.; Mehta, J.S.; Daniels, J.T. Ex-vivo ocular surface stem cell therapies: Current techniques, applications, hurdles and future directions. *Expert Rev. Mol. Med.* **2013**, *15*, e4. [CrossRef]
26. CCG Tseng, S.; Chen, S.Y.; Shen, Y.C.; Chen, W.L.; Hu, F.R. Critical Appraisal of Ex Vivo Expansion of Human Limbal Epithelial Stem Cells. *Curr. Mol. Med.* **2010**, *10*, 841–850. [CrossRef]
27. Dua, H.S.; Miri, A.; Said, D.G. Contemporary limbal stem cell transplantation—A review. *Clin. Exp. Ophthalmol.* **2010**, *38*, 104–117. [CrossRef] [PubMed]
28. Baylis, O.; Figueiredo, F.; Henein, C.; Lako, M.; Ahmad, S. 13 Years of cultured limbal epithelial cell therapy: A review of the outcomes. *J. Cell. Biochem.* **2011**, *112*, 993–1002. [CrossRef] [PubMed]
29. Oie, Y.; Nishida, K. Regenerative medicine for the cornea. *Biomed Res. Int.* **2013**, *2013*, 428247. [CrossRef] [PubMed]
30. Pellegrini, G.; Rama, P.; Di Rocco, A.; Panaras, A.; De Luca, M. Concise review: Hurdles in a successful example of limbal stem cell-based regenerative medicine. *Stem Cells* **2014**, *32*, 26–34. [CrossRef] [PubMed]
31. Sangwan, V.S.; Jain, R.; Basu, S.; Bagadi, A.B.; Sureka, S.; Mariappan, I.; Macneil, S. Transforming ocular surface stem cell research into successful clinical practice. *Indian J. Ophthalmol.* **2014**, *62*, 29–40. [CrossRef] [PubMed]
32. Genicio, N.; Gallo Paramo, J.; Shortt, A.J. Quantum dot labeling and tracking of cultured limbal epithelial cell transplants in vitro. *Investig. Ophthalmol. Vis. Sci.* **2015**, *56*, 3051–3059. [CrossRef] [PubMed]
33. Pedrotti, E.; Passilongo, M.; Fasolo, A.; Nubile, M.; Parisi, G.; Mastropasqua, R.; Ficial, S.; Bertolin, M.; Di Iorio, E.; Ponzin, D.; et al. In Vivo Confocal Microscopy 1 Year after Autologous Cultured Limbal Stem Cell Grafts. *Ophthalmology* **2015**, *122*, 1660–1668. [CrossRef] [PubMed]
34. Ghareeb, A.E.; Lako, M.; Figueiredo, F.C. Recent Advances in Stem Cell Therapy for Limbal Stem Cell Deficiency: A Narrative Review. *Ophthalmol. Ther.* **2020**, *9*, 809–831. [CrossRef]
35. European Medicines Agency. EU/3/08/579. Available online: https://www.ema.europa.eu/en/medicines/human/orphan-designations/eu308579 (accessed on 6 November 2020).
36. Rama, P.; Matuska, S.; Paganoni, G.; Spinelli, A.; De Luca, M.; Pellegrini, G. Limbal Stem-Cell Therapy and Long-Term Corneal Regeneration. *N. Engl. J. Med.* **2010**, *363*, 147–155. [CrossRef]
37. Pellegrini, G.; Ardigò, D.; Milazzo, G.; Iotti, G.; Guatelli, P.; Pelosi, D.; De Luca, M. Navigating Market Authorization: The Path Holoclar Took to Become the First Stem Cell Product Approved in the European Union. *Stem Cells Transl. Med.* **2018**, *7*, 146–154. [CrossRef]
38. López-Paniagua, M.; de la Mata, A.; Galindo, S.; Blázquez, F.; Calonge, M.; Nieto-Miguel, T. Advanced therapy medicinal products for the eye: Definitions and regulatory framework. *Pharmaceutics* **2021**, *13*, 347. [CrossRef]
39. Gay, M.H.; Baldomero, H.; Farge-Bancel, D.; Robey, P.G.; Rodeo, S.; Passweg, J.; Müller-Gerbl, M.; Martin, I. The survey on cellular and tissue-engineered therapies in Europe in 2016 and 2017. *Tissue Eng. Part A* **2021**, *27*, 336–350. [CrossRef] [PubMed]
40. Le, Q.; Chauhan, T.; Yung, M.; Tseng, C.H.; Deng, S.X. Outcomes of Limbal Stem Cell Transplant: A Meta-analysis. *JAMA Ophthalmol.* **2020**, *138*, 660–670. [CrossRef]

41. Mishan, M.A.; Yaseri, M.; Baradaran-Rafii, A.; Kanavi, M.R. Systematic review and meta-analysis investigating autograft versus allograft cultivated limbal epithelial transplantation in limbal stem cell deficiency. *Int. Ophthalmol.* **2019**, *39*, 2685–2696. [CrossRef] [PubMed]
42. Koizumi, N.; Inatomi, T.; Suzuki, T.; Sotozono, C.; Kinoshita, S. Cultivated corneal epithelial stem cell transplantation in ocular surface disorders. *Ophthalmology* **2001**, *108*, 1569–1574. [CrossRef]
43. Regulation (EC) No 1394/2007 of the European Parliament and of the Council of 13 November 2007 on Advance Therapy Medicinal Products and Amending Directive 2001/83/EC and Regulation /EC) N0 726/2004. Available online: https://eur-lex.europa.eu/LexUriServ/LexUriServ.do?uri=OJ:L:2007:324:0121:0137:en:PDF (accessed on 29 July 2021).
44. Commission Directive 2003/94/EC of 8 October 2003 Laying down the Principles and Guidelines of Good Manufacturing Practice in Respect of Medicinal Products for Human Use and Investigational Medicinal Products for Human Use. Available online: https://eur-lex.europa.eu/LexUriServ/LexUriServ.do?uri=OJ:L:2003:262:0022:0026:en:PDF (accessed on 29 July 2021).
45. Zhao, Y.; Ma, L. Systematic review and meta-analysis on transplantation of ex vivo cultivated limbal epithelial stem cell on amniotic membrane in limbal stem cell deficiency. *Cornea* **2015**, *34*, 592–600. [CrossRef]
46. Shortt, A.J.; Secker, G.A.; Notara, M.D.; Limb, G.A.; Khaw, P.T.; Tuft, S.J.; Daniels, J.T. Transplantation of Ex Vivo Cultured Limbal Epithelial Stem Cells: A Review of Techniques and Clinical Results. *Surv. Ophthalmol.* **2007**, *52*, 483–502. [CrossRef] [PubMed]
47. Borderie, V.M.; Ghoubay, D.; Georgeon, C.; Borderie, M.; de Sousa, C.; Legendre, A.; Rouard, H. Long-Term Results of Cultured Limbal Stem Cell Versus Limbal Tissue Transplantation in Stage III Limbal Deficiency. *Stem Cells Transl. Med.* **2019**, *8*, 1230–1241. [CrossRef] [PubMed]
48. Bobba, S.; Chow, S.; Watson, S.; Di Girolamo, N. Clinical outcomes of xeno-free expansion and transplantation of autologous ocular surface epithelial stem cells via contact lens delivery: A prospective case series. *Stem Cell Res. Ther.* **2015**, *6*, 23. [CrossRef] [PubMed]
49. Li, W.; Hayashida, Y.; Chen, Y.T.; Tseng, S.C. Niche regulation of corneal epithelial stem cells at the limbus. *Cell Res.* **2007**, *17*, 26–36. [CrossRef]
50. Shimazaki, J.; Higa, K.; Kato, N.; Satake, Y. Barrier function of cultivated limbal and oral mucosal epithelial cell sheets. *Investig. Ophthalmol. Vis. Sci.* **2009**, *50*, 5672–5680. [CrossRef]
51. Sugiyama, H.; Yamato, M.; Nishida, K.; Okano, T. Evidence of the survival of ectopically transplanted oral mucosal epithelial stem cells after repeated wounding of cornea. *Mol. Ther.* **2014**, *22*, 1544–1555. [CrossRef] [PubMed]
52. Hayashida, Y.; Nishida, K.; Yamato, M.; Watanabe, K.; Maeda, N.; Watanabe, H.; Kikuchi, A.; Okano, T.; Tano, Y. Ocular surface reconstruction using autologous rabbit oral mucosal epithelial sheets fabricated ex vivo on a temperature-responsive culture surface. *Investig. Ophthalmol. Vis. Sci.* **2005**, *46*, 1632–1639. [CrossRef] [PubMed]
53. Nakamura, T.; Endo, K.I.; Cooper, L.J.; Fullwood, N.J.; Tanifuji, N.; Tsuzuki, M.; Koizumi, N.; Inatomi, T.; Sano, Y.; Kinoshita, S. The successful culture and autologous transplantation of rabbit oral mucosal epithelial cells on amniotic membrane. *Investig. Ophthalmol. Vis. Sci.* **2003**, *44*, 106–116. [CrossRef]
54. Nakamura, T.; Inatomi, T.; Sotozono, C.; Amemiya, T.; Kanamura, N.; Kinoshita, S. Transplantation of cultivated autologous oral mucosal epithelial cells in patients with severe ocular surface disorders. *Br. J. Ophthalmol.* **2004**, *88*, 1280–1284. [CrossRef] [PubMed]
55. Cabral, J.V.; Jackson, C.J.; Utheim, T.P.; Jirsova, K. Ex vivo cultivated oral mucosal epithelial cell transplantation for limbal stem cell deficiency: A review. *Stem Cell Res. Ther.* **2020**, *11*, 301. [CrossRef] [PubMed]
56. Duan, C.Y.; Xie, H.T.; Zhao, X.Y.; Xu, W.H.; Zhang, M.C. Limbal niche cells can reduce the angiogenic potential of cultivated oral mucosal epithelial cells. *Cell. Mol. Biol. Lett.* **2019**, *24*, 3. [CrossRef] [PubMed]
57. Chen, H.C.; Chen, H.L.; Lai, J.Y.; Chen, C.C.; Tsai, Y.J.; Kuo, M.T.; Chu, P.H.; Sun, C.C.; Chen, J.K.; Ma, D.H. Persistence of transplanted oral mucosal epithelial cells in human cornea. *Investig. Ophthalmol. Vis. Sci.* **2009**, *50*, 4660–4668. [CrossRef]
58. Wang, J.; Qi, X.; Dong, Y.; Cheng, J.; Zhai, H.; Zhou, Q.; Xie, L. Comparison of the efficacy of different cell sources for transplantation in total limbal stem cell deficiency. *Graefe's Arch. Clin. Exp. Ophthalmol.* **2019**, *257*, 1253–1263. [CrossRef]
59. Samoila, O.; Gocan, D. Clinical Outcomes From Cultivated Allogenic Stem Cells vs. Oral Mucosa Epithelial Transplants in Total Bilateral Stem Cells Deficiency. *Front. Med.* **2020**, *7*, 43. [CrossRef] [PubMed]
60. Nieto-Miguel, T.; Galindo, S.; López-Paniagua, M.; Pérez, I.; Herreras, J.M.; Calonge, M. Cell Therapy Using Extraocular Mesenchymal Stem Cells. In *Corneal Regeneration Therapy and Surgery*; Alió, J., Alió del Barrio, J.L., Arnalich-Montiel, F., Eds.; Springer Nature: Basingstoke, UK, 2019; pp. 231–262. [CrossRef]
61. Oh, J.Y.; Kim, M.K.; Shin, M.S.; Wee, W.R.; Lee, J.H. Cytokine secretion by human mesenchymal stem cells cocultured with damaged corneal epithelial cells. *Cytokine* **2009**, *46*, 100–103. [CrossRef] [PubMed]
62. Hu, N.; Zhang, Y.Y.; Gu, H.W.; Guan, H.J. Effects of bone marrow mesenchymal stem cells on cell proliferation and growth factor expression of limbal epithelial cells in vitro. *Ophthalmic Res.* **2012**, *48*, 82–88. [CrossRef]
63. Tang, Q.; Luo, C.; Lu, B.; Fu, Q.; Yin, H.; Qin, Z.; Lyu, D.; Zhang, L.; Fang, Z.; Zhu, Y.; et al. Thermosensitive chitosan-based hydrogels releasing stromal cell derived factor-1 alpha recruit MSC for corneal epithelium regeneration. *Acta Biomater.* **2017**, *61*, 101–113. [CrossRef]
64. Mittal, S.K.; Omoto, M.; Amouzegar, A.; Sahu, A.; Rezazadeh, A.; Katikireddy, K.R.; Shah, D.I.; Sahu, S.K.; Chauhan, S.K. Restoration of Corneal Transparency by Mesenchymal Stem Cells. *Stem Cell Rep.* **2016**, *7*, 582–590. [CrossRef]

65. Roddy, G.W.; Oh, J.Y.; Lee, R.H.; Bartosh, T.J.; Ylostalo, J.; Coble, K.; Rosa, R.H.; Prockop, D.J. Action at a distance: Systemically administered adult stem/progenitor cells (MSCs) reduce inflammatory damage to the cornea without engraftment and primarily by secretion of TNF-α stimulated gene/protein 6. *Stem Cells* **2011**, *29*, 1572–1579. [CrossRef]
66. Cejka, C.; Holan, V.; Trosan, P.; Zajicova, A.; Javorkova, E.; Cejkova, J. The Favorable Effect of Mesenchymal Stem Cell Treatment on the Antioxidant Protective Mechanism in the Corneal Epithelium and Renewal of Corneal Optical Properties Changed after Alkali Burns. *Oxid. Med. Cell. Longev.* **2016**, *2016*, 5843809. [CrossRef] [PubMed]
67. Mittal, S.K.; Foulsham, W.; Shukla, S.; Elbasiony, E.; Omoto, M.; Chauhan, S.K. Mesenchymal Stromal Cells Modulate Corneal Alloimmunity via Secretion of Hepatocyte Growth Factor. *Stem Cells Transl. Med.* **2019**, *8*, 1030–1040. [CrossRef] [PubMed]
68. Djouad, F.; Charbonnier, L.-M.; Bouffi, C.; Louis-Plence, P.; Bony, C.; Apparailly, F.; Cantos, C.; Jorgensen, C.; Noël, D. Mesenchymal Stem Cells Inhibit the Differentiation of Dendritic Cells through an Interleukin-6-Dependent Mechanism. *Stem Cells* **2007**, *25*, 2025–2032. [CrossRef] [PubMed]
69. Ren, G.; Zhang, L.; Zhao, X.; Xu, G.; Zhang, Y.; Roberts, A.I.; Zhao, R.C.; Shi, Y. Mesenchymal Stem Cell-Mediated Immunosuppression Occurs via Concerted Action of Chemokines and Nitric Oxide. *Cell Stem Cell* **2008**, *2*, 141–150. [CrossRef]
70. Aggarwal, S.; Pittenger, M.F. Human mesenchymal stem cells modulate allogeneic immune cell responses. *Blood* **2005**, *105*, 1815–1822. [CrossRef]
71. Rohaina, C.M.; Then, K.Y.; Ng, A.M.; Wan Abdul Halim, W.H.; Zahidin, A.Z.; Saim, A.; Idrus, R.B. Reconstruction of limbal stem cell deficient corneal surface with induced human bone marrow mesenchymal stem cells on amniotic membrane. *Transl. Res.* **2014**, *163*, 200–210. [CrossRef]
72. Venugopal, B.; Shenoy, S.J.; Mohan, S.; Anil Kumar, P.R.; Kumary, T.V. Bioengineered corneal epithelial cell sheet from mesenchymal stem cells—A functional alternative to limbal stem cells for ocular surface reconstruction. *J. Biomed. Mater. Res. Part B Appl. Biomater.* **2020**, *108*, 1033–1045. [CrossRef]
73. Ma, Y.; Xu, Y.; Xiao, Z.; Yang, W.; Zhang, C.; Song, E.; Du, Y.; Li, L. Reconstruction of Chemically Burned Rat Corneal Surface by Bone Marrow-Derived Human Mesenchymal Stem Cells. *Stem Cells* **2006**, *24*, 315–321. [CrossRef]
74. Ye, J.; Yao, K.; Kim, J.C. Mesenchymal stem cell transplantation in a rabbit corneal alkali burn model: Engraftment and involvement in wound healing. *Eye* **2006**, *20*, 482–490. [CrossRef]
75. Ahmed, S.K.; Soliman, A.A.; Omar, S.M.; Mohammed, W.R. Bone marrow mesenchymal stem cell transplantation in a rabbit corneal alkali burn model (a histological and immune histo-chemical study). *Int. J. Stem Cells* **2015**, *8*, 69–78. [CrossRef]
76. Reinshagen, H.; Auw-Haedrich, C.; Sorg, R.V.; Boehringer, D.; Eberwein, P.; Schwartzkopff, J.; Sundmacher, R.; Reinhard, T. Corneal surface reconstruction using adult mesenchymal stem cells in experimental limbal stem cell deficiency in rabbits. *Acta Ophthalmol.* **2011**, *89*, 741–748. [CrossRef]
77. Espandar, L.; Caldwell, D.; Watson, R.; Blanco-Mezquita, T.; Zhang, S.; Bunnell, B. Application of adipose-derived stem cells on scleral contact lens carrier in an animal model of severe acute alkaline burn. *Eye Contact Lens* **2014**, *40*, 243–247. [CrossRef] [PubMed]
78. Galindo, S.; Herreras, J.M.; López-Paniagua, M.; Rey, E.; de la Mata, A.; Plata Cordero, M.; Calonge, M.; Nieto-Miguel, T. Therapeutic Effect of Human Adipose Tissue-Derived Mesenchymal Stem Cells in Experimental Corneal Failure Due to Limbal Stem Cell Niche Damage. *Stem Cells* **2017**, *35*, 2160–2174. [CrossRef]
79. Zeppieri, M.; Salvetat, M.L.; Beltrami, A.P.; Cesselli, D.; Bergamin, N.; Russo, R.; Cavalleri, F.; Varano, G.P.; Alcalde, I.; Merayo, J.; et al. Human adipose-derived stem cells for the treatment of chemically burned rat cornea: Preliminary Results. *Curr. Eye Res.* **2013**, *38*, 451–463. [CrossRef] [PubMed]
80. Ghazaryan, E.; Zhang, Y.; He, Y.; Liu, X.; Li, Y.; Xie, J.; Su, G. Mesenchymal stem cells in corneal neovascularization: Comparison of different application routes. *Mol. Med. Rep.* **2016**, *14*, 3104–3112. [CrossRef] [PubMed]
81. Zajicova, A.; Pokorna, K.; Lencova, A.; Krulova, M.; Svobodova, E.; Kubinova, S.; Sykova, E.; Pradny, M.; Michalek, J.; Svobodova, J.; et al. Treatment of ocular surface injuries by limbal and mesenchymal stem cells growing on nanofiber scaffolds. *Cell Transplant.* **2010**, *19*, 1281–1290. [CrossRef] [PubMed]
82. Rengasamy, M.; Gupta, P.K.; Kolkundkar, U.; Singh, G.; Balasubramanian, S.; SundarRaj, S.; Chullikana, A.; Majumdar, A. Sen Preclinical safety & toxicity evaluation of pooled, allogeneic human bone marrow-derived mesenchymal stromal cells. *Indian J. Med. Res.* **2016**, *144*, 852–864. [CrossRef] [PubMed]
83. Guess, A.J.; Daneault, B.; Wang, R.; Bradbury, T.; La Perle, K.M.; Fitch, J.; Hedrick, S.L.; Hamelberg, E.; Astbury, C.; White, P.; et al. Safety Profile of Good Manufacturing Practice Manufactured Interferon γ-Primed Mesenchymal Stem/Stromal Cells for Clinical Trials. *Stem Cells Transl. Med.* **2017**, *6*, 1868–1879. [CrossRef] [PubMed]
84. Gramlich, O.W.; Burand, A.J.; Brown, A.J.; Deutsch, R.J.; Kuehn, M.H.; Ankrum, J.A. Cryopreserved mesenchymal stromal cells maintain potency in a retinal ischemia/reperfusion injury model: Toward an off-the-shelf therapy. *Sci. Rep.* **2016**, *6*, 26463. [CrossRef]
85. Tappenbeck, N.; Schröder, H.M.; Niebergall-Roth, E.; Hassinger, F.; Dehio, U.; Dieter, K.; Kraft, K.; Kerstan, A.; Esterlechner, J.; Frank, N.Y.; et al. In vivo safety profile and biodistribution of GMP-manufactured human skin-derived ABCB5-positive mesenchymal stromal cells for use in clinical trials. *Cytotherapy* **2019**, *21*, 546–560. [CrossRef] [PubMed]
86. Labrador Velandia, S.; Di Lauro, S.; Alonso-Alonso, M.L.; Tabera Bartolomé, S.; Srivastava, G.K.; Pastor, J.C.; Fernandez-Bueno, I. Biocompatibility of intravitreal injection of human mesenchymal stem cells in immunocompetent rabbits. *Graefe's Arch. Clin. Exp. Ophthalmol.* **2018**, *256*, 125–134. [CrossRef]

87. Cotsarelis, G.; Cheng, S.Z.; Dong, G.; Sun, T.T.; Lavker, R.M. Existence of slow-cycling limbal epithelial basal cells that can be preferentially stimulated to proliferate: Implications on epithelial stem cells. *Cell* **1989**, *57*, 201–209. [CrossRef]
88. Luetzkendorf, J.; Nerger, K.; Hering, J.; Moegel, A.; Hoffmann, K.; Hoefers, C.; Mueller-Tidow, C.; Mueller, L.P. Cryopreservation does not alter main characteristics of Good Manufacturing Process-grade human multipotent mesenchymal stromal cells including immunomodulating potential and lack of malignant transformation. *Cytotherapy* **2015**, *17*, 186–198. [CrossRef]
89. Calonge, M.; Pérez, I.; Galindo, S.; Nieto-Miguel, T.; López-Paniagua, M.; Fernández, I.; Alberca, M.; García-Sancho, J.; Sánchez, A.; Herreras, J.M. A proof-of-concept clinical trial using mesenchymal stem cells for the treatment of corneal epithelial stem cell deficiency. *Transl. Res.* **2019**, *206*, 18–40. [CrossRef] [PubMed]
90. Shimazaki, J.; Higa, K.; Morito, F.; Dogru, M.; Kawakita, T.; Satake, Y.; Shimmura, S.; Tsubota, K. Factors Influencing Outcomes in Cultivated Limbal Epithelial Transplantation for Chronic Cicatricial Ocular Surface Disorders. *Am. J. Ophthalmol.* **2007**, *143*, 945–953. [CrossRef]
91. Shortt, A.J.; Secker, G.A.; Rajan, M.S.; Meligonis, G.; Dart, J.K.; Tuft, S.J.; Daniels, J.T. Ex Vivo Expansion and Transplantation of Limbal Epithelial Stem Cells. *Ophthalmology* **2008**, *115*, 1989–1997. [CrossRef] [PubMed]
92. Pauklin, M.; Fuchsluger, T.A.; Westekemper, H.; Steuhl, K.P.; Meller, D. Midterm results of cultivated autologous and allogeneic limbal epithelial transplantation in limbal stem cell deficiency. *Dev. Ophthalmol.* **2010**, *45*, 57–70. [CrossRef]
93. Prabhasawat, P.; Ekpo, P.; Uiprasertkul, M.; Chotikavanich, S.; Tesavibul, N. Efficacy of cultivated corneal epithelial stem cells for ocular surface reconstruction. *Clin. Ophthalmol.* **2012**, *6*, 1483–1492. [CrossRef] [PubMed]
94. Zakaria, N.; Possemiers, T.; Dhubhghaill, S.N.; Leysen, I.; Rozema, J.; Koppen, C.; Timmermans, J.P.; Berneman, Z.; Tassignon, M.J. Results of a phase I/II clinical trial: Standardized, non-xenogenic, cultivated limbal stem cell transplantation. *J. Transl. Med.* **2014**, *12*, 58. [CrossRef]
95. Ganger, A.; Vanathi, M.; Mohanty, S.; Tandon, R. Long-term outcomes of cultivated limbal epithelial transplantation: Evaluation and comparison of results in children and adults. *Biomed Res. Int.* **2015**, *2015*, 480983. [CrossRef]
96. Parihar, J.K.; Parihar, A.S.; Jain, V.K.; Kaushik, J.; Nath, P. Allogenic cultivated limbal stem cell transplantation versus cadaveric keratolimbal allograft in ocular surface disorder: 1-Year outcome. *Int. Ophthalmol.* **2017**, *37*, 1323–1331. [CrossRef]
97. Sharma, N.; Mohanty, S.; Jhanji, V.; Vajpayee, R.B. Amniotic membrane transplantation with or without autologous cultivated limbal stem cell transplantation for the management of partial limbal stem cell deficiency. *Clin. Ophthalmol.* **2018**, *12*, 2103–2106. [CrossRef] [PubMed]
98. Campbell, J.D.; Ahmad, S.; Agrawal, A.; Bienek, C.; Atkinson, A.; Mcgowan, N.W.; Kaye, S.; Mantry, S.; Ramaesh, K.; Glover, A.; et al. Allogeneic Ex Vivo Expanded Corneal Epithelial Stem Cell Transplantation: A Randomized Controlled Clinical Trial. *Stem Cells Transl. Med.* **2019**, *8*, 323–331. [CrossRef]
99. Behaegel, J.; Zakaria, N.; Tassignon, M.J.; Leysen, I.; Bock, F.; Koppen, C.; Ní Dhubhghaill, S. Short- and Long-Term Results of Xenogeneic-Free Cultivated Autologous and Allogeneic Limbal Epithelial Stem Cell Transplantations. *Cornea* **2019**, *38*, 1543–1549. [CrossRef] [PubMed]
100. Shimazaki, J.; Satake, Y.; Higa, K.; Yamaguchi, T.; Noma, H.; Tsubota, K. Long-term outcomes of cultivated cell sheet transplantation for treating total limbal stem cell deficiency: Long-term outcomes of cultivated cell sheet transplantation. *Ocul. Surf.* **2020**, *18*, 663–671. [CrossRef] [PubMed]
101. Directive 2001/83/EC of The European Parliament and of the Council of 6 November 2001 on the Community Code Relating to Medicinal Products for Human Use. Available online: https://ec.europa.eu/health/sites/health/files/files/eudralex/vol-1/dir_2001_83_consol_2012/dir_2001_83_cons_2012_en.pdf (accessed on 29 July 2021).
102. Arda, B.; Aciduman, A. An evaluation regarding the current situation of stem cell studies in Turkey. *Stem Cell Rev. Rep.* **2009**, *5*, 130–134. [CrossRef] [PubMed]
103. U.S. Food and Drug Administration. Cellular & Gene Therapy Products. Available online: https://www.fda.gov/vaccinesbloodbiologics/cellular-gene-therapy-products (accessed on 29 July 2021).
104. Jokura, Y.; Yano, K.; Yamato, M. Comparison of the new Japanese legislation for expedited approval of regenerative medicine products with the existing systems in the USA and European Union. *J. Tissue Eng. Regen. Med.* **2018**, *12*, e1056–e1062. [CrossRef]
105. Okada, K.; Koike, K.; Sawa, Y. Consideration of and expectations for the Pharmaceuticals, Medical Devices and Other Therapeutic Products Act in Japan. *Regen. Ther.* **2015**, *1*, 80–83. [CrossRef]
106. Lahiry, S.; Choudhury, S.; Sinha, R.; Chatterjee, S. The national guidelines for stem cell research (2017): What academicians need to know? *Perspect. Clin. Res.* **2019**, *10*, 148–154. [CrossRef]
107. Indian Council of Medical Research & Department of Biotechnology. National Guidelines for Stem Cell Research. 2017. Available online: https://dbtindia.gov.in/sites/default/files/National_Guidelines_StemCellResearch-2017.pdf (accessed on 29 July 2021).
108. Therapeutic Goods Order No. 88—Standards for Donor Selection, Testing, and Minimising Infectious Disease Transmission Via Therapeutic Goods That Are Human Blood and Blood Components, Human Tissues and Human Cellular Therapy Products. Australian Government. Available online: https://www.legislation.gov.au/Details/F2013L00854 (accessed on 29 July 2021).
109. Australian Code of Good Manufacturing Practice for Human Blood and Blood Components, Human Tissues and Human Cellular Therapy Products. Australian Department of Health & Aging Therapeutic Goods Administration; Version 1.0. Available online: https://www.tga.gov.au/si (accessed on 29 July 2013).
110. Jawaheer, L.; Anijeet, D.; Ramaesh, K. Diagnostic criteria for limbal stem cell deficiency—A systematic literature review. *Surv. Ophthalmol.* **2017**, *62*, 522–532. [CrossRef]

111. Banayan, N.; Georgeon, C.; Grieve, K.; Borderie, V.M. Spectral-domain Optical Coherence Tomography in Limbal Stem Cell Deficiency. A Case-Control Study. *Am. J. Ophthalmol.* **2018**, *190*, 179–190. [CrossRef] [PubMed]
112. Zakaria, N.; Dhubhghaill, S.N.; Taal, M.; Berneman, Z.; Koppen, C.; Tassignon, M.J. Optical coherence tomography in cultivated Limbal epithelial stem cell transplantation surgery. *Asia-Pac. J. Ophthalmol.* **2015**, *4*, 339–345. [CrossRef] [PubMed]
113. Liang, Q.; Le, Q.; Cordova, D.W.; Tseng, C.H.; Deng, S.X. Corneal Epithelial Thickness Measured Using Anterior Segment Optical Coherence Tomography as a Diagnostic Parameter for Limbal Stem Cell Deficiency. *Am. J. Ophthalmol.* **2020**, *216*, 132–139. [CrossRef] [PubMed]
114. Nicholas, M.P.; Mysore, N. Corneal neovascularization. *Exp. Eye Res.* **2021**, *202*, 108363. [CrossRef] [PubMed]
115. Yin, J.; Jacobs, D.S. Long-term outcome of using Prosthetic Replacement of Ocular Surface Ecosystem (PROSE) as a drug delivery system for bevacizumab in the treatment of corneal neovascularization. *Ocul. Surf.* **2019**, *17*, 134–141. [CrossRef]
116. Stern, J.H.; Tian, Y.; Funderburgh, J.; Pellegrini, G.; Zhang, K.; Goldberg, J.L.; Ali, R.R.; Young, M.; Xie, Y.; Temple, S. Regenerating Eye Tissues to Preserve and Restore Vision. *Cell Stem Cell.* **2018**, *22*, 834–849. [CrossRef] [PubMed]
117. Sangwan, V.S.; Vemuganti, G.K.; Singh, S.; Balasubramanian, D. Successful Reconstruction of Damaged Ocular Outer Surface in Humans using Limbal and Conjuctival Stem Cell Culture Methods. *Biosci. Rep.* **2003**, *23*, 169–174. [CrossRef]
118. Tsubota, K.; Satake, Y.; Kaido, M.; Shinozaki, N.; Shimmura, S.; Bissen-Miyajima, H.; Shimazaki, J. Treatment of Severe Ocular-Surface Disorders with Corneal Epithelial Stem-Cell Transplantation. *N. Engl. J. Med.* **1999**, *340*, 1697–1703. [CrossRef] [PubMed]
119. Kolli, S.A.; Ahmad, S.; Lako, M.; Figueiredo, F. Successful clinical implementation of corneal epithelial stem cell therapy for treatment of unilateral limbal stem cell deficiency. *Stem Cells* **2010**, *28*, 597–610. [CrossRef]
120. Le, Q.H.; Wang, W.T.; Hong, J.X.; Sun, X.H.; Zheng, T.Y.; Zhu, W.Q.; Xu, J.J. An in vivo confocal microscopy and impression cytology analysis of goblet cells in patients with chemical burns. *Investig. Ophthalmol. Vis. Sci.* **2010**, *51*, 1397–1400. [CrossRef]
121. Lagali, N.; Edén, U.; Utheim, T.P.; Chen, X.; Riise, R.; Dellby, A.; Fagerholm, P. In vivo morphology of the limbal palisades of vogt correlates with progressive stem cell deficiency in aniridia-related keratopathy. *Investig. Ophthalmol. Vis. Sci.* **2013**, *54*, 5333–5342. [CrossRef]
122. Ramírez, B.E.; Victoria, D.A.; Murillo, G.M.; Herreras, J.M.; Calonge, M. In vivo confocal microscopy assessment of the corneoscleral limbal stem cell niche before and after biopsy for cultivated limbal epithelial transplantation to restore corneal epithelium. *Histol. Histopathol.* **2015**, *30*, 183–192. [CrossRef]
123. Mastropasqua, L.; Calienno, R.; Lanzini, M.; Nubile, M.; Colabelli-Gisoldi, R.A.; De Carlo, L.; Pocobelli, A. In vivo confocal microscopy of the sclerocorneal limbus after limbal stem cell transplantation: Looking for limbal architecture modifications and cytological phenotype correlations. *Mol. Vis.* **2016**, *22*, 748–760. [PubMed]
124. Pellegrini, G.; Rama, P.; Matuska, S.; Lambiase, A.; Bonini, S.; Pocobelli, A.; Colabelli, R.G.; Spadea, L.; Fasciani, R.; Balestrazzi, E.; et al. Biological parameters determining the clinical outcome of autologous cultures of limbal stem cells. *Regen. Med.* **2013**, *8*, 553–567. [CrossRef] [PubMed]
125. Fasolo, A.; Pedrotti, E.; Passilongo, M.; Marchini, G.; Monterosso, C.; Zampini, R.; Bohm, E.; Birattari, F.; Franch, A.; Barbaro, V.; et al. Safety outcomes and long-Term effectiveness of ex vivo autologous cultured limbal epithelial transplantation for limbal stem cell deficiency. *Br. J. Ophthalmol.* **2017**, *101*, 640–649. [CrossRef]
126. Parthasarathy, M.; Sasikala, R.; Gunasekaran, P.; Raja, J. Antimicrobial Activity of Human Amniotic and Chorionic Membranes. *J. Acad. Ind. Res.* **2014**, *2*, 545–547.
127. Niknejad, H.; Peirovi, H.; Jorjani, M.; Ahmadiani, A.; Ghanavi, J.; Seifalian, A.M. Properties of the amniotic membrane for potential use in tissue engineering. *Eur. Cells Mater.* **2008**, *15*, 88–99. [CrossRef] [PubMed]
128. Sudha, B.; Sitalakshmi, G.; Iyer, G.K.; Krishnakumar, S. Putative stem cell markers in limal epithelial cells cultured on intact & denuded human amniotic membrane. *Indian J. Med. Res.* **2008**, *128*, 149–156. [PubMed]
129. Schwab, I.R.; Reyes, M.; Isseroff, R.R. Successful transplantation of bioengineered tissue replacements in patients with ocular surface disease. *Cornea* **2000**, *19*, 421–426. [CrossRef]
130. Koizumi, N.; Inatomi, T.; Quantock, A.J.; Fullwood, N.J.; Dota, A.; Kinoshita, S. Amniotic membrane as a substrate for cultivating limbal corneal epithelial cells for autologous transplantation in rabbits. *Cornea* **2000**, *19*, 65–71. [CrossRef] [PubMed]
131. Meller, D.; Pires, R.T.; Tseng, S.C. Ex vivo preservation and expansion of human limbal epithelial stem cells on amniotic membrane cultures. *Br. J. Ophthalmol.* **2002**, *86*, 463–471. [CrossRef] [PubMed]
132. Grueterich, M.; Espana, E.M.; Touhami, A.; Ti, S.E.; Tseng, S.C. Phenotypic study of a case with successful transplantation of ex vivo expanded human limbal epithelium for unilateral total limbal stem cell deficiency. *Ophthalmology* **2002**, *109*, 1547–1552. [CrossRef]
133. Gomes, J.A.; Dos Santos, M.S.; Cunha, M.C.; Mascaro, V.L.; De Nadai Barros, J.N.; De Sousa, L.B. Amniotic membrane transplantation for partial and total limbal stem cell deficiency secondary to chemical burn. *Ophthalmology* **2003**, *10*, 466–473. [CrossRef]
134. Kim, J.C.; Tseng, S.C. Transplantation of preserved human amniotic membrane for surface reconstruction in severely damaged rabbit corneas. *Cornea* **1995**, *14*, 473–484. [CrossRef] [PubMed]
135. Shimazaki, J.; Yang, H.Y.; Tsubota, K. Amniotic membrane transplantation for ocular surface reconstruction in patients with chemical and thermal burns. *Ophthalmology* **1997**, *104*, 2068–2076. [CrossRef]
136. Atrah, H.I. Fibrin glue. *BMJ* **1994**, *308*, 933–934. [CrossRef]

137. Lagoutte, F.M.; Gauthier, L.; Comte, P.R. A fibrin sealant for perforated and preperforated corneal ulcers. *Br. J. Ophthalmol.* **1989**, *73*, 757–761. [CrossRef]
138. Kopp, J.; Jeschke, M.G.; Bach, A.D.; Kneser, U.; Horch, R.E. Applied tissue engineering in the closure of severe burns and chronic wounds using cultured human autologous keratinocytes in a natural fibrin matrix. *Cell Tissue Bank.* **2004**, *5*, 89–96. [CrossRef] [PubMed]
139. Talbot, M.; Carrier, P.; Giasson, C.J.; Deschambeault, A.; Guérin, S.L.; Auger, F.A.; Bazin, R.; Germain, L. Autologous transplantation of rabbit limbal epithelia cultured on fibrin gels for ocular surface reconstruction. *Mol. Vis.* **2006**, *12*, 65–75.
140. Rama, P.; Bonini, S.; Lambiase, A.; Golisano, O.; Paterna, P.; De Luca, M.; Pellegrini, G. Autologous fibrin-cultured limbal stem cells permanently restore the corneal surface of patients with total limbal stem cell deficiency. *Transplantation* **2001**, *72*, 1478–1485. [CrossRef] [PubMed]
141. Di Iorio, E.; Ferrari, S.; Fasolo, A.; Böhm, E.; Ponzin, D.; Barbaro, V. Techniques for culture and assessment of limbal stem cell grafts. *Ocul. Surf.* **2010**, *8*, 146–153. [CrossRef]
142. Di Girolamo, N.; Chui, J.; Wakefield, D.; Coroneo, M.T. Cultured human ocular surface epithelium on therapeutic contact lenses. *Br. J. Ophthalmol.* **2007**, *91*, 459–564. [CrossRef] [PubMed]
143. De la Mata, A.; Mateos-Timoneda, M.A.; Nieto-Miguel, T.; Galindo, S.; López-Paniagua, M.; Planell, J.A.; Engel, E.; Calonge, M. Poly-L/DL-lactic acid films functionalized with collagen IV as carrier substrata for corneal epithelial stem cells. *Colloids Surf. B Biointerfaces* **2019**, *177*, 121–129. [CrossRef]
144. Geggel, H.S.; Friend, J.; Thoft, R.A. Collagen gel for ocular surface. *Investig. Ophthalmol. Vis. Sci.* **1985**, *26*, 901–905.
145. Haagdorens, M.; Cėpla, V.; Melsbach, E.; Koivusalo, L.; Skottman, H.; Griffith, M.; Valiokas, R.; Zakaria, N.; Pintelon, I.; Tassignon, M.J. In vitro cultivation of limbal epithelial stem cells on surface-modified crosslinked collagen scaffolds. *Stem Cells Int.* **2019**, *2019*, 7867613. [CrossRef]
146. Chae, J.J.; McIntosh Ambrose, W.; Espinoza, F.A.; Mulreany, D.G.; Ng, S.; Takezawa, T.; Trexler, M.M.; Schein, O.D.; Chuck, R.S.; Elisseeff, J.H. Regeneration of corneal epithelium utilizing a collagen vitrigel membrane in rabbit models for corneal stromal wound and limbal stem cell deficiency. *Acta Ophthalmol.* **2015**, *93*, 57–66. [CrossRef]
147. Levis, H.; Daniels, J.T. New technologies in limbal epithelial stem cell transplantation. *Curr. Opin. Biotechnol.* **2009**, *20*, 593–597. [CrossRef]
148. Mi, S.; Chen, B.; Wright, B.; Connon, C.J. Plastic compression of a collagen gel forms a much improved scaffold for ocular surface tissue engineering over conventional collagen gels. *J. Biomed. Mater. Res. Part A* **2010**, *95*, 447–453. [CrossRef]
149. Levis, H.J.; Brown, R.A.; Daniels, J.T. Plastic compressed collagen as a biomimetic substrate for human limbal epithelial cell culture. *Biomaterials* **2010**, *31*, 7726–7737. [CrossRef]
150. Mi, S.; Chen, B.; Wright, B.; Connon, C.J. Ex vivo construction of an artificial ocular surface by combination of corneal limbal epithelial cells and a compressed collagen scaffold containing keratocytes. *Tissue Eng. Part A* **2010**, *95*, 447–453. [CrossRef]
151. De La Mata, A.; Nieto-Miguel, T.; López-Paniagua, M.; Galindo, S.; Aguilar, M.R.; García-Fernández, L.; Gonzalo, S.; Vázquez, B.; Román, J.S.; Corrales, R.M.; et al. Chitosan-gelatin biopolymers as carrier substrata for limbal epithelial stem cells. *J. Mater. Sci. Mater. Med.* **2013**, *24*, 2819–2829. [CrossRef]
152. Grolik, M.; Szczubiałka, K.; Wowra, B.; Dobrowolski, D.; Orzechowska-Wylęgała, B.; Wylęgała, E.; Nowakowska, M. Hydrogel membranes based on genipin-cross-linked chitosan blends for corneal epithelium tissue engineering. *J. Mater. Sci. Mater. Med.* **2012**, *23*, 1991–2000. [CrossRef] [PubMed]
153. Zhu, X.; Beuerman, R.W.; Chan-Park, M.B.; Cheng, Z.; Ang, L.P.; Tan, D.T. Enhancement of the mechanical and biological properties of a biomembrane for tissue engineering the ocular surface. *Ann. Acad. Med. Singap.* **2006**, *35*, 210–214.
154. Bray, L.J.; George, K.A.; Ainscough, S.L.; Hutmacher, D.W.; Chirila, T.V.; Harkin, D.G. Human corneal epithelial equivalents constructed on Bombyx mori silk fibroin membranes. *Biomaterials* **2011**, *32*, 5086–5091. [CrossRef]
155. Li, Y.; Yang, Y.; Yang, L.; Zeng, Y.; Gao, X.; Xu, H. Poly(ethylene glycol)-modified silk fibroin membrane as a carrier for limbal epithelial stem cell transplantation in a rabbit LSCD model. *Stem Cell Res. Ther.* **2017**, *8*, 256. [CrossRef] [PubMed]
156. Nishida, K.; Yamato, M.; Hayashida, Y.; Watanabe, K.; Maeda, N.; Watanabe, H.; Yamamoto, K.; Nagai, S.; Kikuchi, A.; Tano, Y.; et al. Functional bioengineered corneal epithellial sheet grafts from corneal stem cells expanded ex vivo on a temperature-responsive cell culture surface. *Transplantation* **2004**, *77*, 379–385. [CrossRef] [PubMed]
157. Yazdanpanah, G.; Haq, Z.; Kang, K.; Jabbehdari, S.; Rosenblatt, M.L.; Djalilian, A.R. Strategies for reconstructing the limbal stem cell niche. *Ocul. Surf.* **2019**, *17*, 230–240. [CrossRef]
158. Oh, J.Y.; Kim, M.K.; Shin, M.S.; Lee, H.J.; Ko, J.H.; Wee, W.R.; Lee, J.H. The Anti-Inflammatory and Anti-Angiogenic Role of Mesenchymal Stem Cells in Corneal Wound Healing Following Chemical Injury. *Stem Cells* **2008**, *26*, 1047–1055. [CrossRef]
159. Galindo, S.; de la Mata, A.; López-Paniagua, M.; Herreras, J.M.; Pérez, I.; Calonge, M.; Nieto-Miguel, T. Subconjunctival injection of mesenchymal stem cells for corneal failure due to limbal stem cell deficiency: State of the art. *Stem Cell Res. Ther.* **2021**, *12*, 60. [CrossRef]
160. Di, G.; Du, X.; Qi, X.; Zhao, X.; Duan, H.; Li, S.; Xie, L.; Zhou, Q. Mesenchymal stem cells promote diabetic corneal epithelial wound healing through TSG-6-dependent stem cell activation and macrophage switch. *Investig. Ophthalmol. Vis. Sci.* **2017**, *58*, 4344–4354. [CrossRef]

161. Zhang, N.; Luo, X.; Zhang, S.; Liu, R.; Liang, L.; Su, W.; Liang, D. Subconjunctival injection of tumor necrosis factor-α pre-stimulated bone marrow-derived mesenchymal stem cells enhances anti-inflammation and anti-fibrosis in ocular alkali burns. *Graefe's Arch. Clin. Exp. Ophthalmol.* **2021**, *259*, 929–940. [CrossRef] [PubMed]
162. Li, G.; Zhang, Y.; Cai, S.; Sun, M.; Wang, J.; Li, S.; Li, X.; Tighe, S.; Chen, S.; Xie, H.; et al. Human limbal niche cells are a powerful regenerative source for the prevention of limbal stem cell deficiency in a rabbit model. *Sci. Rep.* **2018**, *8*, 6566. [CrossRef] [PubMed]
163. Pan, J.; Wang, X.; Li, D.; Li, J.; Jiang, Z. MSCs inhibits the angiogenesis of HUVECs through the miR-211/Prox1 pathway. *J. Biochem.* **2019**, *166*, 107–113. [CrossRef] [PubMed]
164. Shukla, S.; Mittal, S.K.; Foulsham, W.; Elbasiony, E.; Singhania, D.; Sahu, S.K.; Chauhan, S.K. Therapeutic efficacy of different routes of mesenchymal stem cell administration in corneal injury. *Ocul. Surf.* **2019**, *17*, 729–736. [CrossRef]
165. Xiao, Y.T.; Xie, H.T.; Liu, X.; Duan, C.Y.; Qu, J.Y.; Zhang, M.C.; Zhao, X.Y. Subconjunctival Injection of Transdifferentiated Oral Mucosal Epithelial Cells for Limbal Stem Cell Deficiency in Rats. *J. Histochem. Cytochem.* **2021**, *69*, 177–190. [CrossRef] [PubMed]
166. Sohni, A.; Verfaillie, C.M. Mesenchymal stem cells migration homing and tracking. *Stem Cells Int.* **2013**, *2013*, 130763. [CrossRef]
167. Mäkelä, T.; Takalo, R.; Arvola, O.; Haapanen, H.; Yannopoulos, F.; Blanco, R.; Ahvenjärvi, L.; Kiviluoma, K.; Kerkelä, E.; Nystedt, J.; et al. Safety and biodistribution study of bone marrow-derived mesenchymal stromal cells and mononuclear cells and the impact of the administration route in an intact porcine model. *Cytotherapy* **2015**, *17*, 392–402. [CrossRef]
168. Lee, R.H.; Yu, J.M.; Foskett, A.M.; Peltier, G.; Reneau, J.C.; Bazhanov, N.; Oh, J.Y.; Prockop, D.J. TSG-6 as a biomarker to predict efficacy of human mesenchymal stem/progenitor cells (hMSCs) in modulating sterile inflammation in vivo. *Proc. Natl. Acad. Sci. USA* **2014**, *111*, 16766–16771. [CrossRef]
169. Yun, Y.I.; Park, S.Y.; Lee, H.J.; Ko, J.H.; Kim, M.K.; Wee, W.R.; Reger, R.L.; Gregory, C.A.; Choi, H.; Fulcher, S.F.; et al. Comparison of the anti-inflammatory effects of induced pluripotent stem cell–derived and bone marrow–derived mesenchymal stromal cells in a murine model of corneal injury. *Cytotherapy* **2017**, *19*, 28–35. [CrossRef]
170. Haagdorens, M.; Van Acker, S.I.; Van Gerwen, V.; Ní Dhubhghaill, S.; Koppen, C.; Tassignon, M.J.; Zakaria, N. Limbal stem cell deficiency: Current treatment options and emerging therapies. *Stem Cells Int.* **2016**, *2016*, 9798374. [CrossRef]
171. Lachaud, C.C.; Hmadcha, A.; Soria, B. Corneal Regeneration: Use of Extracorneal Stem Cells. In *Corneal Regeneration Therapy and Surgery*; Alió, J., Alió del Barrio, J.L., Arnalich-Montiel, F., Eds.; Springer Nature: Basingstoke, UK, 2019; pp. 123–144. [CrossRef]
172. Nosrati, H.; Alizadeh, Z.; Nosrati, A.; Ashrafi-Dehkordi, K.; Banitalebi-Dehkordi, M.; Sanami, S.; Khodaei, M. Stem cell-based therapeutic strategies for corneal epithelium regeneration. *Tissue Cell* **2021**, *68*, 101470. [CrossRef] [PubMed]
173. Thomson, J.A. Embryonic stem cell lines derived from human blastocysts. *Science* **1998**, *282*, 1145–1147. [CrossRef] [PubMed]
174. Hanson, C.; Hardarson, T.; Ellerström, C.; Nordberg, M.; Caisander, G.; Rao, M.; Hyllner, J.; Stenevi, U. Transplantation of human embryonic stem cells onto a partially wounded human cornea in vitro. *Acta Ophthalmol.* **2013**, *91*, 127–130. [CrossRef]
175. Zhu, J.; Zhang, K.; Sun, Y.; Gao, X.; Li, Y.; Chen, Z.; Wu, X. Reconstruction of functional ocular surface by acellular porcine cornea matrix scaffold and limbal stem cells derived from human embryonic stem cells. *Tissue Eng. Part A* **2013**, *19*, 2412–2425. [CrossRef]
176. Da Mata Martins, T.M.; da Silva Cunha, P.; Rodrigues, M.A.; de Carvalho, J.L.; de Souza, J.E.; de Carvalho Oliveira, J.A.; Gomes, D.A.; de Goes, A.M. Epithelial basement membrane of human decellularized cornea as a suitable substrate for differentiation of embryonic stem cells into corneal epithelial-like cells. *Mater. Sci. Eng. C* **2020**, *116*, 111215. [CrossRef]
177. Ahmad, S.; Stewart, R.; Yung, S.; Kolli, S.; Armstrong, L.; Stojkovic, M.; Figueiredo, F.; Lako, M. Differentiation of Human Embryonic Stem Cells into Corneal Epithelial-Like Cells by In Vitro Replication of the Corneal Epithelial Stem Cell Niche. *Stem Cells* **2007**, *25*, 1145–1155. [CrossRef]
178. Zhang, C.; Du, L.; Pang, K.; Wu, X. Differentiation of human embryonic stem cells into corneal epithelial progenitor cells under defined conditions. *PLoS ONE* **2017**, *12*, e0183303. [CrossRef]
179. Zhang, C.; Du, L.; Sun, P.; Shen, L.; Zhu, J.; Pang, K.; Wu, X. Construction of tissue-engineered full-thickness cornea substitute using limbal epithelial cell-like and corneal endothelial cell-like cells derived from human embryonic stem cells. *Biomaterials* **2017**, *124*, 180–194. [CrossRef] [PubMed]
180. He, J.; Ou, S.; Ren, J.; Sun, H.; He, X.; Zhao, Z.; Wu, H.; Qu, Y.; Liu, T.; Jeyalatha, V.; et al. Tissue engineered corneal epithelium derived from clinical-grade human embryonic stem cells. *Ocul. Surf.* **2020**, *18*, 672–680. [CrossRef] [PubMed]
181. Kiskinis, E.; Eggan, K. Progress toward the clinical application of patient-specific pluripotent stem cells. *J. Clin. Investig.* **2010**, *120*, 51–59. [CrossRef] [PubMed]
182. Takahashi, K.; Tanabe, K.; Ohnuki, M.; Narita, M.; Ichisaka, T.; Tomoda, K.; Yamanaka, S. Induction of Pluripotent Stem Cells from Adult Human Fibroblasts by Defined Factors. *Cell* **2007**, *131*, 861–872. [CrossRef]
183. Casaroli-Marano, R.P. Cell-based Therapy Using Induced Plutipotent Stem Cell. In *Corneal Regeneration Therapy and Surgery*; Alió, J., Alió del Barrio, J.L., Arnalich-Montiel, F., Eds.; Springer Nature: Basingstoke, UK, 2019; pp. 263–273. [CrossRef]
184. Chakrabarty, K.; Shetty, R.; Ghosh, A. Corneal cell therapy: With iPSCs, it is no more a far-sight. *Stem Cell Res. Ther.* **2018**, *9*, 287. [CrossRef]
185. Theerakittayakorn, K.; Nguyen, H.T.; Musika, J.; Kunkanjanawan, H.; Imsoonthornruksa, S.; Somredngan, S.; Ketudat-Cairns, M.; Parnpai, R. Differentiation induction of human stem cells for corneal epithelial regeneration. *Int. J. Mol. Sci.* **2020**, *21*, 7834. [CrossRef]

186. Hayashi, R.; Ishikawa, Y.; Ito, M.; Kageyama, T.; Takashiba, K.; Fujioka, T.; Tsujikawa, M.; Miyoshi, H.; Yamato, M.; Nakamura, Y.; et al. Generation of Corneal Epithelial Cells from Induced Pluripotent Stem Cells Derived from Human Dermal Fibroblast and Corneal Limbal Epithelium. *PLoS ONE* **2012**, *7*, 45435. [CrossRef]
187. Hayashi, R.; Ishikawa, Y.; Sasamoto, Y.; Katori, R.; Nomura, N.; Ichikawa, T.; Araki, S.; Soma, T.; Kawasaki, S.; Sekiguchi, K.; et al. Co-ordinated ocular development from human iPS cells and recovery of corneal function. *Nature* **2016**, *531*, 376–380. [CrossRef]
188. Hayashi, R.; Ishikawa, Y.; Katori, R.; Sasamoto, Y.; Taniwaki, Y.; Takayanagi, H.; Tsujikawa, M.; Sekiguchi, K.; Quantock, A.J.; Nishida, K. Coordinated generation of multiple ocular-like cell lineages and fabrication of functional corneal epithelial cell sheets from human iPS cells. *Nat. Protoc.* **2017**, *12*, 683–696. [CrossRef] [PubMed]
189. Mikhailova, A.; Ilmarinen, T.; Uusitalo, H.; Skottman, H. Small-molecule induction promotes corneal epithelial cell differentiation from human induced pluripotent stem cells. *Stem Cell Rep.* **2014**, *2*, 219–231. [CrossRef] [PubMed]
190. Hongisto, H.; Vattulainen, M.; Ilmarinen, T.; Mikhailova, A.; Skottman, H. Efficient and scalable directed differentiation of clinically compatible corneal limbal epithelial stem cells from human pluripotent stem cells. *J. Vis. Exp.* **2018**, *24*, 58279. [CrossRef]
191. Taylor, C.J.; Peacock, S.; Chaudhry, A.N.; Bradley, J.A.; Bolton, E.M. Generating an iPSC bank for HLA-matched tissue transplantation based on known donor and recipient hla types. *Cell Stem Cell* **2012**, *11*, 147–152. [CrossRef]
192. De Rham, C.; Villard, J. Potential and limitation of HLA-based banking of human pluripotent stem cells for cell therapy. *J. Immunol. Res.* **2014**, *2014*, 518135. [CrossRef]
193. Sullivan, S.; Stacey, G.N.; Akazawa, C.; Aoyama, N.; Baptista, R.; Bedford, P.; Bennaceur Griscelli, A.; Chandra, A.; Elwood, N.; Girard, M.; et al. Quality control guidelines for clinical-grade human induced pluripotent stem cell lines. *Regen Med.* **2018**, *13*, 859–866. [CrossRef]
194. Zhu, J.; Slevin, M.; Guo, B.Q.; Zhu, S.R. Induced pluripotent stem cells as a potential therapeutic source for corneal epithelial stem cells. *Int. J. Ophthalmol.* **2018**, *11*, 2004–2010. [CrossRef] [PubMed]
195. Kelaini, S.; Cochrane, A.; Margariti, A. Direct reprogramming of adult cells: Avoiding the pluripotent state. *Stem Cells Cloning Adv. Appl.* **2014**, *7*, 19–29. [CrossRef]
196. Cieślar-Pobuda, A.; Rafat, M.; Knoflach, V.; Skonieczna, M.; Hudecki, A.; Małecki, A.; Urasińska, E.; Ghavami, S.; Łos, M.J. Human induced pluripotent stem cell differentiation and direct transdifferentiation into corneal epithelial-like cells. *Oncotarget* **2016**, *7*, 42314–42329. [CrossRef]
197. Monteiro, B.G.; Serafim, R.C.; Melo, G.B.; Silva, M.C.; Lizier, N.F.; Maranduba, C.M.; Smith, R.L.; Kerkis, A.; Cerruti, H.; Gomes, J.A.; et al. Human immature dental pulp stem cells share key characteristic features with limbal stem cells. *Cell Prolif.* **2009**, *42*, 587–594. [CrossRef] [PubMed]
198. Gomes, J.Á.; Monteiro, B.G.; Melo, G.B.; Smith, R.L.; da Silva, M.C.; Lizier, N.F.; Kerkis, A.; Cerruti, H.; Kerkis, I. Corneal reconstruction with tissue-engineered cell sheets composed of human immature dental pulp stem cells. *Investig. Ophthalmol. Vis. Sci.* **2010**, *51*, 1408–1414. [CrossRef]
199. Tsai, C.L.; Chuang, P.C.; Kuo, H.K.; Chen, Y.H.; Su, W.H.; Wu, P.C. Differentiation of stem cells from human exfoliated deciduous teeth toward a phenotype of corneal epithelium in vitro. *Cornea* **2015**, *34*, 1471–1477. [CrossRef]
200. Patil, S.; D'Souza, C.; Patil, P.; Patil, V.; Prabhu, M.; Bargale, A.; Kaveeshwar, V.; Kumar, S.; Shetty, P. Culture and characterization of human dental pulp-derived stem cells as limbal stem cells for corneal damage repair. *Mol. Med. Rep.* **2019**, *20*, 4688–4694. [CrossRef]
201. Kushnerev, E.; Shawcross, S.G.; Sothirachagan, S.; Carley, F.; Brahma, A.; Yates, J.M.; Hillarby, M.C. Regeneration of corneal epithelium with dental pulp stem cells using a contact lens delivery system. *Investig. Ophthalmol. Vis. Sci.* **2016**, *57*, 5192–5199. [CrossRef]
202. Monteiro, B.G.; Loureiro, R.R.; Cristovam, P.C.; Covre, J.L.; Gomes, J.Á.; Kerkis, I. Amniotic membrane as a biological scaffold for dental pulp stem cell transplantation in ocular surface reconstruction. *Arq. Bras. Oftalmol.* **2019**, *82*, 32–37. [CrossRef]
203. Taylor, G.; Lehrer, M.S.; Jensen, P.J.; Sun, T.T.; Lavker, R.M. Involvement of follicular stem cells in forming not only the follicle but also the epidermis. *Cell* **2000**, *102*, 451–461. [CrossRef]
204. Ito, M.; Liu, Y.; Yang, Z.; Nguyen, J.; Liang, F.; Morris, R.J.; Cotsarelis, G. Stem cells in the hair follicle bulge contribute to wound repair but not to homeostasis of the epidermis. *Nat. Med.* **2005**, *11*, 1351–1354. [CrossRef] [PubMed]
205. Blazejewska, E.A.; Schlötzer-Schrehardt, U.; Zenkel, M.; Bachmann, B.; Chankiewitz, E.; Jacobi, C.; Kruse, F.E. Corneal Limbal Microenvironment Can Induce Transdifferentiation of Hair Follicle Stem Cells into Corneal Epithelial-like Cells. *Stem Cells* **2009**, *27*, 642–652. [CrossRef] [PubMed]
206. Meyer-Blazejewska, E.A.; Call, M.K.; Yamanaka, O.; Liu, H.; Schlötzer-Schrehardt, U.; Kruse, F.E.; Kao, W.W. From hair to cornea: Toward the therapeutic use of hair follicle-derived stem cells in the treatment of limbal stem cell deficiency. *Stem Cells* **2011**, *29*, 57–66. [CrossRef] [PubMed]
207. Miki, T.; Lehmann, T.; Cai, H.; Stolz, D.B.; Strom, S.C. Stem Cell Characteristics of Amniotic Epithelial Cells. *Stem Cells* **2005**, *23*, 1549–1559. [CrossRef]
208. Miki, T. Stem cell characteristics and the therapeutic potential of amniotic epithelial cells. *Am. J. Reprod. Immunol.* **2018**, *80*, 13003. [CrossRef] [PubMed]
209. He, Y.G.; Alizadeh, H.; Kinoshita, K.; McCulley, J.P. Experimental transplantation of cultured human limbal and amniotic epithelial cells onto the corneal surface. *Cornea* **1999**, *18*, 570–579. [CrossRef]

210. Fatimah, S.S.; Ng, S.L.; Chua, K.H.; Hayati, A.R.; Tan, A.E.; Tan, G.C. Value of human amniotic epithelial cells in tissue engineering for cornea. *Hum. Cell* **2010**, *23*, 141–151. [CrossRef]
211. Yao, M.; Chen, J.; Yang, X.X.; Zhang, X.L.; Ji, Q.S.; Zhou, Q.; Xu, J.T. Differentiation of human amniotic epithelial cells into corneal epithelial-like cells in vitro. *Int. J. Ophthalmol.* **2013**, *6*, 564–572. [CrossRef]
212. Zhou, Q.; Liu, X.Y.; Ruan, Y.X.; Wang, L.; Jiang, M.M.; Wu, J.; Chen, J. Construction of corneal epithelium with human amniotic epithelial cells and repair of limbal deficiency in rabbit models. *Hum. Cell* **2015**, *28*, 22–36. [CrossRef] [PubMed]
213. Ruetze, M.; Gallinat, S.; Lim, I.J.; Chow, E.; Phan, T.T.; Staeb, F.; Wenck, H.; Deppert, W.; Knott, A. Common features of umbilical cord epithelial cells and epidermal keratinocytes. *J. Dermatol. Sci.* **2008**, *50*, 227–231. [CrossRef] [PubMed]
214. Huang, L.; Wong, Y.P.; Gu, H.; Cai, Y.J.; Ho, Y.; Wang, C.C.; Leung, T.Y.; Burd, A. Stem cell-like properties of human umbilical cord lining epithelial cells and the potential for epidermal reconstitution. *Cytotherapy* **2011**, *13*, 145–155. [CrossRef]
215. Saleh, R.; Reza, H.M. Short review on human umbilical cord lining epithelial cells and their potential clinical applications. *Stem Cell Res. Ther.* **2017**, *8*, 222. [CrossRef]
216. Reza, H.M.; Ng, B.Y.; Gimeno, F.L.; Phan, T.T.; Ang, L.P. Umbilical Cord Lining Stem Cells as a Novel and Promising Source for Ocular Surface Regeneration. *Stem Cell Rev. Rep.* **2011**, *7*, 935–947. [CrossRef]

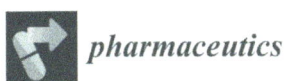

Review

Is the Conjunctiva a Potential Target for Advanced Therapy Medicinal Products?

Yolanda Diebold [1,2,*] **and Laura García-Posadas** [1]

1. Ocular Surface Group, Instituto de Oftalmobiología Aplicada (IOBA), Universidad de Valladolid, 47011 Valladolid, Spain; lgarciap@ioba.med.uva.es
2. Centro de Investigación Biomédica en Red de Bioingeniería, Biomateriales y Nanomedicina (CIBER-BBN), Instituto de Salud Carlos III, 28029 Madrid, Spain
* Correspondence: yol@ioba.med.uva.es

Abstract: The conjunctiva is a complex ocular tissue that provides mechanical, sensory, and immune protection for the ocular surface. It is affected by many diseases through different pathological mechanisms. If a disease is not treated and conjunctival function is not fully restored, the whole ocular surface and, therefore, sight is at risk. Different therapeutic approaches have been proposed, but there are still unsolved conjunctival alterations that require more sophisticated therapeutic options. Advanced therapy medicinal products (ATMPs) comprise a wide range of products that includes cell therapy, tissue engineering, and gene therapy. To the best of our knowledge, there is no commercialized ATMP specifically for conjunctival treatment yet. However, the conjunctiva can be a potential target for ATMPs for different reasons. In this review, we provide an overview of the advances in experimental phases of potential ATMPs that primarily target the conjunctiva. Important advances have been achieved through the techniques of cell therapy and tissue engineering, whereas the use of gene therapy in the conjunctiva is still marginal. Undoubtedly, future research in this field will lead to achieving commercially available ATMPs for the conjunctiva, which may provide better treatments for patients.

Keywords: advanced therapies; cell therapy; conjunctiva; ocular mucosa; gene therapy; tissue engineering

1. Introduction

The human conjunctiva is a complex and fascinating ocular tissue. Traditionally neglected in favor of the cornea, its functions are essential in maintaining ocular surface homeostasis. Over the years, as our knowledge of tear film complexity and the pathophysiology of the ocular surface has increased, the conjunctiva has slowly come to be acknowledged as an essential protective element for ocular surface structures. MUC5AC, a well-known mucin specifically secreted by the conjunctival goblet cells, as well as many other different secretory products, participates in the maintenance of the tear film [1,2].

The conjunctiva is a mucosal tissue that extends from the mucocutaneous junction at the lid margin to the limbal region next to the peripheral cornea and rests on the sclera. In essence, the role of the conjunctiva is to protect the transparency of the cornea, a much more vulnerable tissue that lacks blood and lymphatic vessels, as well as a sufficiently strong in situ immune response for full protection from foreign invaders.

Due to its anatomical features and many roles, the conjunctiva is difficult to study and model in the laboratory. We now know that conjunctival pathophysiology is complex and affects the homeostasis of the so-called lacrimal functional unit [3,4]. Conventional pharmacological treatments are not sufficient or curative in many instances for recovering a functional conjunctiva and/or maintaining healthy ocular surface tissues.

The aim of this review is to present the challenges that the conjunctiva poses from clinical and therapeutic points of view and analyze the reported developments that may become advanced therapies for conjunctival diseases in the future.

1.1. Conjunctival Structure and Functions

From an anatomical point of view, the conjunctiva is generally divisible into three main regions: (1) the tarsal, or palpebral, which lines the inner surface of the eyelids; (2) the forniceal, which lines the upper and lower fornices; and (3) the bulbar, which overlays the sclera on the anterior portion of the globe. These three regions are specialized in different functions, ranging from trapping small foreign objects in a net of secreted mucins and facilitating their removal by blinking to providing immune protection to the cornea by the local presence of lymphoid tissue [5].

The complexity of the conjunctiva relies upon the multiple tissues present in its structure: (1) a non-keratinized stratified squamous epithelium that possesses five reported epithelial cell subtypes, including goblet cells; (2) a basal membrane, where potential autoantigens reside and, subsequently, immune material becomes deposited in certain autoimmune diseases (e.g., mucous membrane pemphigoid), in addition to a loose stroma mainly composed of type IV collagen; (3) an abundant vasculature; (4) a regional lymphoid tissue—namely, conjunctiva-associated lymphoid tissue (CALT) and lymphatic vessels; (5) a melanocyte population; and (6) sensory afferent nerve fibers derived from the ophthalmic (in the bulbar and palpebral areas) and the maxillary (in the inferior forniceal area) branches of the trigeminal nerve. In addition, the conjunctiva possesses the accessory lacrimal glands of Wolfring and Kruse, which are present in the tarsal conjunctiva and in the fornices, respectively, and the pseudoglands of Henle, which are groups of abundant goblet cells that also appear in the tarsal plate.

An amazing variety of cell types are part of the conjunctiva (Figure 1) and account for its functional complexity: mucin-secreting epithelial cells, fibroblasts, melanocytes, dendritic cells, lymphocytes, eosinophils, neutrophils, and mast cells, not to mention mesenchymal stem cells (MSCs). This illustrates how difficult it has been to model conjunctival tissue in the laboratory over the years.

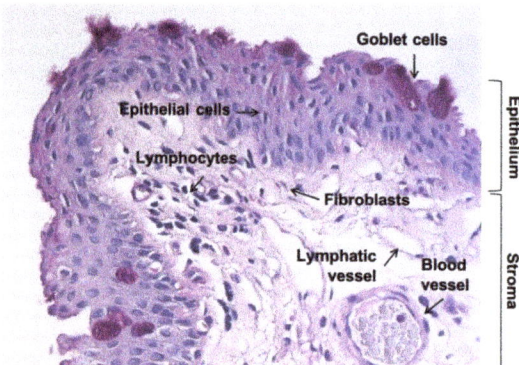

Figure 1. Tissue section of human conjunctiva with periodic acid-Schiff (PAS) staining showing the main cell types present in the epithelium and stroma. Magnification: 200×.

From a functional point of view, the conjunctiva realizes the mechanical, sensory, and immune protection of the ocular surface; the specialized secretion of fluid, electrolytes, and diverse components of the tear film [2], mainly mucins and antimicrobial peptides [6]; the modulation of the local inflammatory state; the regulation of tissue repair and fibrosis; neo-angiogenesis; and pain perception [7]. In addition, epithelial cells can respond to signals derived from the abundant microbiota resident on the ocular surface producing inflammatory cytokines [8]. Further, it is worth mentioning the contribution of the conjunctiva to the antioxidant system protecting the ocular surface with the expression of superoxide dismutase, catalase, glutathione synthetase, and glutathione reductase [9] and peroxiredoxin I [10], in addition to glutathione [11].

This wide range of functions makes the conjunctiva a key element in the maintenance of ocular surface homeostasis and, at the same time, quite reactive to small environmental changes and even prone to alterations. This aspect will be further discussed in this review.

1.2. Regeneration of the Conjunctival Tissue

Tissue regeneration allows the complete functional recovery of damaged tissue, while tissue repair usually leaves structural alterations or even permanent scars associated with collagen deposits, which may lead to disorders. The regeneration process relies upon the local presence of stem cells, whose activation and proliferation lead to the replenishment of lost cells. Ocular surface epithelia are able to self-renew; however, conjunctival regeneration is still debated among experts. The main reasons for this are related to the lack of clarity regarding the presence of human conjunctival stem cells in the different conjunctival regions and their potential to regenerate not only squamous epithelial cells but also conjunctival goblet cells, as discussed below.

There are few published papers for which the potential locations of epithelial stem cells in the human conjunctiva have been studied. The currently accepted locations are the fornix [12,13] and the bulbar conjunctiva [12–16]. In one of the latest papers on this topic published to date, clonogenic ability and stem cell marker expression in both fixed tissue and cultured cells from the same human donors were used to identify conjunctival stem cells, resulting in stem cells being scattered throughout the basal epithelial cell layer of the whole conjunctival tissue. However, the highest levels of stem cell markers are located in the medial canthal and inferior fornieceal areas of the conjunctiva [17] with no apparent organization in a niche, as is the case in the limbus. We still know very little about the mechanism of conjunctival epithelial renewal and how the bipotent cell precursor proposed by Pellegrini et al. in 1999 [14] actually gives rise to either a squamous cell or a goblet cell. What is clear, however, is the fact that conjunctival tissue may fail to regenerate and give rise to pathology, as limbal and corneal tissues do [18,19].

Additionally, the conjunctival stroma possesses multipotent MSCs that express markers of undifferentiated stem cells [20]. Several studies have demonstrated the capacity of these conjunctival MSCs to differentiate into corneal cells [21], photoreceptor cells [22], or insulin-producing cells [23,24], among others, suggesting their utility for tissue engineering and ocular reconstruction [22,25].

1.3. In Vitro/Ex Vivo Systems for Studying Conjunctival Pathophysiology

As mentioned previously, the conjunctiva has long been neglected. The lack of research in this field means that there are few models with which to study the tissue, and fewer models mean less knowledge. This vicious circle needed to be broken, and fortunately, it seems that it actually has been. Although the in vitro models available with which to study the normal functioning of the conjunctiva and the diseases affecting it are limited in number, they have been improved over the last few years. Several new immortalized cells and more complex cell culture models have been added to the "classic" cell lines. The complexity of these models ranges from cell monolayers of a single cell type to complete 3D models that can more faithfully represent the structure of this tissue [26].

The main advantage of cell lines is that they are easy to use and allow the obtaining of large quantities of cells with which to perform many experiments. However, they can show important differences from the native tissue cells [27]. The spontaneously immortalized Wong–Kilbourne derivative of the Chang cell line has been widely used in conjunctival research. However, it lacks the expression of typical markers such as cytokeratin (CK) 4 and the adhesion protein E-cadherin. It also differs from normal primary cultures of the human conjunctiva in its response to inflammatory cytokines [28], and, in addition, it is commonly acknowledged that it is cross-contaminated with HeLa cells [29,30]. For that reason, it is not frequently used today. Another spontaneously immortalized cell line is IOBA-NHC, which was developed by Diebold et al. [31]. It has allowed us to increase our knowledge of the inflammatory response of conjunctival epithelial cells [32–34], but, unfortunately, it has shown signs of senescence, limiting its use in the last few years. Another widely used cell line is telomerase-immortalized human conjunctival epithelial cells (ConjEp-1/p53DD/cdk4R/TERT, abbreviated to HCjE), which were developed by Gipson et al. from primary cultures [35]. HCjE cells express some of the markers typically found in the native conjunctival epithelium, such as CK19 and MUC1, 4 and 16. However, the expression of MUC5AC is sparse. Finally, another immortalized human conjunctival epithelial cell line (IM-HConjEpiC) has been commercialized by Innoprot, Innovative Technologies in Biological Systems, S.L. (Derio, Spain). IM-HConjEpiCs were developed by immortalizing primary human conjunctival epithelial cells with SV40 large T antigens. Although these cells may be a valuable tool, further phenotypic and functional characterization is needed.

Other than the existence of cell lines representing normal conjunctiva, some authors have established cell lines for different diseases, such as conjunctival squamous cell carcinoma [36].

To overcome some of the limitations of cell lines, several authors have described different protocols for isolating and culturing primary cells from the human conjunctival epithelium [37–39] and stroma [39]. Conjunctival goblet cells have also been cultured from rat [40], human [41], and mouse [42] tissues. Finally, to study diseases affecting the conjunctiva, cells can be directly isolated from pathological tissue. These cells can be expanded in vitro and used to study the physiopathology of the pterygium [43–45] or the ocular pemphigoid [46], among others.

All these cell culture systems have allowed researchers to analyze the response of the conjunctiva to inflammatory stimuli, perform the initial screening of different drugs, or study the signaling pathways involved in mucin secretion [47–50]. However, they are limited in their capacity to represent the complex connections between the different cell types that compose the conjunctiva. This can only be partially achieved with the use of more complex 3D models. We recently reviewed the available human 3D cell culture models of the anterior segment of the eye, including the conjunctiva [26]. Some of these models only represent the epithelium [51], and some others also include a fibroblast-containing stroma mimicked by a scaffold made from collagen [52] or fibrin [53]. There is no doubt that more complex and representative 3D models of the conjunctiva will be constructed with the aid of tissue engineering in the near future.

Finally, there are several ex vivo models of the conjunctiva. Tovell et al. described an ex vivo model used to study conjunctival scarring [54]. They maintained ex vivo segments of porcine conjunctiva in culture and analyzed the tissue contraction in response to different substances. Although this model uses the porcine conjunctiva, it could probably be adapted to human tissue.

2. Diseases Affecting the Conjunctiva

The conjunctiva is involved in a wide variety of ocular surface disorders, in which it becomes damaged to different extents. The mechanisms that lead to the development of alterations in conjunctival tissues include infectious, autoimmune and immune-based, cicatrizing, and inflammatory diseases; benign and malignant tumors; and chemical trauma. In some of these conditions, a wide area of the diseased conjunctiva must be removed, and the subsequent wound has to be covered with another tissue. When a conjunctival wound is neglected, serious damage develops; a secondary healing of the conjunctiva occurs and leads to dysfunctional conjunctival scarring. In turn, conjunctival scarring reduces the motility of the eyeball, which can result in severe anatomical and functional impairment, such as the development of diplopia. In addition, there may be a loss of the conjunctival secretory cells, such as goblet cells and accessory lacrimal glands of Wolfring and Kruse, which alters the conjunctiva's contribution to a healthy tear film and leads to additional damage to the ocular surface. This scenario clearly shows how relevant it is to achieve complete functional regeneration of the conjunctival tissues.

Table 1 summarizes the main diseases that can affect conjunctival tissues and may require tissue transplantation in a way that is intended to be informative rather than exhaustive. The ideal conjunctival tissue graft would be healthy conjunctival tissue from the same or the contralateral eye. However, an autologous healthy conjunctiva is not always available, especially in recurrent and/or bilateral cases.

Table 1. Summary of the main conjunctival diseases that may require tissue transplantation.

Disease	Mechanism that May Necessitate Transplantation
Infectious conjunctivitis: - Adenoviral - Streptococcal - Trachoma	Fibrosis of the upper tarsal conjunctiva can lead to corneal pathology when blinking. Surgical removal of cicatrizing tissue may require conjunctival tissue-like transplantation.
Atopy-related conjunctivitis: - Vernal keratoconjunctivitis - Atopic keratoconjunctivitis	Fibrosis is possible, but not frequent. Surgery to remove giant papillae in VKC, rarely needed, could necessitate conjunctival tissue-like transplantation.
Autoimmune cicatrizing conjunctivitis: - Mucous membrane pemphigoid (ocular cicatricial pemphigoid)	Intense progressive fibrosis leading to fornix shortening and symblephara may necessitate reconstructive surgery and, thus, conjunctival tissue-like transplantation, especially if further limbal stem cell therapy-like and/or corneal transplant is needed.
Immune-based conjunctivitis: - Graft vs. host disease - Rosacea-related - Sjögren-associated DED - Stevens–Johnson syndrome (SJS) and its spectrum	Intense fibrosis leading to symblephara and corneal pathology, most likely in SJS, may necessitate conjunctival tissue-like transplantation after its removal. Mostly required if stem cell transplantation and/or corneal transplant is planned.
Multiple mechanisms involved: - Pterygium	Conjunctival tissue-like transplantation is always required after surgical removal.
Extensive benign and malignant tumors: - Epithelial tumors - Lymphoid hyperplasia/lymphoma - Melanocytic tumors	Conjunctival tissue-like transplantation may be required after surgical removal if extensive areas of the conjunctiva are removed.
Trauma- and surgery-related pathology: - Chemical injury - Multiple glaucoma filtering surgeries - Periorbital reconstruction	If extensive fibrosis makes the removal of tissue necessary, then conjunctival tissue-like transplantation can be considered.

The current conventional regenerative treatments for the conjunctiva mainly involve non-ocular tissues, such as the amniotic membrane (AM) and oral/nasal mucosa. The AM is the innermost placental layer and possesses a multilayered structure in which mesenchymal stem cells are present. The main biological properties of the AM include a lack of immunogenicity, as well as anti-fibrotic, anti-inflammatory, anti-angiogenic, and antimicrobial features. The AM can be used as a basement membrane substitute or as a temporary graft. Its use in ocular surface reconstruction has expanded since 1995, mainly because of its transparency and ability to promote epithelialization [55]. When grafted in conjunctival defects, AM supports conjunctival re-epithelialization when conjunctival stem cells remain in the recipient and helps to repopulate the tissue [56].

There are many published examples regarding the use of oral or nasal mucosal tissues for reconstructing conjunctival defects. For a comparative review, see [57]. Oral mucosal grafting remains the most viable option for the replacement of the conjunctiva in the absence of autologous healthy tissue; however, its main limitation is the lack of goblet cells, along with cosmetic issues. Nasal mucosal grafts maintain goblet cells, and, for some indications, they may be preferred to oral mucosal transplants [58].

In many instances, AM is not sufficiently effective; in the most frequent indication—after pterygium removal surgery—a conjunctival autograft is more effective than AM [59], but the conjunctiva is not always available, as mentioned before. As another example, when the entire conjunctival fornices and palpebral conjunctiva need to be reconstructed, the oral or buccal mucosa is used if there is no other option. However, the results are not functionally or esthetically optimal, and, in many of the indications, the oral mucosa is also compromised with the same background disease; in this case, if the eyelid mucosa is not satisfactorily reconstructed, all attempts to restore vision by corneal transplant are doomed to fail [60].

Therefore, it is clear that there is a clinical need for human healthy conjunctival tissue that regular tissue sources cannot satisfy. Considering this fact, the development of advanced therapy medicinal products (ATMPs) may have enormous potential to help in conjunctival functional regeneration.

Other than the need to cover an extensive conjunctiva tissue area after the removal of diseased tissue, there is a common biological situation in most of the conjunctival pathologies included in Table 1: The presence of fibrosis.

Fibrosis is a complex biological process that is related to different diseases that potentially cause blindness. Fibrotic diseases are characterized by tissue contraction as a result of fibroblast activation and the excess accumulation of the extracellular matrix. Different cells can be involved in the process; however, myofibroblasts, which are activated fibroblasts, play a pivotal role. Scarring is an aberrant wound healing process that results in the formation of a permanent scar that affects not only the tissue morphology but also the functional recovery of wounded tissues. The cytokine transforming growth factor-beta (TGFβ) is the main fibrogenic signal that modulates the fibrotic process [61,62].

The conjunctiva, along with the cornea, is susceptible to fibrotic disease [63]. We can find fibrovascular scarring underlying different situations, such as pterygium, ocular pemphigoids, Stevens–Johnson syndrome, ocular graft versus host disease, or glaucoma filtering surgery (trabeculectomy) [64]. In these, there is an underlying inflammatory or wound healing alteration that triggers the formation of fibrotic tissue. For instance, it is well-established that TGFβ mediates scarring in the conjunctiva, which, in turn, can lead to a reduction in filtration efficacy after trabeculectomy [65]. Another example is pterygium, a very common multifactorial disorder of the conjunctiva that includes an ingrowth of fibrovascular subconjunctival connective tissue, among other features [66,67]. Currently acknowledged as a proliferative disorder more than a degeneration of the conjunctival stroma, pterygium involves a cicatricial fibrotic alteration that can eventually become very severe and impair globe motility and even vision.

For those reasons, the development of effective anti-scarring therapies could represent a revolution in the management of ocular surface diseases and tissue injuries, including surgery.

3. Potential of Advanced Therapy Medicinal Products (ATMPs) to Improve Conjunctival Treatment

The conjunctival diseases listed in Table 1, in addition to their specific pharmacological therapies, may be candidates for advanced therapies.

To the best of our knowledge, there is no commercialized ATMP specifically for conjunctival treatment yet. There are several developments that have the potential to become ATMPs in the near future, as explained below. In general, the term ATMPs groups somatic cell therapy medicinal products, tissue engineering products, gene therapy medicinal products, and the combination of any of the previous with a medical device (combined ATMP) [68].

3.1. Cell-Based Therapies

Tissue engineering and cell therapy are emerging disciplines that combine biomaterials, bioengineering, and cell biology to repair or regenerate biological tissues [69]. Tissue engineering involves developing polymeric scaffolds and assembling them together with cells and/or biologically active molecules to construct bioengineered tissues with features similar to those of the original tissue so that they are able to renew, regenerate, or replace damaged tissues [70,71]. Different cell types, including stem cells, can be expanded ex vivo and stimulated in different ways to achieve the differentiation of several cell types or allow better performance to be obtained.

Regenerative medicines for eye tissues focused on tissue engineering techniques have been developed and established as a new clinical field with enormous potential. In particular, the regeneration of ocular surface tissues such as the cornea or the limbus has greatly benefited from diverse tissue engineering developments (for a recent review, see [72,73]). Regarding human conjunctival tissue regeneration, some examples have been described in preclinical studies, but most of them have not yet been investigated in clinical studies. However, it is clear that there is a clinical need for healthy human conjunctival tissue that regular tissue sources cannot satisfy. Bioengineered tissues are considered an appealing solution for use as ATMPs for severe ocular surface disorders involving the conjunctiva. Additionally, the in vitro recapitulation of conjunctival tissues for transplantation seems to be a promising strategy along with their ex vivo expansion [74]. Two clinical studies have analyzed the efficiency of using human conjunctival tissue expanded ex vivo to regenerate the ocular surface [75,76].

Ricardo et al. expanded a forniceal conjunctiva biopsy on the basement membrane surface of denuded AM [75]. After two weeks in culture, conjunctival epithelial cells were transplanted on the corneal surfaces of 12 eyes from 10 patients with chemical burns, idiopathic ocular surface disease, or Stevens–Johnson syndrome, among other conditions. After the transplantation, the authors observed re-epithelialization with the transparent and regular epithelium, achieving partial or total success in 10 out of 12 eyes. This study demonstrates the capacity of cultured conjunctival epithelial cells to restore the ocular surface.

In 2014, Vasania et al. published the results of a multicentric clinical trial performed in India with the purpose of establishing "the efficacy and safety of ex vivo cultured autologous human conjunctival epithelial cell transplantation for treatment of pterygia" [76]. Similar to the procedure described by Ricardo et al., they obtained superior fornix biopsies and seeded them on AM. Cells were cultured for 14–21 days before using them as grafts to cover the conjunctival defect performed during pterygium surgery. No significant complications were reported, and the pterygium recurrence rate was 21.7%. Interestingly, 82.6% of the patients showed adequate goblet cells present at the site of transplantation.

Di Girolamo et al. developed a method to expand and transplant autologous conjunctival stem cells onto the ocular surface by using contact lenses as carriers [77,78]. A biopsy was obtained from the superior forniceal conjunctiva, placed on the concave surface of a siloxane-hydrogel contact lens, and cultured until the cells reached confluence. Then, the contact lens was inserted into the patient's eye. With this technique, the authors achieved a successful reconstitution of the ocular surface using autologous cells even in cases of bilateral disease. Interestingly, more successful outcomes were obtained with conjunctival cells (78%) than with limbal cells (43%) [78]. Another advantage of this method is that transplanted cells are not exposed to foreign human biological or xenogeneic materials.

These examples highlight the potential of using ex vivo expanded conjunctival epithelial cells to successfully treat different pathological conditions affecting the ocular surface. Nevertheless, there are other examples of using non-ocular engineered cells that have achieved promising results. Kobayashi et al. engineered ex vivo-expanded nasal mucosal epithelial cells from biopsy-derived human nasal mucosal tissues on AM [79]. Interestingly, the bioengineered tissue was stratified and included a high density of functional goblet cells. When transplanted onto defective conjunctival areas surgically created in rabbits, the generated tissues survived and remained clear and smooth two weeks after transplantation, without signs of extensive inflammation. The expression of several markers, including MUC5AC mucin, was detected in the transplanted tissue. Although this study did not elucidate the molecular pathway involved in the differentiation of transplanted nasal tissue, the results were quite promising, as it is difficult to maintain functional goblet cells in culture.

An early attempt was published by Yang et al. in 2015, in which the feasibility of the directed differentiation of human amniotic epithelial cells into the conjunctival epithelium was tested [80]. The transformation of conjunctival epithelial cells after AM transplantation to repair conjunctival damage due to burns had previously been reported [81,82]. Amniotic epithelial cells at passage 3 were used to inoculate a human decellularized conjunctival matrix and left for five days to differentiate. They differentiated into cells with the phenotype of conjunctival goblet and non-goblet epithelial cells expressing markers such as cytokeratin (CK 4, CK 13) and the goblet cell-associated mucin MUC5AC. Then, the authors constructed an engineered conjunctiva using a decellularized amniotic membrane as a scaffold and amniotic epithelial cells differentiated into the conjunctival epithelium. When transplanted to the eyes of rabbits with defective conjunctivas, the bioengineered conjunctivas, including PAS-positive goblet cells, were completely grafted, showing good tissue biocompatibility. The transplanted cells survived and maintained an aligned regular morphology. However, this study did not report for how long the transplanted cells remained viable and expressed conjunctival markers. Although this pilot study showed promising results, they were far from demonstrating a truly functional ocular surface reconstruction.

Another more recent example was published by Bertolin et al. in 2019 [83]. They presented a protocol for preparing autologous tissue-engineered conjunctival epithelial sheets free of all animal components. They used AM and fibrin tissue gel as scaffolds to culture human conjunctival cells obtained from different conjunctival areas. Cells biopsied from the inferior forniceal area demonstrated higher percentages of stem cells, resulting in the best area for isolating cells having a high regenerative capacity in terms of the expression of specific markers and growing on the scaffolds. The authors found variability depending on the AM batch. This, along with the difficulties in accomplishing quality control before releasing the graft, is the main hurdle the authors identified in standardizing a medical product composed of conjunctival cells grown on AM. In addition, they also observed holes in the AM while cells were growing, which could affect the integrity of the surface. Regarding the fibrin glue gel, the authors considered it the ideal scaffold, as it is already a transparent pharmaceutical product, and the quality control tests could be performed without affecting the final product, although low numbers of goblet cells were identified and small amounts of MUC5AC were measured. The impact of this paper is limited, as no in vivo experiments for regenerating conjunctival defects were carried out.

Finally, there was a recent study [84] in which a 3D-printed gelatin/elastin/hyaluronic acid membrane was designed for conjunctival reconstruction. The overall aim was to replace the use of AM as a graft in ocular surface reconstruction because of its well-known limitations. An in vivo evaluation was conducted that involved implanting the bioprinted membranes and AM on induced conjunctival defects in rabbits. Although the constructs showed physical and mechanical characteristics adequate for successful ocular surface defect reconstruction, and the authors claimed that their membrane could be considered a promising alternative to AM, this first attempt had an important limitation: it completely lacked the cellular component. The endpoint of the study was only the morphological quality of the healed conjunctiva after the membrane transplant. Although the bioengineered membrane may work as a wound dressing, the functional regeneration of conjunctival tissue would not be achieved.

We are still far from achieving a bioengineered complete human conjunctival tissue replacement, but these promising studies are paving the way towards that goal.

3.2. Gene Therapy

Gene therapy has great potential to prevent conjunctival bleb fibrosis associated with the failure of glaucoma filtering surgery. However, there are very few examples of gene therapy developments for treating this problem. We next mention several published papers related to this topic using animal or human-derived materials.

The use of antimetabolites, such as mitomycin-C and 5-fluorouracil, as conjunctival anti-scarring agents in glaucoma filtering surgery began in the 1990s; however, their potentially blinding side-effects, such as wound leakage, hypotony, and infection, along with their indiscriminate effects on cells render conjunctival scarring a not-yet-resolved problem of high clinical relevance.

As TGFβ is the main fibrogenic signal that modulates the fibrotic process [61,62], interfering with the signaling pathway that TGFβ1–β3 use to induce fibrosis could be a good strategy for preventing or treating conjunctival fibrosis. Smad7 gene transfer, a member of the Smad signaling pathway, was reported as a potential strategy with which to modulate the fibrotic reaction that occurs in an incision-injured mouse conjunctiva during the healing process [85,86]. The authors first showed that Smad7 overexpression delivered using an adenoviral vector inhibited the TGFβ1-driven upregulation of both fibrogenic and inflammatory components in cultured human subconjunctival fibroblasts [85]. All this suggests the therapeutic potential of adenovirus-based Smad7 gene transfer to prevent excess scarring from trabeculectomy.

A recent review published by Komáromy et al. [87] clearly summarizes the more advanced developments in this field. There have been several successful examples in experimental models, but few techniques have reached the clinical trial stage in humans. An example is the development of a small interfering RNA to silence transcription factors involved in conjunctival tissue fibrosis, such as the myocardin-related transcription factor/serum response factor (MRTF/SRF) pathway or secreted protein acidic and rich in cysteine (SPARC) [88–90]. Another example is the presurgical subconjunctival injection or topical administration onto the surgical field of recombinant adenovirus with the human p21 transgene (encoding the CDKN1A protein) in rabbits [91]. The modulation of wound healing after trabeculectomy would be achieved in this case by the cell cycle arrest of surrounding cells rather than their destruction using conventional mitomycin-C. Finally, the adenovirus-mediated blockage of p38 mitogen-activated protein kinase (MAPK) resulted in the inhibition of the fibrogenic reaction induced by the subconjunctival fibroblasts in mice with conjunctival scarring [86].

In humans, one strategy studied was gene delivery using an anti-sense oligonucleotide that specifically inhibits the gene expression of TGFβ2(ISTH0036) [92], which has shown promising results in open-angle glaucoma patients undergoing trabeculectomy. Patients received a single dose of ISTH0036 at the end of surgery by intravitreal injection. The results of the study showed that ISTH0036 was safe, as there were no adverse events directly related to the ISTH0036 injection. Additionally, single-dose ISTH0036 administration resulted in intraocular pressure values < 10 mmHg that were maintained over the three-month postoperative observation period. This is the first clinical study that shows the clinically relevant results of a gene therapy product that displays a potent anti-fibrotic effect in the conjunctiva. It may be worth exploring its application in other forms of fibrotic diseases in which the conjunctiva is involved.

4. Concluding Remarks

The conjunctiva is an essential tissue for maintaining a healthy ocular surface. The great complexity of this tissue, along with the effect of neglecting it in favor of the cornea and limbus, accounts for the delay in the development of ATMPs that target the conjunctiva. Nevertheless, as described in this review, important advances have been made in the last few years, especially in the field of tissue engineering. Further interesting studies in this field are anticipated in the next few years.

Author Contributions: Y.D. conceived the review; Y.D. and L.G.-P. wrote the manuscript. All authors have read and agreed to the published version of the manuscript.

Funding: This research was funded by the Ministerio de Ciencia, Innovación y Universidades (MCIU, Government of Spain), Agencia Estatal de Investigación (AEI, Government of Spain), and the Fondo Europeo de Desarrollo Regional (FEDER), grant number RTI2018–094071-B-C2. L.G.-P. is funded by the Postdoctoral contracts 2017 call (University of Valladolid, Spain).

Institutional Review Board Statement: Not applicable.

Informed Consent Statement: Not applicable.

Acknowledgments: The authors wish to thank Margarita Calonge for providing clinical advice about conjunctival diseases.

Conflicts of Interest: The authors declare no conflict of interest.

References

1. Hori, Y. Secreted mucins on the ocular surface. *Investig. Ophthalmol. Vis. Sci.* **2018**, *59*, DES151–DES156. [CrossRef]
2. Dartt, D.A. Regulation of mucin and fluid secretion by conjunctival epithelial cells. *Prog. Retin. Eye Res.* **2002**, *21*, 555–576. [CrossRef]
3. Stern, M.E.; Beuerman, R.W.; Fox, R.I.; Gao, J.; Mircheff, A.K.; Pflugfelder, S.C. The pathology of dry eye: The interaction between the ocular surface and lacrimal glands. *Cornea* **1998**, *17*, 584–589. [CrossRef]
4. Stern, M.E.; Gao, J.; Siemasko, K.F.; Beuerman, R.W.; Pflugfelder, S.C. The role of the lacrimal functional unit in the pathophysiology of dry eye. *Exp. Eye Res.* **2004**, *78*, 409–416. [CrossRef] [PubMed]
5. Knop, N.; Knop, E. Conjunctiva-associated lymphoid tissue in the human eye. *Investig. Ophthalmol. Vis. Sci.* **2000**, *41*, 1270–1279.
6. McDermott, A.M. Defensins and other antimicrobial peptides at the ocular surface. *Ocul. Surf.* **2004**, *2*, 229–247. [CrossRef]
7. Aiello, F.; Gallo Afflitto, G.; Li, J.-P.O.; Martucci, A.; Cesareo, M.; Nucci, C. CannabinEYEds: The endocannabinoid system as a regulator of the ocular surface nociception, inflammatory response, neovascularization and wound healing. *J. Clin. Med.* **2020**, *9*, 4036. [CrossRef] [PubMed]
8. Galdiero, M.; Petrillo, F.; Pignataro, D.; Lavano, M.A.; Santella, B.; Folliero, V.; Zannella, C.; Astarita, C.; Gagliano, C.; Franci, G.; et al. Current evidence on the ocular surface microbiota and related diseases. *Microorganisms* **2020**, *8*, 1033. [CrossRef]
9. Corrales, R.M.; Galarreta, D.; Herreras, J.; Calonge, M.; Chaves, F. Antioxidant enzyme mRNA expression in conjunctival epithelium of healthy human subjects. *Can. J. Ophthalmol.* **2011**, *46*, 35–39. [CrossRef]
10. Klebe, S.; Callahan, T.; Power, J.H.T. Peroxiredoxin I and II in human eyes: Cellular distribution and association with pterygium and DNA damage. *J. Histochem. Cytochem.* **2014**, *62*, 85–96. [CrossRef]
11. Gukasyan, H.J.; Kim, K.J.; Lee, V.H.L.; Kannan, R. Glutathione and its transporters in ocular surface defense. *Ocul. Surf.* **2007**, *5*, 269–279. [CrossRef]
12. Budak, M.T.; Alpdogan, O.S.; Zhou, M.; Lavker, R.M.; Akinci, M.A.M.; Wolosin, J.M. Ocular surface epithelia contain ABCG2-dependent side population cells exhibiting features associated with stem cells. *J. Cell Sci.* **2005**, *118*, 1715–1724. [CrossRef]
13. Pauklin, M.; Thomasen, H.; Pester, A.; Steuhl, K.P.; Meller, D. Expression of pluripotency and multipotency factors in human ocular surface tissues. *Curr. Eye Res.* **2011**, *36*, 1086–1097. [CrossRef]
14. Pellegrini, G.; Golisano, O.; Paterna, P.; Lambiase, A.; Bonini, S.; Rama, P.; De Luca, M. Location and clonal analysis of stem cells and their differentiated progeny in the human ocular surface. *J. Cell Biol.* **1999**, *145*, 769–782. [CrossRef] [PubMed]
15. Vascotto, S.G.; Griffith, M. Localization of candidate stem and progenitor cell markers within the human cornea, limbus and bulbar conjunctiva in vivo and in cell culture. *Anat. Rec. Part A Discov. Mol. Cell. Evol. Biol.* **2006**, *288*, 921–931. [CrossRef]
16. Qi, H.; Zheng, X.; Yuan, X.; Pflugfelder, S.C.; Li, D.Q. Potential localization of putative stem/progenitor cells in human bulbar conjunctival epithelium. *J. Cell. Physiol.* **2010**, *225*, 180–185. [CrossRef]
17. Stewart, R.M.K.; Sheridan, C.M.; Hiscott, P.S.; Czanner, G.; Kaye, S.B. Human conjunctival stem cells are predominantly located in the medial canthal and inferior forniceal areas. *Investig. Ophthalmol. Vis. Sci.* **2015**, *56*, 2021–2030. [CrossRef]
18. Sorsby, A.; Symons, H.M. Amniotic membrane grafts in caustic burns of the eye (burns of the second degree). *Br. J. Ophthalmol.* **1946**, *30*, 337–345. [CrossRef] [PubMed]
19. Meller, D.; Pauklin, M.; Thomasen, H.; Westekemper, H.; Steuhl, K.-P. Amniotic membrane transplantation in the human eye. *Dtsch. Aerzteblatt Online* **2011**, *108*, 243–248. [CrossRef]
20. Nadri, S.; Soleimani, M.; Kiani, J.; Atashi, A.; Izadpanah, R. Multipotent mesenchymal stem cells from adult human eye conjunctiva stromal cells. *Differentiation* **2008**, *76*, 223–231. [CrossRef] [PubMed]
21. Soleimanifar, F.; Mortazavi, Y.; Nadri, S.; Soleimani, M. Conjunctiva derived mesenchymal stem cell (CJMSCs) as a potential platform for differentiation into corneal epithelial cells on bioengineered electrospun scaffolds. *J. Biomed. Mater. Res. Part A* **2017**, *105*, 2703–2711. [CrossRef] [PubMed]

22. Soleimannejad, M.; Ebrahimi-Barough, S.; Soleimani, M.; Nadri, S.; Tavangar, S.M.; Roohipoor, R.; Yazdankhah, M.; Bayat, N.; Riazi-Esfahani, M.; Ai, J. Fibrin gel as a scaffold for photoreceptor cells differentiation from conjunctiva mesenchymal stem cells in retina tissue engineering. *Artif. Cells Nanomed. Biotechnol.* **2018**, *46*, 805–814. [CrossRef] [PubMed]
23. Nadri, S.; Barati, G.; Mostafavi, H.; Esmaeilzadeh, A.; Enderami, S.E. Differentiation of conjunctiva mesenchymal stem cells into secreting islet beta cells on plasma treated electrospun nanofibrous scaffold. *Artif. Cells Nanomed. Biotechnol.* **2018**, *46*, 178–187. [CrossRef] [PubMed]
24. Barati, G.; Rahmani, A.; Nadri, S. In vitro differentiation of conjunctiva mesenchymal stem cells into insulin producing cells on natural and synthetic electrospun scaffolds. *Biologicals* **2019**, *62*, 33–38. [CrossRef]
25. Soleimanifar, F.; Mortazavi, Y.; Nadri, S.; Islami, M.; Vakilian, S. Coculture of conjunctiva derived mesenchymal stem cells (CJMSCs) and corneal epithelial cells to reconstruct the corneal epithelium. *Biologicals* **2018**, *54*, 39–43. [CrossRef]
26. García-Posadas, L.; Diebold, Y. Three-dimensional human cell culture models to study the pathophysiology of the anterior eye. *Pharmaceutics* **2020**, *12*, 1215. [CrossRef] [PubMed]
27. Tong, L.; Diebold, Y.; Calonge, M.; Gao, J.; Stern, M.E.; Beuerman, R.W. Comparison of gene expression profiles of conjunctival cell lines with primary cultured conjunctival epithelial cells and human conjunctival tissue. *Gene Expr.* **2009**, *14*, 265–278. [CrossRef]
28. De Saint Jean, M.; Baudouin, C.; Di Nolfo, M.; Roman, S.; Lozato, P.; Warnet, J.M.; Brignole, F. Comparison of morphological and functional characteristics of primary-cultured human conjunctival epithelium and of Wong-Kilbourne derivative of Chang conjunctival cell line. *Exp. Eye Res.* **2004**, *78*, 257–274. [CrossRef]
29. Lavappa, K.S. Survey of ATCC stocks of human cell lines for hela contamination. *In Vitro* **1978**, *14*, 469–475. [CrossRef] [PubMed]
30. Brasnu, E.; Brignole-Baudouin, F.; Riancho, L.; Warnet, J.M.; Baudouin, C. Comparative study on the cytotoxic effects of benzalkonium chloride on the Wong-Kilbourne derivative of Chang conjunctival and IOBA-NHC cell lines. *Mol. Vis.* **2008**, *14*, 394–402.
31. Diebold, Y.; Calonge, M.; De Salamanca, A.E.; Callejo, S.; Corrales, R.M.; Sáez, V.; Siemasko, K.F.; Stern, M.E. Characterization of a spontaneously immortalized cell line (IOBA-NHC) from normal human conjunctiva. *Investig. Ophthalmol. Vis. Sci.* **2003**, *44*, 4263–4274. [CrossRef] [PubMed]
32. Enríquez-de-Salamanca, A.; Calder, V.; Gao, J.; Galatowicz, G.; García-Vázquez, C.; Fernández, I.; Stern, M.E.; Diebold, Y.; Calonge, M. Cytokine responses by conjunctival epithelial cells: An in vitro model of ocular inflammation. *Cytokine* **2008**, *44*, 160–167. [CrossRef]
33. Soriano-Romaní, L.; Contreras-Ruiz, L.; García-Posadas, L.; López-García, A.; Masli, S.; Diebold, Y. Inflammatory cytokine-mediated regulation of thrombospondin-1 and CD36 in conjunctival cells. *J. Ocul. Pharmacol. Ther.* **2015**, *31*, 419–428. [CrossRef] [PubMed]
34. Redfern, R.L.; Barabino, S.; Baxter, J.; Lema, C.; McDermott, A.M. Dry eye modulates the expression of toll-like receptors on the ocular surface. *Exp. Eye Res.* **2015**, *134*, 80–89. [CrossRef]
35. Gipson, I.K.; Spurr-Michaud, S.; Argüeso, P.; Tisdale, A.; Ng, T.F.; Russo, C.L. Mucin gene expression in immortalized human corneal-limbal and conjunctival epithelial cell lines. *Investig. Ophthalmol. Vis. Sci.* **2003**, *44*, 2496–2506. [CrossRef] [PubMed]
36. Thomasen, H.; Müller, B.; Poetsch, M.; Steuhl, K.P.; Meller, D. Establishment of a cell line from conjunctival squamous cell carcinoma: Peca-UkHb-01. *Investig. Ophthalmol. Vis. Sci.* **2015**, *56*, 4460–4469. [CrossRef]
37. Diebold, Y.; Calonge, M. Characterization of epithelial primary cultures from human conjunctiva. *Graefe's Arch. Clin. Exp. Ophthalmol.* **1997**, *235*, 268–276. [CrossRef] [PubMed]
38. Marsh, R.B.C.; Massaro-Giordano, M.; Marshall, C.M.; Lavker, R.M.; Jensen, P.J. Initiation and characterization of keratinocyte cultures from biopsies of normal human conjunctiva. *Exp. Eye Res.* **2002**, *74*, 61–69. [CrossRef] [PubMed]
39. García-Posadas, L.; Arranz-Valsero, I.; López-García, A.; Soriano-Romaní, L.; Diebold, Y. A new human primary epithelial cell culture model to study conjunctival inflammation. *Invest. Ophthalmol. Vis. Sci.* **2013**, *54*, 7143–7152. [CrossRef] [PubMed]
40. Shatos, M.A.; Rios, J.D.; Tepavcevic, V.; Kano, H.; Hodges, R.; Dartt, D.A. Isolation, characterization and propagation of rat conjunctival goblet cells in vitro. *Investig. Ophthalmol. Vis. Sci.* **2001**, *42*, 1455–1464.
41. Shatos, M.A.; Ríos, J.D.; Horikawa, Y.; Hodges, R.R.; Chang, E.L.; Bernardino, C.R.; Rubin, P.A.D.; Dartt, D.A. Isolation and characterization of cultured human conjunctival goblet cells. *Investig. Ophthalmol. Vis. Sci.* **2003**, *44*, 2477–2486. [CrossRef] [PubMed]
42. Contreras-Ruiz, L.; Ghosh-Mitra, A.; Shatos, M.A.; Dartt, D.A.; Masli, S. Modulation of conjunctival goblet cell function by inflammatory cytokines. *Mediat. Inflamm.* **2013**, *2013*, 636812. [CrossRef] [PubMed]
43. Di Girolamo, N.; Tedla, N.; Kumar, R.K.; McCluskey, P.; Lloyd, A.; Coroneo, M.T.; Wakefield, D. Culture and characterisation of epithelial cells from human pterygia. *Br. J. Ophthalmol.* **1999**, *83*, 1077–1082. [CrossRef]
44. Di Girolamo, N.; McCluskey, P.; Lloyd, A.; Coroneo, M.T.; Wakefield, D. Expression of MMPs and TIMPs in human pterygia and cultured pterygium epithelial cells. *Investig. Ophthalmol. Vis. Sci.* **2000**, *41*, 671–679.
45. Chui, J.; Di Girolamo, N.; Coroneo, M.T.; Wakefield, D. The role of substance P in the pathogenesis of pterygia. *Investig. Ophthalmol. Vis. Sci.* **2007**, *48*, 4482–4489. [CrossRef] [PubMed]
46. Saw, V.P.J.; Schmidt, E.; Offiah, I.; Galatowicz, G.; Zillikens, D.; Dart, J.K.G.; Calder, V.L.; Daniels, J.T. Profibrotic phenotype of conjunctival fibroblasts from mucous membrane pemphigoid. *Am. J. Pathol.* **2011**, *178*, 187–197. [CrossRef]

47. Dartt, D.A.; Hodges, R.R.; Li, D.; Shatos, M.A.; Lashkari, K.; Serhan, C.N. Conjunctival goblet cell secretion stimulated by leukotrienes is reduced by resolvins D1 and E1 To promote resolution of inflammation. *J. Immunol.* **2011**, *186*, 4455–4466. [CrossRef]
48. García-Posadas, L.; Hodges, R.R.; Li, D.; Shatos, M.A.; Storr-Paulsen, T.; Diebold, Y.; Dartt, D.A. Interaction of IFN-γ with cholinergic agonists to modulate rat and human goblet cell function. *Mucosal Immunol.* **2015**, *9*, 206–217. [CrossRef]
49. Henriksson, J.T.; Coursey, T.G.; Corry, D.B.; De Paiva, C.S.; Pflugfelder, S.C. IL-13 stimulates proliferation and expression of mucin and immunomodulatory genes in cultured conjunctival goblet cells. *Investig. Ophthalmol. Vis. Sci.* **2015**, *56*, 4186–4197. [CrossRef]
50. García-Posadas, L.; Hodges, R.R.; Diebold, Y.; Dartt, D.A. Context-dependent regulation of conjunctival goblet cell function by allergic mediators. *Sci. Rep.* **2018**, *8*, 12162. [CrossRef]
51. Chung, S.H.; Lee, J.H.; Yoon, J.H.; Lee, H.K.; Seo, K.Y. Multi-layered culture of primary human conjunctival epithelial cells producing MUC5AC. *Exp. Eye Res.* **2007**, *85*, 226–233. [CrossRef]
52. Tsai, R.J.F.; Ho, Y.S.; Chen, J.K. The effects of fibroblasts on the growth and differentiation of human bulbar conjunctival epithelial cells in an in vitro conjunctival equivalent. *Investig. Ophthalmol. Vis. Sci.* **1994**, *35*, 2865–2875.
53. García-Posadas, L.; Soriano-Romaní, L.; López-García, A.; Diebold, Y. An engineered human conjunctival-like tissue to study ocular surface inflammatory diseases. *PLoS One* **2017**, *12*, e0171099. [CrossRef] [PubMed]
54. Tovell, V.E.; Dahlmann-Noor, A.H.; Khaw, P.T.; Bailly, M. Advancing the treatment of conjunctival scarring: A novel ex vivo model. *Arch. Ophthalmol.* **2011**, *129*, 619–627. [CrossRef] [PubMed]
55. Jirsova, K.; Jones, G.L.A. Amniotic membrane in ophthalmology: Properties, preparation, storage and indications for grafting—A review. *Cell Tissue Bank.* **2017**, *18*, 193–204. [CrossRef] [PubMed]
56. Tseng, S.C.G. Amniotic membrane transplantation for ocular surface reconstruction. *Biosci. Rep.* **2001**, *21*, 481–489. [CrossRef]
57. Mai, C.; Bertelmann, E. Oral mucosal grafts: Old technique in new light. *Ophthalmic Res.* **2013**, *50*, 91–98. [CrossRef]
58. Kim, J.H.; Chun, Y.S.; Lee, S.H.; Mun, S.K.; Jung, H.S.; Lee, S.H.; Son, Y.; Kim, J.C. Ocular surface reconstruction with autologous nasal mucosa in cicatricial ocular surface disease. *Am. J. Ophthalmol.* **2010**, *149*, 45–53. [CrossRef]
59. Clearfield, E.; Hawkins, B.S.; Kuo, I.C. Conjunctival autograft versus amniotic membrane transplantation for treatment of pterygium: Findings from a cochrane systematic review. *Am. J. Ophthalmol.* **2017**, *182*, 8–17. [CrossRef]
60. Buonavoglia, A.; Leone, P.; Dammacco, R.; Di Lernia, G.; Petruzzi, M.; Bonamonte, D.; Vacca, A.; Racanelli, V.; Dammacco, F. Pemphigus and mucous membrane pemphigoid: An update from diagnosis to therapy. *Autoimmun. Rev.* **2019**, *18*, 349–358. [CrossRef]
61. Roberts, A.B.; Russo, A.; Felici, A.; Flanders, K.C. Smad3: A key player in pathogenetic mechanisms dependent on TGF-β. *Ann. N.Y. Acad. Sci.* **2003**, *995*, 1–10. [CrossRef] [PubMed]
62. Flanders, K.C. Smad3 as a mediator of the fibrotic response. *Int. J. Exp. Pathol.* **2004**, *85*, 47–64. [CrossRef]
63. Saika, S.; Yamanaka, O.; Sumioka, T.; Miyamoto, T.; Miyazaki, K.I.; Okada, Y.; Kitano, A.; Shirai, K.; Tanaka, S.I.; Ikeda, K. Fibrotic disorders in the eye: Targets of gene therapy. *Prog. Retin. Eye Res.* **2008**, *27*, 177–196. [CrossRef] [PubMed]
64. Khaw, P.T.; Bouremel, Y.; Brocchini, S.; Henein, C. The control of conjunctival fibrosis as a paradigm for the prevention of ocular fibrosis-related blindness. "Fibrosis has many friends." *Eye* **2020**, *34*, 2163–2174.
65. Jinza, K.; Saika, S.; Kin, K.; Ohnishi, Y. Relationship between formation of a filtering bleb and an intrascleral aqueous drainage route after trabeculectomy: Evaluation using ultrasound biomicroscopy. *Ophthalmic Res.* **2000**, *32*, 240–243. [CrossRef]
66. Coroneo, M.T.; Di Girolamo, N.; Wakefield, D. The pathogenesis of pterygia. *Curr. Opin. Ophthalmol.* **1999**, *10*, 282–288. [CrossRef] [PubMed]
67. Torres, J.; Enríquez-de-Salamanca, A.; Fernández, I.; Rodríguez-Ares, M.T.; Quadrado, M.J.; Murta, J.; Benítez del Castillo, J.M.; Stern, M.E.; Calonge, M. Activation of MAPK signaling pathway and NF-κB activation in pterygium and ipsilateral pterygium-free conjunctival specimens. *Investig. Ophthalmol. Vis. Sci.* **2011**, *52*, 5842–5852. [CrossRef]
68. Regulation (EC) No 1394/2007 of the European parliament and of the council of 13 November 2007 on advanced therapy medicinal products and amending directive 2001/83/EC and regulation (EC) No 726/2004. Off. J. Eur. Union L 324 121–137. Available online: https://eur-lex.europa.eu/LexUriServ/LexUriServ.do?uri=OJ:L:2007:324:0121:0137:en:PDF (accessed on 27 June 2021).
69. Hassanzadeh, P.; Atyabi, F.; Dinarvand, R. Tissue engineering: Still facing a long way ahead. *J. Control Release* **2018**, *279*, 181–197. [CrossRef]
70. Pearson, R.G.; Bhandari, R.; Quirk, R.A.; Shakesheff, K.M. Recent advances in tissue engineering. *J. Long-Term Eff. Med Implant.* **2017**, *27*, 199–231. [CrossRef] [PubMed]
71. Reddy, R.; Reddy, N. Biomimetic approaches for tissue engineering. *J. Biomater. Sci. Polym. Ed.* **2018**, *29*, 1667–1685. [CrossRef]
72. Nosrati, H.; Alizadeh, Z.; Nosrati, A.; Ashrafi-Dehkordi, K.; Banitalebi-Dehkordi, M.; Sanami, S.; Khodaei, M. Stem cell-based therapeutic strategies for corneal epithelium regeneration. *Tissue Cell* **2021**, *68*, 101470. [CrossRef] [PubMed]
73. Nosrati, H.; Abpeikar, Z.; Mahmoudian, Z.G.; Zafari, M.; Majidi, J.; Alizadeh, A.; Moradi, L.; Asadpour, S. Corneal epithelium tissue engineering: Recent advances in regeneration and replacement of corneal surface. *Regen. Med.* **2020**, *15*, 2029–2044. [PubMed]
74. Schrader, S.; Notara, M.; Beaconsfield, M.; Tuft, S.J.; Daniels, J.T.; Geerling, G. Tissue engineering for conjunctival reconstruction: Established methods and future outlooks. *Curr. Eye Res.* **2009**, *34*, 913–924. [CrossRef]

75. Ricardo, J.R.S.; Cristovam, P.C.; Filho, P.A.N.; Farias, C.C.; De Araujo, A.L.; Loureiro, R.R.; Covre, J.L.; De Barros, J.N.; Barreiro, T.P.; Dos Santos, M.S.; et al. Transplantation of conjunctival epithelial cells cultivated ex vivo in patients with total limbal stem cell deficiency. *Cornea* **2013**, *32*, 221–228. [CrossRef] [PubMed]
76. Vasania, V.S.; Hari, A.; Tandon, R.; Shah, S.; Haldipurkar, S.; Shah, S.; Sachan, S.; Viswanathan, C. Transplantation of autologous Ex vivo expanded human conjunctival epithelial cells for treatment of pterygia: A prospective open-label single arm multicentric clinical trial. *J. Ophthalmic Vis. Res.* **2014**, *9*, 407–416. [CrossRef] [PubMed]
77. Di Girolamo, N.; Bosch, M.; Zamora, K.; Coroneo, M.; Wakefield, D.; Watson, S. A contact lens-based technique for expansion and transplantation of autologous epithelial progenitors for ocular surface reconstruction. *Transplantation* **2009**, *87*, 1571–1578. [CrossRef]
78. Bobba, S.; Chow, S.; Watson, S.; Di Girolamo, N. Clinical outcomes of xeno-free expansion and transplantation of autologous ocular surface epithelial stem cells via contact lens delivery: A prospective case series. *Stem Cell Res. Ther.* **2015**, *6*, 23. [CrossRef]
79. Kobayashi, M.; Nakamura, T.; Yasuda, M.; Hata, Y.; Okura, S.; Iwamoto, M.; Nagata, M.; Fullwood, N.J.; Koizumi, N.; Hisa, Y.; et al. Ocular surface reconstruction with a tissue-engineered nasal mucosal epithelial cell sheet for the treatment of severe ocular surface diseases. *Stem Cells Transl. Med.* **2015**, *4*, 99–109. [CrossRef] [PubMed]
80. Yang, S.P.; Yang, X.Z.; Cao, G.P. Conjunctiva reconstruction by induced differentiation of human amniotic epithelial cells. *Genet. Mol. Res.* **2015**, *14*, 13823–13834. [CrossRef]
81. Eidet, J.R.; Utheim, O.A.; Raeder, S.; Dartt, D.A.; Lyberg, T.; Carreras, E.; Huynh, T.T.; Messelt, E.B.; Louch, W.E.; Roald, B.; et al. Effects of serum-free storage on morphology, phenotype, and viability of exvivo cultured human conjunctival epithelium. *Exp. Eye Res.* **2012**, *94*, 109–116. [CrossRef]
82. Zhang, Z.D.; Ma, H.X.; Chen, D.; Li, M.; Liu, J.B.; Lu, F.; Qu, J. A novel technique of modified continuous blanket suture for amnioticmembrane fixation in severe ocular surface diseases. *JAMA Ophthalmol.* **2013**, *131*, 941–947. [CrossRef] [PubMed]
83. Bertolin, M.; Breda, C.; Ferrari, S.; Van Acker, S.I.; Zakaria, N.; Di Iorio, E.; Migliorati, A.; Ponzin, D.; Ferrari, B.; Lužnik, Z.; et al. Optimized protocol for regeneration of the conjunctival epithelium using the cell suspension technique. *Cornea* **2019**, *38*, 469–479. [CrossRef] [PubMed]
84. Dehghani, S.; Rasoulianboroujeni, M.; Ghasemi, H.; Keshel, S.H.; Nozarian, Z.; Hashemian, M.N.; Zarei-Ghanavati, M.; Latifi, G.; Ghaffari, R.; Cui, Z.; et al. 3D-Printed membrane as an alternative to amniotic membrane for ocular surface/conjunctival defect reconstruction: An in vitro & in vivo study. *Biomaterials* **2018**, *174*, 95–112. [CrossRef] [PubMed]
85. Yamanaka, O.; Ikeda, K.; Saika, S.; Miyazaki, K.I.; Ooshima, A.; Ohnishi, Y. Gene transfer of Smad7 modulates injury-induced conjunctival wound healing in mice. *Mol. Vis.* **2006**, *12*, 841–851.
86. Yamanaka, O.; Saika, S.; Ohnishi, Y.; Kim-Mitsuyama, S.; Kamaraju, A.K.; Ikeda, K. Inhibition of p38MAP kinase suppresses fibrogenic reaction in conjunctiva in mice. *Mol. Vis.* **2007**, *13*, 1730–1739.
87. Komáromy, A.M.; Koehl, K.L.; Park, S.A. Looking into the future: Gene and cell therapies for glaucoma. *Vet. Ophthalmol.* **2021**, *24* (Suppl. 1), 16–33. [CrossRef]
88. Yu-Wai-Man, C.; Tagalakis, A.D.; Manunta, M.D.; Hart, S.L.; Khaw, P.T. Receptor-targeted liposome-peptide-siRNA nanoparticles represent an efficient delivery system for MRTF silencing in conjunctival fibrosis. *Sci. Rep.* **2016**, *6*, 21881. [CrossRef]
89. Fernando, O.; Tagalakis, A.D.; Awwad, S.; Brocchini, S.; Khaw, P.T.; Hart, S.L.; Yu-Wai-Man, C. Development of targeted siRNA nanocomplexes to prevent fibrosis in experimental glaucoma filtration surgery. *Mol. Ther.* **2018**, *26*, 2812–2822. [CrossRef]
90. Seet, L.F.; Tan, Y.F.; Toh, L.Z.; Chu, S.W.; Lee, Y.S.; Venkatraman, S.S.; Wong, T.T. Targeted therapy for the post-operative conjunctiva: SPARC silencing reduces collagen deposition. *Br. J. Ophthalmol.* **2018**, *102*, 1460–1470. [CrossRef]
91. Perkins, T.W.; Faha, B.; Ni, M.; Kiland, J.A.; Poulsen, G.L.; Antelman, D.; Atencio, I.; Shinoda, J.; Sinha, D.; Brumback, L.; et al. Adenovirus-mediated gene therapy using human p21WAF-1/Cip-1 to prevent wound healing in a rabbit model of glaucoma filtration surgery. *Arch. Ophthalmol.* **2002**, *120*, 941–949. [CrossRef]
92. Pfeiffer, N.; Voykov, B.; Renieri, G.; Bell, K.; Richter, P.; Weigel, M.; Thieme, H.; Wilhelm, B.; Lorenz, K.; Feindor, M.; et al. First-in-human phase I study of ISTH0036, an antisense oligonucleotide selectively targeting transforming growth factor beta 2 (TGF-β2), in subjects with open-angle glaucoma undergoing glaucoma filtration surgery. *PLoS One* **2017**, *12*, e0188899. [CrossRef] [PubMed]

Review

Cell Replacement Therapy for Retinal and Optic Nerve Diseases: Cell Sources, Clinical Trials and Challenges

Rosa M. Coco-Martin [1,2,*], Salvador Pastor-Idoate [1,2,3] and Jose Carlos Pastor [1,2,3,4]

1. Instituto de Oftalmobiologia Aplicada (IOBA), Medical School, Universidad de Valladolid, 47011 Valladolid, Spain; pastoridoate.salvador@gmail.com (S.P.-I.); pastor@ioba.med.uva.es (J.C.P.)
2. National Institute of Health Carlos III (ISCIII), (RETICS) Cooperative Health Network for Research in Ophthalmology (Oftared), 28040 Madrid, Spain
3. Department of Ophthalmology, Hospital Clinico Universitario de Valladolid, 47003 Valladolid, Spain
4. Centro en Red de Medicina Regenerativa y Terapia Celular de Castilla y León, Fundacion del Instituto de Estudios de Ciencias de la Salud de Castilla y León (ICSCYL), 42002 Soria, Spain
* Correspondence: rosa@ioba.med.uva.es; Tel.: +34-983423559

Abstract: The aim of this review was to provide an update on the potential of cell therapies to restore or replace damaged and/or lost cells in retinal degenerative and optic nerve diseases, describing the available cell sources and the challenges involved in such treatments when these techniques are applied in real clinical practice. Sources include human fetal retinal stem cells, allogenic cadaveric human cells, adult hippocampal neural stem cells, human CNS stem cells, ciliary pigmented epithelial cells, limbal stem cells, retinal progenitor cells (RPCs), human pluripotent stem cells (PSCs) (including both human embryonic stem cells (ESCs) and human induced pluripotent stem cells (iPSCs)) and mesenchymal stem cells (MSCs). Of these, RPCs, PSCs and MSCs have already entered early-stage clinical trials since they can all differentiate into RPE, photoreceptors or ganglion cells, and have demonstrated safety, while showing some indicators of efficacy. Stem/progenitor cell therapies for retinal diseases still have some drawbacks, such as the inhibition of proliferation and/or differentiation in vitro (with the exception of RPE) and the limited long-term survival and functioning of grafts in vivo. Some other issues remain to be solved concerning the clinical translation of cell-based therapy, including (1) the ability to enrich for specific retinal subtypes; (2) cell survival; (3) cell delivery, which may need to incorporate a scaffold to induce correct cell polarization, which increases the size of the retinotomy in surgery and, therefore, the chance of severe complications; (4) the need to induce a localized retinal detachment to perform the subretinal placement of the transplanted cell; (5) the evaluation of the risk of tumor formation caused by the undifferentiated stem cells and prolific progenitor cells. Despite these challenges, stem/progenitor cells represent the most promising strategy for retinal and optic nerve disease treatment in the near future, and therapeutics assisted by gene techniques, neuroprotective compounds and artificial devices can be applied to fulfil clinical needs.

Keywords: stem cells; retinal diseases; optic nerve diseases; cell replacement; cell sources

1. Introduction

Retinal degenerative diseases (RDs) have been largely characterized and are considered leading causes of blindness worldwide. They include age-related macular degeneration (AMD) and inherited retinal dystrophies (IRDs) such as retinitis pigmentosa (RP) and Stargardt's disease [1,2]. There is also some retinal degeneration associated with ischemic disorders such as diabetic retinopathy (DR) and retinal vascular occlusion (RVO), which are also relevant to this review [3,4]. All these disorders share some common pathophysiology pathways that lead to the early loss or dysfunction of photoreceptors and/or neural apoptosis. As part of the central nervous system (CNS), the retina has very low regenerative capability, which can result in untreatable blindness [1–4]. The available therapies for some

RDs can protect retinal neurons, rescue or slow disease progression or relieve symptoms, but currently there are hardly any treatments to restore vision, because at present, lost cells cannot be replaced. Stem cell-based therapy is an exciting, rapidly advancing area of translational research that has already entered the clinic. Some of the advantages of the eye as a target organ for cell-based therapy—mainly for the retina—are the following. Its anatomy and physiology are very well known; surgical techniques to access the retina are well established and are reasonably safe (in fact, they are routine clinical procedures everywhere); the subretinal space is a relatively immune-privileged site; the number of cells needed to restore vision may be relatively small; retinal imaging in the living human eye is available with high resolution noninvasive techniques; fellow eye can be used as a control; finally, electrodiagnostic and psychophysical testing to assess functional recovery are also available and well characterized [5].

Rescue strategies seeking a trophic effect from stem/progenitor cell treatment have been investigated, but their efficacy and efficiency are generally restricted by the low rate of proliferation and/or differentiation of cells in vitro and by poor cellular survival, migration, integration and function in vivo, excluding RPE-based therapy for RD. Nevertheless, cell therapy assisted by gene techniques, neuroprotective compounds and artificial devices can be used in these diseases to fulfil clinical needs.

Regarding cell therapy in optic nerve diseases (ONDs), the situation has progressed little in the last five years, compared to a review carried out by our group [6]. We believe there are several reasons. On the one hand, this is due to the heterogenicity of the pathologies that researchers have tried to treat with cell therapy, which in many cases affect some other parts of the CNS too, and it is also due to the obvious difficulties of access in delivering any treatment to some anatomic sections of the optic nerve. It should not be forgotten that the optic nerve (ON) is "born" in the retinal ganglion cells (RGCs) and extends to the lateral geniculate nucleus [7]. The category of so-called optic neuropathies includes a broad spectrum of diseases with various causes, including ischemia, inflammation, toxicity, nutritional deficiencies, glaucoma, trauma, congenital problems and hereditary diseases, in most cases as part of wider neurodegenerative processes [8]. The ON is basically composed of RGC axons, and like other adult neurons of the CNS, they do not have the ability to regenerate after injury. Many factors limit the regeneration of RGC axons. Some are derived from the inhibitory environment created after RGCs suffer axonal damage. Furthermore, oligodendrocytes secrete inhibitory proteins and other molecules which impede axon regrowth, unlike myelinating Schwann cells that promote axon regeneration in the peripheral nervous system, but these cells are not present in the ON. Astrocytes also release inhibitory molecules and proliferate, creating glial scars acting as physical barriers to axonal regeneration [9–11]. Moreover, many genes which are necessary for cellular proliferation and axon growth, although active in embryonic cells, are deeply suppressed in mature ones [9,10]. Finally, axonal injury also interrupts the transport of neurotrophic factors, resulting in an increase in proapoptotic proteins in RGCs [12–14].

Reviews on the use of intravitreal cell therapy to confer neuroprotection through their paracrine properties have been published by our group [6,15]. Several phase I and II clinical trials (CTs) have demonstrated the safety of many types of stem cells, and this fact has prompted researchers to continue to progress in the exploration of the efficacy of this approach [15,16]. However, there are still many unknowns to be solved, such as the best source of cells, the best route of administration, the possible means of inducing the regeneration of lost cells and above all how to maintain the possible beneficial effects in the long term [16]. These unknowns have to be resolved before any of the treatments become a regular part of clinical therapies. In this review, we provide an update on the potential of cell therapies to restore or replace damaged and/or lost cells in RD and OND, reviewing the available data on published CTs and describing the available cell sources and the challenges involved in applying such treatments in real clinical practice.

2. Search Strategy and Selection Criteria

This review cited CTs performed on cell therapy published in the PubMed, Web of Science, Scopus and ClinicalTrials.gov (accessed on 2 May 2021) electronic databases in the most recent years up to December 2020. Potentially relevant papers were obtained using the following search terms in combination as Medical Subject Headings and text words: human, stem cell, cell therapy, clinical trials, intraocular injection, intravitreal injection, subretinal injection, retina, retinal diseases, optic nerve and optic nerve diseases. Only English papers or those with an English abstract were preselected. The reference lists of the selected publications were also scanned to identify additional relevant papers and the MEDLINE option "Related Articles" was also used.

3. Cell Sources

Embryonic cells within the first couple of cell divisions after fertilization are the only cells that are totipotent and they can form all the cell types in a body, plus the extraembryonic or placental cells. Pluripotent cells can give rise to all of the cell types that make up the body; embryonic stem cells are considered pluripotent. Finally, multipotent cells can develop into more than one cell type but are more limited than pluripotent cells; adult stem cells and cord blood stem cells are considered multipotent. Retinal progenitor stem cells (RPCs) are also multipotent cells that can give rise to all the six neurons of the retina and the Müller glial cells.

The main sources of stem cells for transplantation are summarized in Table 1. They include human fetal retinal stem cells, allogenic cadaveric human cells, adult hippocampal neural stem cells, human CNS stem cells, ciliary pigmented epithelial cells, limbal stem cells, RPCs, human pluripotent stem cells (hPSCs) including both human embryonic stem cells (ESCs) and human induced pluripotent stem cells (iPSCs), and mesenchymal stem cells (MSCs) [17,18]. Finally, cells extracted from the adult human RPE, obtained from eye banks and activated in vitro into a stem cell state (RPESCs), are a potential source of such cells [19]. Of these, RPCs, PSCs and MSCs have demonstrated their ability to assume some of the functions of native tissue and have all been used in an increasing number of CTs, since they all can differentiate into RPE, photoreceptors or ganglion cells [20].

Routes of delivery (suprachoroidal, intravitreal and subretinal) are presented in Figure 1.

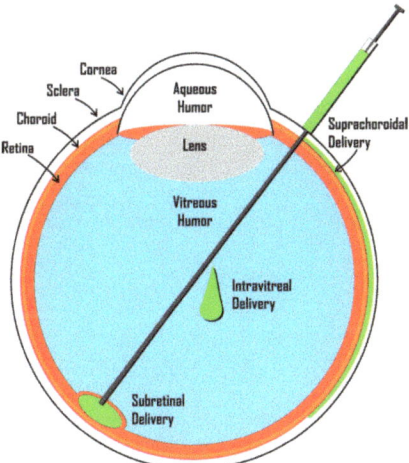

Figure 1. Cell delivery can be either suprachoroidal, intravitreal or subretinal.

Table 1. Stem cell sources and their potential for the treatment of retinal and optic nerve diseases.

Stem Cell Source	Main Advantages and Disadvantages	Cell Type	Potential Applications
Retinal Progenitor Cells			
Fetal stem cells	• Simple accessibility, safety and effectiveness • Shortage of sufficient donor cells • Limited proliferative capacity • Restricted ability to differentiate into specific types of cells • Relatively low risk of immune rejection and tumorigenesis	Retinal progenitor cells (RPCs)	• Paracrine neuroprotection • Exogenous cell replacement
		Cortical progenitor cells (CPCs)	• Paracrine neuroprotection
Pluripotent Stem Cells			
Human embryonic stem cells	• Ability to differentiate into photoreceptors under certain circumstances, but presenting difficulties in obtaining a specific targeted cell type • Shortage of sufficient donor cells • Limited proliferative capacity • Restricted ability to differentiate into specific targeted cells • Potential of tumor formation • Requires immunosuppressive treatment increasing risks and burden • Ethical concerns	Human embryonic stem cell derived retinal pigment epitheliums (hESC-RPE)	• Exogenous cell replacement • Non-cell-based therapy screening
Adult induced pluripotent stem cells	• Able to provide large number of cells for treatments • Low risk of immune reaction (autologous) • Ameliorate the ethical issues of hESCs • Low differentiation efficiency • Relatively high risk of gene mutation	Adult induced pluripotent stem cells (iPSC)	• Exogenous cell replacement • Disease modeling • Non-cell-based therapy screening
Multipotent Stem Cells			
Mesenchymal stem cells	• Able to provide large number of cells for treatments • ADRCs obtained in less invasive procedures and higher immunomodulatory capacity than BMSCs • Anti-inflammatory immunosuppressive antiangiogenic and antiapoptotic or neuroprotective effects • Ability to differentiate into damaged cells • Low rate of cell migration and differentiation • Reported to differentiate into photoreceptors and retinal pigment epithelial (RPE) cells	Bone marrow-derived stem cells (BMSCs)	• Paracrine neuroprotection
		Adipose-derived stem cells (ADRCs)	• Paracrine neuroprotection
	• Higher antiapoptotic effect • Strong rescue effect on retinal function • Potential RPE cell differentiation capacity	Human umbilical multipotent stem cells retrieved from donor umbilical cords (hUTSCs)	• Paracrine neuroprotection
Other sources		Ciliary epithelium-derived stem cells (CESCs)	• Exogenous cell replacement • Endogenous cell replacement?
		Cells extracted from the adult human RPE, obtained from eye banks and activated in vitro into a stem cell state (RPESCs)	• Exogenous cell replacement • Endogenous cell replacement?
		Reprogrammed endogenous Müller glia into RGCs (hMSCs)	• Exogenous cell replacement • Endogenous cell replacement?

RPCs are obtained from the fetal and postnatal retina. Their main advantages are their simple accessibility, safety and effectiveness, the fact that they are widely studied, they avoid ethical issues and have low risk of immune rejection and tumorigenesis. Their main disadvantages are the shortage of sufficient donor cells due to their limited proliferative capacity and their restricted ability to differentiate into specific types of cells [21].

MSCs may originate from amniotic fluid or the umbilical cord, although they are mainly obtained from two developmentally mature organs: bone marrow mesenchymal stem cells (BMMSCs) and adipose mesenchymal stem cells (ADMSCs). The latter are much more abundant and easier to harvest from alive donors, with less invasive procedures. Moreover, they expand faster and demonstrate a higher immunomodulatory capacity than BMMSCs. MSCs have been shown to have anti-inflammatory, immunosuppressive, angiogenic and antiapoptotic or neuroprotective effects [22,23]. Furthermore, they are multipotent; thus, they have some ability to differentiate into damaged cells, although this is somewhat limited. They have a low rate of cell migration and differentiation, though have been reported to differentiate into photoreceptors and RPE cells. Nevertheless, it remains unclear if the newly observed cells may represent the fusion of MSCs with pre-existing photoreceptors [21,24].

Human ESCs come from developing embryos. Their main advantage is their ability to differentiate into photoreceptors under certain circumstances, creating an unlimited source of cells for RD treatment, whereas their main disadvantages are their limited proliferation and multidifferentiation into various cell types, thus presenting difficulties in obtaining the specific targeted cell type; their potential for tumor formation; the requirement of lifelong immunosuppressive therapies that increase risks and economic burdens; finally, since ESCs are isolated from fetal tissues, they raise ethical concerns [25].

The need to provide large numbers of replacement cells has tipped the process toward the use of iPSCs. Various groups have developed protocols to induce and reprogram these cells since their introduction in 2006, and the next challenge will be to establish guidelines to determine their quality [26]. They are obtained from terminally differentiated tissues, which ameliorate the ethical issues of ESCs. They also have a low risk of immune rejection through autologous transplantation, with the disadvantage of a low differentiation efficiency despite their similarity to ESCs, as well as biosafety concerns (e.g., the high risk of gene mutations) [21]. Furthermore, iPSCs have been critical in advancing our understanding of the underlying mechanisms (ontogenesis and pathology) of numerous retinal and optic nerve disorders such as AMD, RP and glaucoma. Cell models have been developed using iPSCs, and these are also important in the study of retinal disease, as well as in developing drug screening and gene therapy approaches. Finally, a new iPSC-based therapy for RD in humans was first reported by a Japanese group in 2017 [26].

On the other hand, stratified neural retina and RPE in a single complex could also be a potential tool in the development of a dual RPE/photoreceptor graft that could be used in individuals with end-stage RD. Recent studies have shown the formation of entire optic cups from ESCs in minimal media conditions [27]. Given the difficulty of the derivation of photoreceptors, especially for producing mature outer segments in 2D cultures [27], approaches using 3D retinal organoid cultures have been attempted. Considerable progress has been shown in the growth of self-organized 3D optic cups from human ESCs, which showed the formation of photoreceptors with reasonable inner segments and connecting cilia [27]. Other methods used for 3D organoid formation have been reported, mechanically picking them up from 2D cultures during differentiation and further optimizing them using a two-step culture system for human iPSCs [28]. Finally, there are also protocols for generating 3D optic vesicle-like structures from human iPSCs showing axon growth [29].

In the case of retinal vasculopathies, direct tissue replacement might be more challenging, as different cells are involved in their pathogenesis, such as the vascular endothelium cells, vascular pericytes, vascular smooth muscle cells, inner retinal neurons, photoreceptors and the retinal glia and microglia cells. Most researchers used MSCs and RPCs, which are considered to have some (although limited) ability to differentiate into the various cells damaged in the context of retinal vascular disease [30,31]. Thus, circulating vascular precursor cells CD34+ and endothelial progenitor cells (EPCs) have been used for tissue regeneration and angiogenesis following ischemia due to the fact that they may play a role in functional collateralization and secrete neurotrophic cytokines and proangiogenic factors [30,32]. CD34+ may differentiate into endothelial cells and because of this they are being explored in CTs as a potential therapy for various ischemic disorders, including ischemic cardiomyopathy, peripheral ischemia, cerebrovascular accidents, DR, ischemic retinal vein occlusion and ischemic optic neuropathy [33–35]. Another potential cell source is a subpopulation of EPCs named outgrowth endothelial cells (OECs), which have significant proliferative potential, but which need to be explored further as a therapy for ischemic retinopathies [36]. In addition, within the stromal vascular fraction of ADSCs there is a distinct population of cells that are thought to represent resident pericytes or their precursors. When these cells were administered intravitreally and intravenously into animal models of oxygen-induced retinopathy (OIR) and DR, the perivascular integration of these cells was observed producing the rescue of damaged retinal capillaries [37]. One more approach would be to use subretinal transplantation of iPSCs (without c-Myc to minimize teratogenicity), because in rat eyes they were able to rescue the ischemic damaged retina through trophic paracrine effects. Moreover, researchers differentiated ESCs or iPSCs into endothelial precursor cells (particularly, endothelial colony unit-forming cells), and these showed some efficacy in treating an animal model of OIR [38]. Nevertheless, in a murine model of ischemia-reperfusion injury, vascular progenitor cells derived from ESCs and iPSCs from cord blood showed engraftment, homing and repair capabilities, whereas those derived from fibroblasts did not [39]. Lastly, extracellular stem cell-derived exosomes (MSC-Exos) may have a positive role in anatomical and functional restoration of the retina in retinal ischemia and DR by modulating angiogenesis and inflammation pathways, through immunomodulation or even through tissue regeneration [40,41].

4. Direct Cell Replacement Therapy for Retinal and Optic Nerve Diseases

4.1. RPE Replacement

Human RPE cells were first isolated and characterized over 30 years ago, and since that time, cell replacement has been tested as a potential treatment for RD. The second attempt at these cells' replacement occurred during the last decade, when RPE derivation from ESCs and iPSCs was established in many laboratories. The RPE cell layer does not require synaptic connections, unlike other cell types in the retina, but its ability to perform its essential functions depends on the RPE being a confluent monolayer with tight junctions and maintaining polarity for ion transport with a healthy Bruch's membrane [42,43]. Nevertheless, subretinal injection of healthy RPE cells allows them to maintain or improve the health of the outer nuclear, outer plexiform and photoreceptor inner/out segment layers [44]. An advantage of this is, as was mentioned before, that the subretinal space is a unique target for cell-based therapy because it is an immune-privileged environment in normal conditions. Therefore, direct cell replacement is being explored as a potential therapy for macular atrophy, using stem cells injected into the submacular space, since RPE dysfunction and death in the macula is the main devastating feature of AMD and Stargardt's disease. This kind of cell therapy has also been launched for RP patients with monogenic mutations affecting RPE65, LRAT and MERTK, genes involved in visual signaling process dysfunction, specifically at the RPE level [45].

Clinical trials on RPE replacement are numerous and a great number of them have succeeded (Table 2). A cell product named CNTO2476, consisting of a suspension of human umbilical multipotent stem cells retrieved from donor umbilical cords (hUTSCs), has also been subretinally injected in patients with geographic atrophy due to AMD in a clinical trial (NCT01226628). The trial has been completed but its results have not been posted. Moreover, there are two open labeled CTs evaluating the safety and efficacy of autologous BMMNCs in the subretinal space of patients with RP (NCT01914913 and NCT02280135). These studies have not yet provided definitive data, but the preclinical results are promising in RPE diseases, in which the morphology of photoreceptors has seemed to improve. Two more CTs using BMMSC intravitreally are ongoing for RP patients (NCT01560715 and NCT01531348). However, another CT has raised concerns about the safety of BMMSCs, as one out of three patients with advanced RP developed severe fibrous tissue proliferation at the injection site, in the vitreous cavity and in the retrolental space, which led to tractional retinal detachment [46]. One more ongoing CT in Saudi Arabia (NCT02016508) is investigating the safety and efficacy of the unilateral intravitreal injection of autologous BMMSC in subjects with geographic atrophy secondary to AMD [47].

Table 2. RPE replacement clinical trials.

Reference	Cell Type	Title	Disease	Administration Procedure	Status
NCT01226628 Phase I/IIa Study	Human umbilical multipotent stem cells retrieved from donor umbilical cords (hUTSCs)	A Safety Study of CNTO 2476 in Patients With Age-Related Macular Degeneration	Geographic atrophy due to age-related macular Degeneration	Subretinal with the iTrack Model 275 micro catheter	Completed
NCT01914913 Phase I/II Study	Autologous bone marrow derived mono nuclear stem cells (BMMNCs)	Clinical Study to Evaluate Safety and Efficacy of BMMNC in Retinitis Pigmentosa	Retinitis pigmentosa	Intravitreal	Unknown
NCT02280135 Phase I Study	Autologous bone marrow stem cells	Clinical Trial of Intravitreal Injection of Autologous Bone Marrow Stem Cells in Patients With Retinitis Pigmentosa	Retinitis pigmentosa	Intravitreal	Completed
NCT01560715 Phase II Study	Autologous bone marrow stem cells	Autologous Bone Marrow-Derived Stem Cells Transplantation For Retinitis Pigmentosa	Retinitis pigmentosa	Intravitreal	Completed
NCT01531348 Phase I Study	Human bone marrow-derived mesenchymal stem cells	Feasibility and Safety of Human Bone Marrow-derived Mesenchymal Stem Cells by Intravitreal Injection in Patients With Retinitis Pigmentosa	Retinitis pigmentosa	Subretinal	Unknown
NCT02016508 Phase I/II Study	Autologous bone marrow derived stem cells	Safety Study of Use of Autologous Bone Marrow Derived Stem Cell in Treatment of Age Related Macular Degeneration	Age-related macular degeneration	Intravitreal	Unknown
NCT03944239 Phase I Study	Retinal pigment epithelial (RPE) cells derived from human embryonic stem cells (hESC)	Safety and Efficacy of Subretinal Transplantation of Clinical Human Embryonic Stem Cell Derived Retinal Pigment Epitheliums in Treatment of Retinitis Pigmentosa	Retinitis pigmentosa	Subretinal	Recruiting
NCT02749734 Phase I/II Study	Human embryonic stem cell derived retinal pigment epitheliums (hESC-RPE)	Clinical Study of Subretinal Transplantation of Human Embryo Stem Cell Derived Retinal Pigment Epitheliums in Treatment of Macular Degeneration Diseases	Macular degeneration and Stargardt's macular dystrophy	Subretinal	Unknown
NCT03046407 Phase I/II Study	Human embryonic stem cell derived retinal pigment epitheliums (hESC-RPE)	Treatment of Dry Age Related Macular Degeneration Disease With Retinal Pigment Epithelium Derived From Human Embryonic Stem Cells	Dry age-related macular degeneration	Subretinal	Unknown
NCT03167203 Phase I/II Study	Human embryonic stem cell derived retinal pigment epitheliums (hESC-RPE)	A Safety Surveillance Study in Subjects With Macular Degenerative Disease Treated With Human Embryonic Stem Cell-derived Retinal Pigment Epithelial Cell Therapy	Macular degenerative disease	Subretinal	Enrolling by invitation
NCT02941991 Follow up Study	Human embryonic stem cell derived retinal pigment epitheliums (hESC-RPE)	A Follow up Study to Determine the Safety and Tolerability of Sub-retinal Transplantation of Human Embryonic Stem Cell Derived Retinal Pigmented Epithelial (hESC-RPE) Cells in Patients With Stargardt's Macular Dystrophy (SMD)	Stargardt's macular dystrophy	Biological: hESC-RPE	Completed

Table 2. Cont.

Reference	Cell Type	Title	Disease	Administration Procedure	Status
NCT02903576 Phase I/II Study	• Procedure: injection of hESC-RPE in suspension • Procedure: injection hESC-RPE seeded in a substrate	Stem Cell Therapy for Outer Retinal Degenerations	• Age-related macular degeneration • Stargardt's disease • Exudative age-related macular degeneration	Subretinal	Completed
NCT01345006 Phase I/II Study	Human embryonic stem cell derived retinal pigment epithelium cells Biological: (MA09-hRPE)	Sub-retinal Transplantation of hESC Derived RPE(MA09-hRPE) Cells in Patients With Stargardt's Macular Dystrophy	Stargardt's macular dystrophy	Subretinal	Completed
NCT01469832 Phase I/II Study	Human embryonic stem cell derived retinal pigment epithelium cells Biological: (MA09-hRPE)	Safety and Tolerability of Sub-retinal Transplantation of Human Embryonic Stem Cell Derived Retinal Pigmented Epithelial (hESC-RPE) Cells in Patients With Stargardt's Macular Dystrophy (SMD)	Stargardt's macular dystrophy	Subretinal	Completed
NCT01344993 Phase I/II Study	Human embryonic stem cell derived retinal pigment epithelium cells Biological: (MA09-hRPE)	Safety and Tolerability of Sub-retinal Transplantation of hESC Derived RPE (MA09-hRPE) Cells in Patients With Advanced Dry Age Related Macular Degeneration	Dry age-related macular degeneration	Subretinal	Completed
NCT01344993 Phase I/II Study	Human embryonic stem cell derived retinal pigment epithelium cells Biological: (MA09-hRPE)	Safety and Tolerability of Sub-retinal Transplantation of hESC Derived RPE (MA09-hRPE) Cells in Patients With Advanced Dry Age Related Macular Degeneration	Dry age-related macular degeneration	Subretinal	Completed
NCT02463344 Phase I/II Study	Human embryonic stem cell derived retinal pigment epithelium cells Biological: (MA09-hRPE)	Long Term Follow Up of Sub-retinal Transplantation of hESC Derived RPE Cells in Patients With AMD	Age-related macular degeneration	Subretinal	Completed
NCT01345006 Phase I/II Study	Human embryonic stem cell derived retinal pigment epithelium cells Biological: (MA09-hRPE)	Sub-retinal Transplantation of hESC Derived RPE(MA09-hRPE)Cells in Patients With Stargardt's Macular Dystrophy	Stargardt's macular dystrophy	Subretinal	Completed
NCT02445612 Long term follow up	Human embryonic stem cell derived retinal pigment epithelium cells Biological: (MA09-hRPE)	Long Term Follow Up of Sub-retinal Transplantation of hESC Derived RPE Cells in Stargardt Macular Dystrophy Patients	Stargardt's macular dystrophy	Subretinal	Completed
NCT01469832 Phase I/II Study	Human embryonic stem cell derived retinal pigment epithelium cells Biological: (MA09-hRPE)	Safety and Tolerability of Sub-retinal Transplantation of Human Embryonic Stem Cell Derived Retinal Pigmented Epithelial (hESC-RPE) Cells in Patients With Stargardt's Macular Dystrophy (SMD)	Stargardt's macular dystrophy	Subretinal	Completed
NCT01625559 Phase I/II Study	Human embryonic stem cell derived retinal pigment epithelium cells Biological: (MA09-hRPE)	Safety and Tolerability of MA09-hRPE Cells in Patients With Stargardt's Macular Dystrophy(SMD)	Stargardt's macular dystrophy	Subretinal	Unknown
NCT01674829 Phase I/II Study	Human embryonic stem cell derived retinal pigment epithelium cells Biological: (MA09-hRPE)	A Phase I/IIa, Open-Label, Single-Center, Prospective Study to Determine the Safety and Tolerability of Sub-retinal Transplantation of Human Embryonic Stem Cell Derived Retinal Pigmented Epithelial(MA09-hRPE) Cells in Patients With Advanced Dry Age-related Macular Degeneration(AMD)	Dry age-related macular degeneration	Subretinal	Active, not recruiting

Table 2. Cont.

Reference	Cell Type	Title	Disease	Administration Procedure	Status
NCT02286089 Phase I/II Study	Retinal pigment epithelial (RPE) cells derived from human embryonic stem cells (hESC) Biological: OpRegen: cell suspension either in ophthalmic Balanced Salt Solution Plus (BSS Plus) or in CryoStor® 5 (Thaw-and-Inject, TAI)	Safety and Efficacy Study of OpRegen for Treatment of Advanced Dry-Form Age-Related Macular Degeneration	Age-related macular degeneration	Subretinal	Active, not recruiting
NCT03963154 Phase I/II Study	Human embryonic stem cell derived retinal pigment epithelium (RPE) Investigational Medicinal Product: ISTEM-01	Interventional Study of Implantation of hESC-derived RPE in Patients With RP Due to Monogenic Mutation	Retinitis pigmentosa	Subretinal	Recruiting
NCT02590692 Phase I/II Study	Human embryonic stem cell-derived RPE cells Biological: CPCB-RPE1	Study of Subretinal Implantation of Human Embryonic Stem Cell-Derived RPE Cells in Advanced Dry AMD	• Dry macular degeneration • Geographic atrophy	Subretinal	Active, not recruiting
NCT03102138 Safety follow up Study	Human embryonic stem cell-derived RPE cells Biological: PF-05206388	Retinal Pigment Epithelium Safety Study For Patients In B4711001	Age-related macular degeneration	Intravitreal	Active, not recruiting
NCT01691261 Phase I Study	Human embryonic stem cell derived retinal pigment epithelium (RPE) living tissue equivalent Biological: PF-05206388: monolayer of RPE cells immobilized on a polyester membrane	A Study Of Implantation Of Retinal Pigment Epithelium In Subjects With Acute Wet Age Related Macular Degeneration	Age-related macular degeneration	Intraocular	Active, not recruiting
NCT02464956 Feasibility of production of these cells	Induced pluripotent stem cell (iPSC)-derived RPE cells from a patient's own skin or blood	Production of iPSC Derived RPE Cells for Transplantation in AMD	Age-related macular degeneration	None	Unknown

Concerning hESCs, two cell products are being tested in CTs for macular diseases, one from Pfizer (NCT01691261) and the other from the Astellas Institute for Regenerative Medicine (formerly Ocata/Advanced Cell Technology). The latter is currently completing a phase I/IIa CT designed to test the tolerability of transplanted RPE cells derived from hESCs for the treatment of patients with Stargardt's disease (NCT01345006) and advanced dry AMD (NCT01344993) without a control group and using systemic immunosuppression. Indications of effectiveness have been shown, as 10 out of 18 patients improved their vision. There was no evidence of proliferation, rejection or serious systemic adverse events, but one patient had staphylococcus endophthalmitis, and cataract progression. Localized RPE damage and intraocular inflammation were reported [48,49]. In addition, transplantation of hESM-derived RPE cells in the subretinal space with systemic immunosuppressive therapy for 13 weeks has been tested in 12 patients with Stargardt's disease (NCT01469832) using the same biological. In that trial, focal areas of subretinal hyperpigmentation were observed in all participants in a dose-dependent manner and no evidence of uncontrolled proliferation or inflammatory responses were found. Borderline improvements in best-corrected visual acuity (BCVA) in four participants either were unstained or showed a similar improvement in the untreated contralateral eye. Quality of life questionnaires and microperimetry demonstrated no evidence of a benefit at 12 months, and in one case, localized retinal thinning and reduced sensitivity in the area of hyperpigmentation suggested potential harm [50]. Lineage cell therapeutics has developed a similar study in patients with the advanced atrophic-form of AMD (still recruiting) that has the objective of evaluating the safety and tolerability of a cell product named OpRegen® (hESC-RPE cells) transplanted subretinally via the suprachoroidal approach through a microinjection using the Orbit Subretinal Delivery System (Orbit SDS) developed by Gyroscope Therapeutics (formerly Orbit Biomedical, Ltd.), which avoids the need to create a retinal hole and aims to provide precise and consistent dosing. The study will also assess the ability of transplanted OpRegen® cells to engraft, survive and moderate disease progression (NCT02286089) and results will be presented later this year. Furthermore, there are several recruiting phase I/II clinical trials using hEMS in AMD and/or Stargardt's disease in China (NCT02749734, NCT03046407 and NCT02755428), the United States (NCT01344993, NCT02463344, NCT03167203, NCT01345006 and NCT02445612), France (NCT02941991 and NCT01469832) and Korea (NCT01625559 and NCT01674829) aiming to verify the overall safety and feasibility of hESC-RPE cell-based therapies, providing some promising early visual results, in which any major complications could be primarily attributed to the use of immunosuppressants during allogenic transplantation [45,51,52]. In addition, for RP a trial using hESC-derived-RPE cells is recruiting 10 patients to test the safety and efficacy of its subretinal transplantation technique (NCT03944239). Finally, a phase I/II, open-label, prospective CT tried to determine the safety and tolerability of the subretinal transplantation of hESC-derived RPE cells (MA09-hRPE) in patients with patchy atrophy secondary to myopic macular degeneration (NCT02122159), but the study was withdrawn in 2016 and no results have been posted.

RPE cells obtained from human autologous somatic cells (hiPSCs) were used in a phase I CT in 2013 in Japan (UMIM000011929) in which the first patient improved without adverse effects, but the study was put on hold because oncogenic genetic mutations were found in the second patient, probably due to the documented genomic instability of iPSCs. The CT since resumed, using HLA-matched allogenic iPSCS-derived RPE cells in suspension compared with autologous iPSCs, the first being safer and more likely to succeed economically. The transplanted sheet remained intact and BCVA was stable one year after surgery, although cystoid macular edema was present [53]. More recently, another two ongoing CTs have commenced in England and the USA (NCT02464956) to test the efficiency of creating iPSC-derived RPE cells from the patient's own skin or blood. This trial started in 2015 in 10 patients with AMD and is not yet recruiting [54]. At the same time, many scientists are studying the safety concerns surrounding the iPSCs obtained through the reprogramming process.

Recently, a combination of gene and cell therapy has been implemented using the CRISPR/Cas9 system applied to the production of iPSCs with selective HLA gene disruption [55]. One example is a recent CT for a specific type of RP with mutations in disease-causing genes that affect RPE function (NCT03963154), aiming to restore RPE function and protect photoreceptors from degeneration at a relatively early stage.

However, the delivery strategy of a cell suspension might not be sufficient, and more complex reconstructed tissue formulations are probably required, both to improve functionality and to target pathological conditions with altered Bruch's membrane-like AMD. For clinical applications, Kamao et al. developed a protocol for an RPE monolayer sheet obtained from hiPSC-RPE cells without using any synthetic scaffold, but rather self-producing their basement membrane consisting of collagen IV and laminin. This was shown to be functional in vivo when used in neovascular AMD after the removal of the choroidal neovascularization, with no sign of rejection and no patients needing additional anti-VEGF injections. The major problem was the cost and extensive preparation time needed for each individual patient (more than 10 months) [56,57]. Likewise, more complex reconstructed tissue formulations have been proposed in order to improve functionality and replace the damaged Bruch's membrane in AMD using 3D bioengineered tissues amenable for regenerative medicine, developing RPE sheets or substrates to make the technical transfer more tolerable to the cells during surgery and to increase survival compared to cells in suspension, as well as increasing the chance of the cells forming an organized orientation tissue reminiscent of the endogenous cellular structure [58]. An example of this new strategy is a recruiting phase I/II CT (NCT02903576) that is trying to determine whether the surgical implantation of an hESC-derived RPE cell monolayer seeded onto a polymeric substrate versus hESC-derived RPE cell injections alone into the subretinal space are safe procedures. This has been planned in patients with dry AMD, disciform scarring due to wet AMD and Stargardt's disease. Thus, Kashani et al. have designed an implant using a scaffold, termed the California Project to Cure Blindness–Retinal Pigment Epithelium 1 (CPCB-RPE1), which consists of a polarized monolayer of hESC-derived RPE cells on an ultrathin synthetic parylene (plastic) substrate designed to mimic Bruch's membrane. This group has published data on a cohort of 16 patients with advanced dry AMD (NCT02590692), which demonstrate the technique's safety and suggest that it may improve visual function, since none of the implanted eyes showed the progression of vision loss, one eye improved by 17 letters and two eyes demonstrated improved fixation [59]. The group led by da Cruz et al. is investigating a similar RPE patch in severe exudative AMD as a part of The London Project to Cure Blindness (NCT03102138). Finally, a phase I CT used an engineered RPE patch comprising a fully differentiated hESC-derived RPE monolayer on a coated, synthetic basement membrane, delivered using a purpose-designed microsurgical tool into the subretinal space of one eye in two patients with severe exudative AMD. Only local immunosuppression was used long-term. The authors reported the successful delivery and survival of the RPE patch by means of biomicroscopy and optical coherence tomography (OCT), and a BCVA gain of 29 and 21 letters in the two patients, respectively, over 12 months. They also presented the preclinical surgical, cell safety and tumorigenicity studies, leading to the trial's approval [60].

4.2. Photoreceptor Replacement

To treat IRD, and mainly RP, it is necessary to replace dysfunctional or dead rods and cones, creating a therapeutic "slot" for cell therapies between gene therapy (for early stages of the disease) and retinal microchips (for advanced stages of the disease). One of the difficulties in treating advanced stages is that most of these conditions affect the entire retina. Replacing photoreceptors has been tried when these are the major cell type involved in retinal degeneration. In this case, the introduced precursors would have to form a polarized outer nuclear layer with the formation of light-sensitive outer segments, and then would have to reconnect synaptically with downstream retinal neurons in order to send information down the visual pathway.

To do this, various forms of transplant have been applied, including a full-thickness retina; photoreceptor sheets (sliced using a laser or vibratome); dissociated cells, including photoreceptors or the retinal progenitor cells (RPCs) that are able to produce them; hPSC-derived cells [61]. Patients may also benefit from a combined RPE and photoreceptor transplant, but whether this would be a stepwise approach with RPE replacement followed by photoreceptor transplantation or whether the two could be transplanted together needs to be explored, as Zhu et al. showed that the survival of photoreceptor progenitor cells was increased when they were cocultured with hESC-derived RPE [62].

The first publications on this issue indicated the potential benefit of transplanting fetal retinal cells or tissue in patients with retinal degeneration and its safety, but these grafts were limited due to ethical concerns and reduced availability [63]. Furthermore, the surgical techniques used to perform the subretinal transplantation of full-thickness retina or photoreceptor sheets are difficult to perform, and cell integration and synaptic reconnection are also challenging [64]. However, with the advent of well-established protocols to differentiate substantial quantities of retinal cells from hESCs and iPSCs, regenerative retinal therapies have become a practical goal in clinical practice [65].

RPCs have been demonstrated to become mature and express photoreceptor markers when injected into the subretinal space, and they are also able to integrate into the host inner retina and rescue degenerated photoreceptors [66]. RPCs and hESC-derived photoreceptor precursor cells have been shown to integrate into the host retina and improve light sensitivity, although the effect was reversed in months [66,67]. Another source could be hiPSC-derived photoreceptor precursors—results have demonstrated that adult fibroblast-derived iPSCs can differentiate into retinal precursors to be used for the transplantation and treatment of retinal degeneration diseases [68–70]. The main question is whether transplanted photoreceptors actually integrate. They may instead fuse with existing photoreceptors, since in recent years a phenomenon known as "material transfer" has been proposed, whereby biomaterial such as proteins and/or mRNA is transferred from donor to host photoreceptors, thereby restoring some visual function by rescuing remaining photoreceptor cells [71,72]. An important point is that more progress in preclinical studies is needed in order to better understand and optimize cell integration in order to plan future CTs.

CTs on photoreceptor replacement are summarized in Table 3. One of them is implementing the use of subretinally transplanted hRPCs derived from the fetal retina. This is a phase I/IIa, open-label, prospective study aiming to test their safety and tolerability in patients with advanced RP and has been sponsored by ReNeuron (NCT02464436).

Table 3. Photoreceptor replacement clinical trials.

Reference	Cell Type	Title	Disease	Administration Procedure	Status
NCT02464436 Phase I/IIa Study	Human retinal progenitor cells (hRPC)	Safety and Tolerability of hRPC in Retinitis Pigmentosa	Retinitis pigmentosa	Subretinal	Recruiting
NCT01068561 Phase I Study	Autologous bone marrow-derived stem cells	Autologous Bone Marrow-Derived Stem Cells Transplantation For Retinitis Pigmentosa	Retinitis pigmentosa	Intravitreal	Completed
NCT01560715 Phase II Study	Autologous bone marrow stem cells	Autologous Bone Marrow-Derived Stem Cells Transplantation For Retinitis Pigmentosa	Retinitis pigmentosa	Intravitreal	Completed
NCT01518127 Phase I/II Study	Autologous bone marrow stem cells	Intravitreal Bone Marrow-Derived Stem Cells in Patients With Macular Degeneration	Age-related macular degeneration and Stargartd	Intravitreal	Completed
NCT03437759 Phase I Study	Biological: exosomes derived from mesenchymal stem cells (MSC-Exo)	MSC-Exos Promote Healing of MHs	Macular holes	Intravitreal during a vitrectomy and the aid of endotamponades	Active, not recruiting
NCT03853252 Not applicable (proof of concept)	Autologous skin biopsy to get cells from choroideremia patients	iPS Cells of Patients for Models of Retinal Dystrophies	Retinal dystrophies: choroideremia	Other: create cell models of disease	Recruiting

Mesenchymal stem cells have a reduced ability of cell differentiation when compared to embryonic stem cells although they may differ in some cells such as retinal pigmented epithelium cells and retinal glial cells. However, these cells secrete large amounts of trophic factors that could theoretically increase the longevity of retinal cells in distress and also to produce a recovery of function. With this goal, Siqueira et al. at the University of Sao Paulo have primarily investigated the use of autologous BMMSCs intravitreally injected to treat patients with advanced degenerative retinopathies (one RP patient and two affected by cone-rod dystrophy) in a phase I CT (NCT01068561), without detecting serious adverse events. In a phase II study, they started to confirm the efficacy of this technique (NCT1560715) in 20 RP patients, showing a transitory improvement of vision that lasted no longer than one year [73,74]. The same group has investigated the safety and effectiveness of their cell product in AMD and Stargardt's patients (NCT01518127). Nevertheless, this is not real photoreceptor replacement but rescue.

Another approach is to use iPSCs, but in the particular case of IRD, patient-derived iPSCs carry pathogenic gene mutations that may affect the survival and function of autologous transplanted cells. Thus, the cell replacement strategy can utilize patient-specific photoreceptor precursor cells that have been genetically corrected through conventional gene therapy using viral vectors or via gene editing, using both the clustered regularly interspaced short palindromic repeats-associated protein 9 (CRISPR/Cas9) system or the transcription activator-like effector nucleases (TALEN) system [75,76]. However, the phenotypic correction of iPSCs is not efficient enough (because of transgene silencing), so it may be more advantageous to correct somatic cells "ex vivo" before reprogramming. The advantage of this approach is that it could be used to treat IRD, regardless of the clinical stage or prevalence of the disease, and of the size of the causative gene [77]. Further work is required to ensure safety regarding off-target mutations due to gene editing and mutagenesis that may occur during the derivation and differentiation of iPSCs, although despite these challenges, gene editing technology has made rapid advances and is a valuable tool in understanding and treating RD [78]. CRISPR/Cas9 can be also used to turn genes on, instead of snipping them via epigenetics, by modulating histone marks, rather than editing DNA sequences, thus obtaining improvements or the amelioration of symptoms. Nevertheless, some challenges remain before this can be implemented in the clinic [79]. Additionally, a drug-tunable gene therapy, which led to the expression of a neurotrophic factor-destabilization domain fusion protein, preserved cone vision in preclinical studies, suggesting its potential use against broad-spectrum RD and its possible use as an adjunct therapy along with stem-cell therapy [80]. In this respect, Cereso et al. used AAV2/5 as a carrying vector to effectively transduce iPSC-derived RPE cells from a choroideremia patient, thus illustrating the potential of patient iPSC-derived RPE cells to provide a proof-of-concept model for gene replacement when there is no appropriate animal model [81]. Furthermore, Burnight et al. transduced patient-specific, iPSC-derived, photoreceptor precursor cells with lentiviral vectors carrying full-length CEP290 in order to correct a causing mutation of Leber's congenital amaurosis, which affects the cilia formation of the photoreceptors. Their results showed the expression of full-length transcripts and functional rescue of the ciliogenesis defect in patient cells [82]. Bassuk et al. used the CRISPR/Cas9 system to precisely repair an RPGR point mutation that causes X-linked RP (XLRP) [83]. Lastly, another CT using iPSCs to develop cell models of different retinal dystrophies is also recruiting (NCT03853252) to evaluate the efficiency of gene therapy approaches.

An additional approach to cell-based therapy is to introduce optical sensors into grafted photoreceptor cells to make them function stably and independently of the RPE [84].

Finally, mesenchymal stem cell-derived exosomes are also being tested in a clinical trial (NCT03437759) because they seem to the promote healing of large and refractory macular holes.

4.3. Ganglion Cell Replacement and Cell Therapy for Optic Nerve Diseases (ONDs)

Among the studies registered in ClinicalTrials.gov (accessed on 2 May 2021), only 18 are related to OND, and six have not shown results for a long time, so it is presumable that they have failed or have been interrupted (Table 4). The rest are phase I or II CTs related to a few diseases (Table 5).

Table 4. Optic nerve regeneration: failed cell therapy clinical trials for optic nerve disorders.

Reference	Disease	Cell Type	Administration Route	Study Start Date	Status
NCT01364246 Phase I/II Study	Multiple sclerosis and neuromyelitis optica	Human umbilical multipotent stem cells retrieved from donor umbilical cords (hUTSCs)	Transplantation	January 2010	Unknown
NCT01834079 Phase I/II Study	Optic nerve atrophy	Autologous bone marrow derived stem cells	Intrathecal injection	September 2014	Unknown
NCT02249676 Phase II Study	Progressive and refractory neuromyelitis optica spectrum disorders	Autologous mesenchymal stem cells	Intravenous infusion of MSC a day-case 2.0 $\times 10^6$ cells/kg	January 2013	Unknown
NCT03605238 Phase I Study	Relapsed and/or refractory AQP4-IgG seropositive neuromyelitis optica spectrum disorders	CD19/CD20 tanCAR T Cells	Intravenous infusion	August 2018	Withdrawn

Table 4. Cont.

Reference	Disease	Cell Type	Administration Route	Study Start Date	Status
NCT02976441 Phase I Study	High grade gliomas	Autologous stem cell collection	Stem cell intravenous infusion prior chemoradiation and reinfused back after treatment	January 2017	Withdrawn
NCT02144103 Phase I/II Study	Retinal degeneration and primary open-angle glaucoma	Autologous adipose-derived regenerative cells (ADRC)	Subtenon	May 2014	Unknown
NTC 01339455 Phase I/II Study	Neuromyelitis optica	Autologous hematopoietic stem cells	Intravenous infusion	April 2011	Terminated (recruitment failure)

Table 5. Optic nerve regeneration: cell therapy clinical trials for optic nerve disorders.

Reference	Disease	Cell Type	Administration Route	Sponsor	Study Start Date	Status
NTC 02638714 Phase I/II Study	Optic nerve atrophy	Autologous bone marrow CD 34+, 133+, and 271+ stem cells	No site declared	Stem Cells Arabia	April 2013	Recruiting
NTC 03173638 Phase II Study	Acute ischemic optic neuropathy nonarteritic	Allogenic mesenchymal stem (MSV) cells from bone marrow	Intravitreal injection	IOBA, Spain	March 2018	Recruiting
NCT 022836771 Phase I Study	Neuromyelitis optica	Tolerogenic dendritic cells loaded with myelin peptides	Intravenous administration	Hospital Clinic of Barcelona, Spain	September 2015	Completed
NTC 01920867 Phase (n/a)	Various ocular diseases including optic neuritis	Bone marrow derived stem cells (BMSC). Study I	Injections of BMSC retrobulbar, subtenon and intravenous	MD Stem Cells, USA	August 2012	Enrolling by invitation
NTC 03011541 Phase (n/a)	Various ocular diseases including optic neuropathy Nonarteritic ischemic optic neuropathy Optic atrophy, optic nerve disease, glaucoma, Leber hereditary optic neuropathy	Bone marrow derived stem cells (BMSC). Study II	Injections of BMSC retrobulbar, subtenon and intravenous	MD Stem Cells, USA	January 2016	Recruiting
NTC 00787722 Phase I/II Study	Devic neuromyelitis	High dose immunosuppressive therapy with hematopoietic stem cells transplantation	Intravenous infusion	Northwestern University, USA	October 2009	Completed
NTC 00716066 Phase II Study	Neurologic autoimmune diseases, including neuromyelitis optica	High dose immunosuppressive therapy with autologous hematopoietic stem cell transplantation	Intravenous infusion	Fred Hutchinson Cancer Research Center National Cancer Institute, USA	June 2008	Recruiting
NTC 04577300 Phase II Study	Glaucoma	Dual NT-501 CNTF encapsulated cell therapy	Intravitreal NT-501 implants	Stanford University, USA	October 2020	Not yet recruiting
NTC 02862938 Phase II Study	Glaucoma	NT-501 CNTF encapsulated cell therapy	Intravitreal NT-501 implants	Stanford University, USA	August 2016	Active, not recruiting
NTC 02330978 Phase I Study	Glaucoma	Autologous bone marrow-derived mesenchymal stem cell	Intravitreal	University of Sao Paulo, Brazil	July 2019	Completed

(n/a): not applicable; (CNTF): soluble ciliary neurotrophic factor.

Three of them are focused on optic nerve atrophy, which is the end result of many pathologies with different pathogeneses. Four included patients with optic neuromyelitis (Devic's disease), an autoimmune disorder predominantly characterized by severe optic neuritis and transverse myelitis. For many years this disease was considered a variant of multiple sclerosis, but the discovery that most patients have autoantibodies against aquaporin-4 (AQP4) or NMO-IgG changed the understanding of the disease [85].

In one of the CTs, dominant optic atrophies and Leber's hereditary optic neuropathy (LHON) are included, although many other ocular pathologies are also included. This trial will be discussed below.

Three of the CTs are focused on glaucoma. This disease has traditionally been viewed as a primary OND, in which the optic nerve is damaged as a result of high intraocular pressure (IOP). Glaucomatous optic neuropathy is characterized by significant death of RGCs. According to global surveys, the second leading cause of blindness after cataracts is glaucoma. However, there is a substantial group of people (up to 20%) with typical glaucomatous disc changes, progressive visual field defects and open anterior chamber angles associated with intraocular pressure (IOP) constantly below 21 mmHg, a condition known as normal tension glaucoma [86]. Currently the main goal of glaucoma treatment is IOP reduction. The Early Manifest Glaucoma Trial showed that glaucoma progression was decreased by 10% with the reduction of each mmHg of IOP but according to the Collaborative Normal Tension Glaucoma Study Group, an IOP reduction of 30% is required to slow the progression of normal tension glaucoma—a goal that is difficult to achieve with the currently available glaucoma treatments [86]. Therefore, treatment should be ideally targeted at neuroprotection to improve the RGCs or optic nerve head function by means of drugs such as calcium channel blockers or by means of cell therapy. In this case, cell transplantation is still at an early stage of preclinical study, compared with RPE or photoreceptor transplantation. Finally, a CT sponsored by our group (NCT03173638) is focused on the acute phases of acute nonarteritic anterior ischemic optic neuropathy [6].

Regarding the types of cells, six CTs use BMMSCs. Three of these—all of them directed at optic neuromyelitis—use a combination of a high dose of immunosuppressive therapy, followed by autologous hematopoietic cell transplantation.

Two CTs use encapsulated cell technology. They use ARPE19, a retinal pigmented human cell line, genetically modified to produce ciliary neurotrophic factor (CNTF). Cells are encapsulated in a semipermeable polymer capsule which is introduced into the vitreous cavity. The idea seems very attractive and in theory it would open up many possibilities. It was primarily designed for treating retinal degenerative diseases [87], but initial results in diseases such as RP did not show any clinically relevant benefit, and since 2013 there have been no novel results in retinal pathologies [88] associated with the use of this technology. The company now seems to be concentrating on glaucoma, although no results have yet been reported.

However, regarding CNTF, there is a question that must be investigated in depth and that is the action of this factor on the glia cells. At least the acute administration of CNTF appears to be related to glial reactivity, which would not be desirable in the context of diseases either of the retina or of the optic nerve [89].

Returning to the CT sponsored by our Eye Institute (NCT03173638), our hypothesis is that ischemic neuropathy can resemble an ischemic stroke, and it should be possible for there to be a series of ganglion cell axons in the so-called penumbra zone. Thus, some of the growth factors released by BMDMSC could "rescue" these fibers, minimizing the damage. Without the presence of growth factors released by mesenchymal stem cells, many of those axons in the "penumbra zone" will die and the functional damage will be greater. A differential fact, in comparison with other CTs, that may be of great relevance is that our cells are from allogeneic sources.

The so-called Stem Cell Ophthalmology Treatment Study (SCOTS) and SCOTS-2 (NCT01920867 and NCT03011541) are especially deserving of interest. They are considered the largest stem cell studies for ocular diseases [90]. The research subjects include dominant optic atrophy and LHON. As in our CT, the stem cell approach is based on the use of BMDMSCs, but in this case the cells are of autologous origin. This is a multicentric study (involving the USA and the United Arab Emirates), and the principal investigators are using mesenchymal stem cells to take advantage of their neuroprotective effects, which have been reported in a variety of animal models of optic nerve damage [91]. Although they are able to differentiate into neurons and glial cells [92], the use of these cells in these CTs is based on their ability to release neurotrophic agents. These neuroprotective properties have been experimentally proven in retinal layers by our group [93,94]. In the SCOTS-2 CT, five patients with LHON reported improvements in visual acuity and peripheral vision. In 2019, in the first SCOTS report, six patients with dominant optic atrophy were included. Five of them experienced visual improvement. The authors speculated that mitochondrial transfer exosome and neuroprotective exosome secretion from mesenchymal stem cells could contribute to this improvement [95]. Nevertheless, these results must be taken with caution, as there was great variability in the treated conditions, including degenerative, ischemic and physical damage of the retina and/or optic nerve. Moreover, the eyes were treated through the injection of BMMSCs, using many different routes of administration—retrobulbar; sub-Tenon and intravenous together, or a combination of retrobulbar, sub-Tenon, intravitreal and intravenous, making the interpretation of their results difficult and creating certain doubts about the quality of the methodology used in the study's design. Thus, the scientific basis of cell therapy in hereditary optic neuropathies is still under investigation and validation [90].

Regarding the topic of administration routes, those studies that have focused on hematopoietic cell transplantation have obviously used intravenous application, whereas the rest, with two exceptions, have used the intravitreal route. These exceptions are the already mentioned CTs NCT01920867 and NCT03011541, sponsored by the same company, MD Stem Cells (Coral Springs, Florida, USA). This is an interventional, nonmasked, parallel, nonrandomized clinical study, including several retinal conditions and optic nerve diseases (such as glaucoma, optic nerve compression, ischemic optic neuropathy and optic atrophy). The routes for the administration of cells include retrobulbar, subtenon, intravitreal and intravenous routes (alone or as supplements after other routes). The study started in 2016, and the expected date for completion is 2023.

A final reflection can be made on the possibility of using a multimodal therapy for diseases both of the retina and the optic nerve, which are complex and in which perhaps a single therapeutic approach would not work. In a recent paper [96], researchers from Brazil and Florida proposed an interesting combination of gene and cell therapy to increase RGC survival and their axon regrowth. This was an experimental study on a model of optic nerve crush, analyzing the neuroprotective and neuroregenerative potential of pigment epithelium-derived factor (PEDF) gene therapy alone and combined with human mesenchymal stem cell (hMSC) therapy. The authors found a synergistic effect in the combination of gene and cell therapy.

A final point concerns the safety of intravitreal stem cell injections. In a recent paper [97], researchers investigated the vascular outcomes after intravitreal mesenchymal stem cell (MSC) administration in rats, with or without damage to the neurovascular unit (transgenic rats). The authors used rat BMDMSCs and human ADMSCs and found that the intravitreal administration of MSCs induced cataract, retinal vaso-regression, activation of retinal glial cells and an inflammatory response even in normal rat eyes. Our group analyzed the safety of human bone marrow-derived MSCs [98] and these cells were safe and well-tolerated when administered intravitreally at a dose of 15×10^6 cells/mL in pigmented rabbits.

In view of the information analyzed in this review and comparing it with that obtained in our 2016 review [6], it does not appear that there has been much real progress in this field, and it seems that, in the very short term, none of the approaches that are being made in CTs seem to have been transferred to established clinical human treatments.

Ideal cell therapy involves several requisites, such as a source of viable cells, the management of cells under good manufacturing practices (GMPs), reliable delivery methods, long-term survival and functioning of grafted cells without severe adverse effects on the host, and of course a clear objective benefit in terms of the improvement or stabilization of the disease [16].

The main obstacles in this process are derived from the lack of adequacy of the host environment, and the time of use of the cells, which requires the production source close to be close to the clinical place of use. In addition, the short time of release of growth factors by the implanted cells forces us to look for alternatives such as genetically modified cells, which then pose other serious safety problems.

The rescue of RGCs in glaucomatous patients by means of the neuroprotective properties of pluripotent stem cells is a plausible and experimentally proven option. However, the difficulties mentioned above probably influence its very slow development from preclinical research to routine clinical use.

4.4. Cell Therapy for Retinal Vascular Diseases

In 2014, Park et al. injected for the first time autologous CD34+ BMMSCs into the vitreous cavities of six patients with retinal vascular occlusion or RD, finding a good safety profile that merits further exploration (NCT01736059) [99]. To date, autologous BMMSCs have been applied by means of intravenous infusion in 34 patients with DR (No. ChiCTR-ONC-16008055; chictr.org. cn). BCVA and central macular thickness, measured with OCT, improved without severe adverse events, mainly in the nonproliferative stage of the disease [100]. Another CT has proposed one intravitreal injection of bone marrow mononuclear stem cells in 30 patients with ischemic retinopathy, including DR with severe loss of retinal capillaries (NCT01518842). This trial is active but not recruiting. Furthermore, a phase I/II, prospective, randomized, sham-controlled, double-masked CT (NCT03981549) is ongoing, aiming to determine whether intravitreal autologous CD34+ stem cell therapy is safe, feasible and potentially beneficial in minimizing or reversing vision loss in eyes with ischemia due to central retinal vein occlusion. Lastly, the combination of CD34+CD45+ cells derived from iPSCs with iPSCs derived from the mesoderm (vascular wall-derived progenitor cells or endothelial colony forming cells—ECFCs) administered into the vitreous cavity is being evaluated in a clinical trial, assessing their potential beneficial effect in preventing microvascular complications in DR (NCT03403699) due to their antioxidative and anti-inflammatory effects.

Finally, a CT intending to evaluate the function of serum exosomal miRNA in the pathogenesis of DR is ongoing (NCT03264976) but not yet recruiting patients [101]. In fact, researchers will try to validate a diagnostic test sequencing these miRNAs and see if they can serve as a prognostic factor. However, according to the available information, it seems that stem cell-derived exosomes may play an important role in RD treatment in the future too. CTs on cell replacement for retinal vascular diseases are presented in Table 6.

Table 6. Cell replacement clinical trials for retinal vascular diseases.

Reference	Cell Type	Title	Disease	Administration Procedure	Status
NCT01518842 Not applicable	Bone marrow stem cells	Effect of Intravitreal Bone Marrow Stem Cells on Ischemic Retinopathy (RetinaCell)	Ischemic retinopathy, including diabetic retinopathy with severe loss of retinal capillaries	Intravitreal	Unknown
NCT01736059 Phase I Study	CD34+ autologous adult bone marrow stem cells intravitreal	Clinical Trial of Autologous Intravitreal Bone-marrow CD34+ Stem Cells for Retinopathy	Non-exudative age-related macular degeneration Diabetic retinopathy Retina vein occlusion Retinitis pigmentosa hereditary macular degeneration	Intravitreal	Enrolling by invitation
NCT03981549 Phase I/II Study	CD34+ autologous bone marrow stem cells versus sham therapy	Treatment of Central Retinal Vein Occlusion Using Stem Cells Study (TRUST)	Central retinal vein occlusion	Intravitreal	Recruiting

Table 6. Cont.

Reference	Cell Type	Title	Disease	Administration Procedure	Status
NCT03403699 Not applicable	Combination of CD34+CD45+ cells derived from human inducible pluripotent stem cells (iPSCs) with iPSCs derived from the mesoderm: vascular wall-derived progenitor cells or endothelial colony forming cells (ECFCs) subset (SSEA5-KNA+)	Human iPSC for Repair of Vasodegenerative Vessels in Diabetic Retinopathy	Diabetes complications Diabetic retinopathy	Others: to test if the hiPSC-derived-mesoderm subset (SSEA5-KNA+) can revascularize vasodegenerative capillaries and if their reparative action can be enhanced by coinjection of CD34+CD45+ cells intravitreally.	Recruiting
NCT03264976 Not applicable	None	Role of the Serum Exosomal miRNA in Diabetic Retinopathy (DR)	Diabetic retinopathy	Validation of a diagnostic test based on exosomal miRNAs in serum samples that will be sequenced	Not yet recruiting

5. Challenges

Several issues remain to be solved concerning the clinical translation of cell-based therapies, including (1) the ability to enrich for specific retinal subtypes; (2) cell survival; (3) cell delivery, which may need to incorporate a scaffold to induce correct cell polarization, which increases the size of the retinotomy in surgery and, therefore, the chance of severe complications compared to the delivery of isolated cells; (4) the need to induce retinal detachment to perform the subretinal placement of the transplanted cell, which could disrupt the first synapse of the visual pathway and is thought to affect larger areas outside the iatrogenic detachment; (5) the evaluation of the risk of tumor formation caused by undifferentiated stem cells and prolific progenitor cells, which increases when using genome-integrating viruses or gene editing to produce iPSCs because this can cause insertional mutagenesis and unpredictable genetic dysfunction and some transcription factors may have oncogenic properties [5].

The development of surgical techniques for delivering the cells to the right place is one of these challenges. Intravitreal injections have been used, as they are a common procedure in retina patient clinics and are associated with few complications. However, with this route of administration, the concern is that the host retina, mainly the inner limiting membrane, may act as a barrier and prevent the transplanted cells from migrating and integrating into the retinal tissue in the correct location [102]. Therefore, subretinal transplantation is the more commonly used technique when trying to obtain cell replacement, as the cells are delivered to the intended location and therefore better integration and differentiation is observed. However, this is a complex surgical procedure, requiring a skilled retinal surgeon with experience in subretinal surgery, as it has a high risk of surgical complications, including hemorrhage, PVR, graft dislocation and neovascularization [103,104]. If more than one type of cell is needed to restore the natural retinal cell layers, the question will then be whether the layers should be transplanted sequentially or if a retinal complex including the necessary layers would be optimal for the restoration of visual function. When using a cell sheet or an RPE-photoreceptor-scaffold complex, a subretinal approach would be especially necessary, since transplants of this size could not traverse the inner retina, and a purpose-designed microsurgical tool has been proposed to perform these transplants via the suprachoroidal approach, as we have already mentioned [60].

Furthermore, contact with the RPE is essential for photoreceptor cells to properly function. Therefore, new strategies should be found to prevent rosette formation, like transplanting photoreceptors and RPE at the same time [45]. Other attempt to facilitate efficient network formation with host retinal cells is to seed purified photoreceptor cells onto biomaterial sheets and then to transplant them [105].

It is also important to point out that cell survival and transplantation success are determined also by the extent of immune rejection, although we would be working in a relatively immune-privileged site [106]. ESCs do not express major histocompatibility complex (MHC) II and only a low level (although upregulated) of MHC I after transplantation [107]. iPSC-derived cells show less of an immune response [108], but produce an immune response when retroviruses are used to reprogram them [61]. Finally, MHC matching may be beneficial for successful allogeneic stem cell transplantation [109]. All these aspects will be crucial in order to establish the optimal immunosuppression regime for future clinical applications. Moreover, the Center for iPS Cell Research and Application (CiRA) started offering iPSCs stocks for regenerative medicine in 2015, based on the idea that only 10 cell lines carry the three most frequent HLA homologous loci (HLA-A, -B and -DR), thus reducing the possibility of rejection [110]. Therefore, a CT recruited patients suffering from RPE atrophy, who were transplanted with this product without needing systemic immunosuppression, and although one patient showed mild signs of rejection, this was well controlled through the local administration of steroids. However, it resulted in an insufficient number of cells being delivered to the targeted area, which is another problem that should be addressed [111].

On the other hand, future research in regenerative medicine for vascular ischemic retinal diseases must focus on the following issues—(1) whether endothelial precursor cells or MSCs derived from cord blood or pluripotent sources are more pluripotent and therapeutic than adult cells; (2) although adult stem cell therapies are in early I/IIa phase CTd, efficacy and safety results are still pending, and there is a long way to go before their findings can be applied to clinical practice; (3) understanding the interplay between various precursor cells is important in developing the ideal cell therapy for vascular regeneration, since the optimal cell therapy may involve a combination of stem cells or precursor cells; (4) pharmacologic methods aiming to overcome the potential host factors may enhance the regenerative potential of stem cells [112]; (5) understanding the molecular basis for the regenerative effect of stem cells in retinal vascular conditions might shed light on new pharmacologic or genetic approaches to treating retinal vascular disorders and new approaches to enhancing the therapeutic effects of currently available stem cell therapies [113].

As mentioned, the main challenge in OND is the maintenance of RGCs and stimulating the re-growth of their axons [114]. Optic nerve regeneration can be experimentally induced through different approaches, such as by delivering neurotrophic factors, increasing ocular inflammation and manipulating genes targeting growth-related inhibitors, such as phosphatase and tensin homolog (PTEN), Kruppel-like family (KLF) transcription factors and the suppressor of cytokine signaling 3 (SOCS3) [115]. Interestingly, many of these proregenerative pathways are at least indirectly associated with tumor growth, raising concerns about the clinical feasibility of their manipulation [115]. In addition, complex combinatorial approaches are still far from translation.

In 2019, Mesentier et al. [116] showed that intravitreally injected BMMCs promote RGC survival and regeneration after optic nerve crush but RGC survival declined over time. Therefore, one of the challenges is how to maintain the neuroprotective effect over time, especially in diseases in which the etiological treatment is not addressed. The same authors have demonstrated, using an optic nerve crush model, that the intravitreal injection of MSCs sustained RGC neuroprotection and long-distance regeneration, with transient target reconnection, but also with the progressive loss of the axon regenerative effect—an event that is not solely attributed to the clearance of MSCs but also to a limitation of cell therapy alone in achieving permanent neuronal reconnection to its targets. Thus, they suggest that the combination of MSCs or of their secretome with additional therapeutic approaches is more likely to sustain therapeutic effects for a longer time.

The lack of endogenous RGC replacement in mammals differs from what happens in fish and amphibians, which add new RGCs throughout their lifespan, a feature that is thought to arise at least in part from the presence of a specific proneural transcriptional factor, Ascl1, made by retinal Müller glia in cold blooded vertebrates but not by mammalian Müller glia. Three general approaches to replacing RGCs include (i) syngeneic transplantation of adult induced pluripotent stem cells (iPSs) that have been programmed to assume RGC phenotypes, (ii) allogeneic transplantation of RGCs from healthy eyes into host eyes, and (iii) possible reprogramming of endogenous Müller glia into RGCs. Thus, the isolation of RGCs from the retinas of recently deceased humans for transplantation into recipient humans may actually represent a clinically viable strategy for curing otherwise irreversible forms of blindness [10].

As mentioned in the retinal diseases section, another approach could be the possible use of exosomes. Recent evidence has shown that MSCs secrete exosomes, membrane-enclosed vesicles (30–100 nm) containing proteins, mRNA and miRNA, which can be delivered to nearby cells. A recent experimental study in a rat optic nerve crush model demonstrated that exosomes from BMMSCs showed neuroprotective and neuritogenic effects [116]. In this model, BMSC-derived exosomes promoted statistically significant survival of RGCs and regeneration of their axons, while partially preventing RGC axonal loss and RGC dysfunction, opening a treatment possibility as a cell-free therapy for traumatic optic nerve disease, which nevertheless requires further confirmation.

Finally—and since some of the current CTs are directed at the involvement of the optic nerve in multiple sclerosis—it is worth reviewing an experimental approach that may be interesting. Recently, Gramlich et al. [117] aimed to determine the efficacy of MSC therapy on rescuing the visual system in the experimental autoimmune encephalomyelitis (EAE) model of multiple sclerosis (MS). Systemic MSC treatment (intraperitoneally) was found to positively affect RGC function and survival in EAE mice.

In summary, much progress has been made towards translating stem/progenitor cell technology into optimized therapies for retinal and optic nerve diseases, but the road to the clinic will be undeniably long. More defined differentiation protocols are required to improve efficiency and to obtain high-quality enriched retinal cells at the desire state. Notably, insights into human retinal development with the advent of 3D cell culture techniques that mimic in vivo development may help in this regard. Moreover, the genetic modification of stem cells may prove to be a viable approach to generating specific populations of retinal cells that are able to produce some desirable cell products or to be used after correcting a disease-causing mutation. In addition, stem/progenitor cell therapies have already entered early-stage CTs and have demonstrated safety and some indicators of efficacy. Furthermore, the challenge of the immune rejection of transplants needs to be addressed. Currently, stem/progenitor cell therapies for retinal diseases still have some drawbacks, such as inhibition of proliferation and/or differentiation in vitro (with the exception of the RPE) and limited long-term survival and functioning of grafts in vivo. Despite these challenges, stem/progenitor cells represent the most promising strategy for retinal and optic nerve disease treatment in the near future, as therapeutic strategies assisted by gene techniques, neuroprotective compounds and artificial devices can be applied to fulfil clinical needs. Finally, the collaboration of various experts in engineering, cell biology, genetics and clinical medicine is essential for the development of successful cell therapies.

6. Conclusions

Much progress has been made towards translating stem/progenitor cell technology into optimized therapies for retinal and optic nerve diseases demonstrating safety and efficacy. However, scientists need to work in more defined differentiation protocols and immune rejection of transplants, as well as provide insights into human retinal development and genetic modification of stem cells.

Author Contributions: R.M.C.-M. and J.C.P. contributed to the conceptualization and methodology; R.M.C.-M. to writing the part of retinal diseases; S.P.-I. and J.C.P. to writing the part of optic nerve diseases—original draft preparation; R.M.C.-M., to final supervision and editing. All authors have read and agreed to the published version of the manuscript.

Funding: This research received no external funding.

Institutional Review Board Statement: The study was conducted according to the guidelines of the Declaration of Helsinki.

Informed Consent Statement: Not applicable.

Data Availability Statement: Not applicable.

Conflicts of Interest: The authors declare no conflict of interest.

References

1. de Jong, P.T. Age-related macular degeneration. *N. Engl. J. Med.* **2006**, *355*, 1474–1485. [CrossRef] [PubMed]
2. Ferrari, S.; Di Iorio, E.; Barbaro, V.; Ponzin, D.; Sorrentino, F.S.; Parmeggiani, F. Retinitis pigmentosa: Genes and disease mechanisms. *Curr. Genom.* **2011**, *12*, 238–249. [CrossRef]
3. Osborne, N.N.; Casson, R.J.; Wood, J.P.; Chidlow, G.; Graham, M.; Melena, J. Retinal ischemia: Mechanisms of damage and potential therapeutic strategies. *Prog. Retin Eye Res.* **2004**, *23*, 91–147. [CrossRef] [PubMed]
4. Barber, A. A new view of diabetic retinopathy: A neurodegenerative disease of the eye. *Prog. Neuro-Psychopharmacol. Biol. Psychiatry* **2003**, *27*, 283–290. [CrossRef]
5. Zarbin, M. Cell-Based Therapy for Retinal Disease: The New Frontier. *Methods Mol. Biol.* **2019**, *1834*, 367–381. [CrossRef]
6. Labrador-Velandia, S.; Alonso-Alonso, M.L.; Alvarez-Sanchez, S.; González-Zamora, J.; Carretero-Barrio, I.; Pastor, J.C.; Fernandez-Bueno, I.; Srivastava, G.K. Mesenchymal stem cell therapy in retinal and optic nerve diseases: An update of clinical trials. *World J. Stem Cells* **2016**, *8*, 376–383. [CrossRef]
7. Fu, L.; Kwok, S.S.; Chan, Y.K.; Lai, J.S.; Pan, W.; Nie, L.; Shih, K.C. Therapeutic Strategies for Attenuation of Retinal Ganglion Cell Injury in Optic Neuropathies: Concepts in Translational Research and Therapeutic Implications. *BioMed Res. Int.* **2019**, *11*, 1–10. [CrossRef]
8. DeBusk, A.; Moster, M.L. Gene therapy in optic nerve disease. *Curr. Opin. Ophthalmol.* **2018**, *29*, 234–238. [CrossRef]
9. Moore, D.L.; Goldberg, J.L. Four steps to optic nerve regeneration. *J. Neuroophthalmol.* **2010**, *30*, 347–360. [CrossRef] [PubMed]
10. Laha, B.; Stafford, B.K.; Huberman, A.D. Regenerating optic pathways from the eye to the brain. *Science* **2017**, *356*, 1031–1034. [CrossRef] [PubMed]
11. Chun, B.Y.; Cestari, D.M. Advances in experimental optic nerve regeneration. *Curr. Opin. Ophthalmol.* **2017**, *28*, 558–563. [CrossRef] [PubMed]
12. Cenni, M.C.; Bonfanti, L.; Martinou, J.C.; Ratto, G.M.; Strettoi, E.; Maffei, L. Long-term survival of retinal ganglion cells following optic nerve section in adult bcl-2 transgenic mice. *Eur. J. Neurosci.* **1996**, *8*, 1735–1745. [CrossRef]
13. Bonfanti, L.; Strettoi, E.; Chierzi, S.; Cenni, M.C.; Liu, X.H.; Martinou, J.-C.; Maffei, L.; Rabacchi, S.A. Protection of retinal ganglion cells from natural and axotomy-induced cell death in neonatal transgenic mice overexpressing bcl-2. *J. Neurosci.* **1996**, *16*, 4186–4194. [CrossRef]
14. Maes, M.E.; Schlamp, C.L.; Nickells, R.W. BAX to basics: How the BCL2 gene family controls the death of retinal ganglion cells. *Prog. Retin Eye Res.* **2017**, *57*, 1–25. [CrossRef]
15. Puertas-Neyra, K.; Usategui-Martín, R.; Coco, R.M.; Fernandez-Bueno, I. Intravitreal stem cell paracrine properties as a potential neuroprotective therapy for retinal photoreceptor neurodegenerative diseases. *Neural Regen. Res.* **2020**, *15*, 1631–1638. [CrossRef]
16. Shen, Y. Stem cell therapies for retinal diseases: From bench to bedside. *J. Mol. Med.* **2020**, *98*, 1347–1368. [CrossRef] [PubMed]
17. Huang, S.S. Future vision 2020 and beyond. 5 critical trends in eye research. *Asia Pac. J. Ophthalmol.* **2020**, *9*, 180–185. [CrossRef] [PubMed]
18. Kannabiran, C.; Mariappan, I. Therapeutic avenues for hereditary forms of retinal blindness. *J. Genet.* **2018**, *97*, 341–352. [CrossRef]
19. Salero, E.; Blenkinsop, T.A.; Corneo, B.; Harris, A.; Rabin, D.; Stern, J.H.; Temple, S. Adult human RPE can be activated into a multipotent stem cell that produces mesenchymal derivatives. *Cell Stem Cell* **2012**, *10*, 88–95. [CrossRef]
20. Wang, Y.; Tang, Z.; Gu, P. Stem/progenitor cell-based transplantation for retinal degeneration: A review of clinical trials. *Cell Death Dis.* **2020**, *11*, 793. [CrossRef]
21. Tang, Z.; Zhang, Y.; Wang, Y.; Zhang, D.; Shen, B.; Luo, M.; Gu, P. Progress of stem/progenitor cell-based therapy for retinal degeneration. *J. Transl. Med.* **2017**, *15*, 99. [CrossRef] [PubMed]
22. Caplan, A.; Deniis, J. Mesenchymal stem cells as trophic mediators. *J. Cell Biochem.* **2006**, *98*, 1076–1084. [CrossRef] [PubMed]
23. Chamberlian, G.; Fox, J.; Ashton, B.; Middleton, J. Concise review: Mesenchymal stem cells: Their phenotype, differentiation capacity, immunological features, and potential for homing. *Stem Cells* **2007**, *25*, 2739–2749. [CrossRef] [PubMed]
24. Megaw, R.; Dhillon, B. Stem cell therapies in the management of diabetic retinopathy. *Curr. Diab. Rep.* **2014**, *14*, 498. [CrossRef]
25. Alvarez-Palomo, A.B.; McLenachan, S.; Chen, F.K.; Da Cruz, L.; Dilley, R.J.; Requena, J.; Lucas, M.; Lucas, A.; Drukker, M.; Edel, M.J. Prospects for clinical use of IPCS. *Fibrogenesis Tissue Repair* **2015**, *8*, 9. [CrossRef]
26. Mandai, M.; Kurimoto, Y.; Takahashi, M. Comment: Autologous induced stem-cell-derived retinal cells for macular degeneration. *N. Engl. J. Med.* **2017**, *377*, 792–793. [CrossRef] [PubMed]
27. Nakano, T.; Ando, S.; Takata, N.; Kawada, M.; Muguruma, K.; Sekiguchi, K.; Saito, K.; Yonemura, S.; Eiraku, M.; Sasai, K. Self-formation of optic cups and storable stratified neural retina from human ESCs. *Cell Stem Cell* **2012**, *10*, 771–785. [CrossRef]

28. Reichman, S.; Slembrouck, A.; Gagliardi, G.; Chaffiol, A.; Terray, A.; Nanteau, C.; Potey, A.; Belle, M.; Rabesandratana, O.; Duebel, J.; et al. Generation of Storable Retinal Organoids and Retinal Pigmented Epithelium from Adherent Human iPS Cells in Xeno-Free and Feeder-Free Conditions. *Stem Cells* **2017**, *35*, 1176–1188. [CrossRef]
29. Tanaka, T.; Yokoi, T.; Tamalu, F.; Watanabe, S.-I.; Nishina, S.; Azuma, N. Generation of retinal ganglion cells with functional axons from human induced pluripotent stem cells. *Sci. Rep.* **2015**, *5*, 8344. [CrossRef]
30. Kim, H.; Kim, J.J.; Yoon, Y.S. Emerging therapy for diabetic neuropathy: Cell therapy targeting vessels and nerves. *Endocr. Metab. Immune Disord. Drug Targets* **2012**, *12*, 168–178. [CrossRef] [PubMed]
31. Park, S.S. Cell Therapy Applications for Retinal Vascular Diseases: Diabetic Retinopathy and Retinal Vein Occlusion. *Investig. Ophthalmol. Vis. Sci.* **2016**, *57*, ORSFj1–ORSFj10. [CrossRef]
32. Asahara, T.; Murohara, T.; Sullivan, A.; Silver, M.; van der Zee, R.; Li, T.; Witzenbichler, B.; Schatteman, G.; Isner, J.M. Isolation of putative progenitor endothelial cells for angiogenesis. *Science* **1997**, *275*, 964–967. [CrossRef]
33. Mackie, A.R.; Losordo, D.W. CD34 positive stem cells in the treatment of heart and vascular disease in human beings. *Tex. Heart Inst. J.* **2011**, *38*, 474–485. [PubMed]
34. Caballero, S.; Sengupta, N.; Afzal, A.; Chang, K.H.; Li Calzi, S.; Guberski, D.L.; Kern, T.S.; Grant, M.B. Ischemic vascular damage can be repaired by healthy, but not diabetic, endothelial progenitor cells. *Diabetes* **2007**, *56*, 960–967. [CrossRef] [PubMed]
35. Goldenberg-Cohen, N.; Avraham-Lubin, B.C.; Sadikov, T.; Askenasy, N. Effect of co-administration of neuronal growth factors on neuroglial differentiation of bone marrow-derived stem cells in the ischemic retina. *Investig. Ophthalmol. Vis. Sci.* **2014**, *55*, 502–512. [CrossRef] [PubMed]
36. Medina, R.J.; O'Neill, C.L.; Humphreys, M.W.; Gardiner, T.A.; Stitt, A.W. Outgrowth endothelial cells: Characterization and their potential for reversing ischemic retinopathy. *Investig. Ophthalmol. Vis. Sci.* **2010**, *51*, 5906–5913. [CrossRef]
37. Mendel, T.A.; Clabough, E.B.; Kao, D.S.; Demidova-Rice, T.N.; Durham, J.T.; Zotter, B.C.; Seaman, S.A.; Cronk, S.M.; Rakoczy, E.P.; Katz, A.J.; et al. Pericytes derived from adipose-derived stem cells protect against retinal vasculopathy. *PLoS ONE* **2013**, *8*, e65691. [CrossRef]
38. Prasain, N.; Lii, M.R.; Vemula, S.; Meador, J.L.; Yoshimoto, M.; Ferkowicz, M.J.; Fett, A.; Gupta, M.; Rapp, B.M.; Saadatzadeh, M.R.; et al. Differentiation of human pluripotent stem cells to cells similar to cord-blood endothelial colony-forming cells. *Nat. Biotechnol.* **2014**, *32*, 1151–1157. [CrossRef]
39. Park, T.S.; Bhutto, I.; Zimmerlin, L.; Huo, J.S.; Nagaria, P.; Miller, D.; Rufaihah, A.J.; Talbot, C.; Aguilar, J.; Grebe, R.; et al. Vascular progenitors from cord blood-derived induced pluripotent stem cells possess augmented capacity for regenerating ischemic retinal vasculature. *Circulation* **2014**, *129*, 359–372. [CrossRef]
40. Moisseiev, E.; Anderson, J.D.; Oltjen, S.; Goswami, M.; Zawadzki, R.J.; Nolta, J.A.; Park, S.S. Protective Effect of Intravitreal Administration of Exosomes Derived from Mesenchymal Stem Cells on Retinal Ischemia. *Curr. Eye Res.* **2017**, *42*, 1358–1367. [CrossRef]
41. Safwat, A.; Sabry, D.; Ragiae, A.; Amer, E.; Mahmoud, R.H.; Shamardan, R.M. Adipose mesenchymal stem cells-derived exosomes attenuate retina degeneration of streptozotocin-induced diabetes in rabbits. *J. Circ. Biomark.* **2018**, *7*, 1849454418807827. [CrossRef] [PubMed]
42. Alexander, P.; Thomson, H.A.; Luff, A.J.; Lotery, A.J. Retinal pigment epithelium transplantation: Concepts, challenges, and future prospects. *Eye* **2015**, *29*, 992–1002. [CrossRef] [PubMed]
43. Binder, S.; Stolba, U.; Krebs, I.; Kellner, L.; Jahn, C.; Feichtinger, H.; Povelka, M.; Frohner, U.; Kruger, A.; Hilgers, R.D.; et al. Transplantation of autologous retinal pigment epithelium in eyes with foveal neovascularization resulting from age-related macular degeneration: A pilot study. *Am. J. Ophthalmol.* **2002**, *133*, 215–225. [CrossRef]
44. Li, L.X.; Turner, J.E. Inherited retinal dystrophy in the RCS rat: Prevention of photoreceptor degeneration by pigment epithelial cell transplantation. *Exp. Eye Res.* **1988**, *47*, 911–917. [CrossRef]
45. Uyama, H.; Mandai, M.; Takahashi, M. Stem Cell-Based Therapies for Retinal Degenerative Diseases: Current Challenges in the Establishment of New Treatment Strategies. *Dev. Growth Differ.* **2020**, *63*, 59–71. [CrossRef]
46. Satarian, L.; Nourinia, R.; Safi, S.; Kanavi, M.R.; Jarughi, N.; Daftarian, N.; Arab, L.; Aghdami, N.; Ahmadieh, H.; Baharvand, H. Intravitreal injection of bone marrow mesenchymal stem cells in patients with advanced retinitis pigmentosa; a safety study. *J. Ophthalmic Vis. Res.* **2017**, *12*, 58–64. [CrossRef]
47. Egypt Al-Azhar University. Safety Study of Use of Autoluguous Bone Marrow Derived Stem Cell in Treatment of Age Related Macular Degeneration. Available online: https://clinicaltrials.gov/ct2/show/study/NCT02016508 (accessed on 2 May 2021).
48. Schwartz, S.D.; Hubschman, J.-P.; Heilwell, G.; Franco-Cardenas, V.; Pan, C.K.; Ostrick, R.M.; Mickunas, E.; Gay, R.; Klimanskaya, I.; Lanza, R.; et al. Embryonic stem cell trials for macular degeneration: A preliminary report. *Lancet* **2012**, *379*, 713–720. [CrossRef]
49. Schwartz, S.; Regillo, C.; Lam, B.; Eliott, D.; Rosenfeld, P.; Gregori, N.; Hubschman, J.-P.; Davis, J.; Heilwell, G.; Spirn, M. Human embryonic stem cell-derived retinal pigment epithelium in patients with age related macular degeneration and Stargardt's macular dystrophy: Follow-up of two open-label phase 1/2 studies. *Lancet* **2015**, *385*, 509–516. [CrossRef]
50. Mehat, M.S.; Sundaram, V.; Ripamonti, C. Transplantation of Human Embryonic Stem Cell-Derived Retinal Pigment Epithelial Cells in Macular Degeneration. *Ophthalmology* **2018**, *125*, 1765–1775. [CrossRef]
51. Song, W.K.; Park, K.M.; Kim, H.J.; Lee, J.H.; Choi, J.; Chong, S.Y.; Shim, S.H.; Del Priore, L.V.; Lanza, R. Treatment of macular degeneration using embryonic stem cell-derived retinal pigment epithelium: Preliminary results in Asian patients. *Stem Cell Rep.* **2015**, *4*, 860–872. [CrossRef]

52. Liu, Y.; Xu, H.W.; Wang, L.; Li, S.Y.; Zhao, C.J.; Hao, J.; Li, Q.Y.; Zhao, T.T.; Wu, W.; Wang, Y.; et al. Human embryonic stem cell-derived retinal pigment epithelium transplants as a potential treatment for wet age-related macular degeneration. *Cell Discov.* **2018**, *4*, 50. [CrossRef] [PubMed]
53. Mandai, M.; Watanabe, A.; Kurimoto, Y.; Hirami, Y.; Morinaga, C.; Daimon, T.; Fujihara, M.; Akimaru, H.; Sakai, N.; Shibata, Y.; et al. Autologous induced stem-cell–derived retinal cells for macular degeneration. *N. Engl. J. Med.* **2017**, *376*, 1038–1046. [CrossRef]
54. Production of iPSC Derived RPE Cells for Transplantation in AMD. ClinicalTrials.gov. Identifier: NCT02464956. Last Updated: 8 June 2015. Available online: https://clinicaltrials.gov/ct2/show/NCT02464956 (accessed on 2 May 2021).
55. Xu, H.; Wang, B.; Ono, M.; Kagita, A.; Fujii, K.; Sasakawa, N.; Ueda, T.; Gee, P.; Nishikawa, M.; Nomura, M.; et al. Targeted Disruption of HLA Genes via CRISPR-Cas9 Generates iPSCs with Enhanced Immune Compatibility. *Cell Stem Cell* **2019**, *24*, 566–578. [CrossRef]
56. Maeda, T.; Lee, M.J.; Palczewska, G.; Marsili, S.; Tesar, P.J.; Palczewski, K.; Takahashi, M.; Maeda, A. Retinal pigmented epithelial cells obtained from human induced pluripotent stem cells possess functional visual cycle enzymes in vitro and in vivo. *J. Biol. Chem.* **2013**, *288*, 34484–34493. [CrossRef]
57. Kamao, H.; Mandai, M.; Okamoto, S.; Sakai, N.; Suga, A.; Sugita, S.; Kiryu, J.; Takahashi, M. Characterization of Human Induced Pluripotent Stem Cell-Derived Retinal Pigment Epithelium Cell Sheets Aiming for Clinical Application. *Stem Cell Rep.* **2014**, *2*, 205–218. [CrossRef] [PubMed]
58. Ben M'Barek, K.; Habeler, W.; Monville, C. Stem Cell-Based RPE Therapy for Retinal Diseases: Engineering 3D Tissues Amenable for Regenerative Medicine. *Adv. Exp. Med. Biol.* **2018**, *1074*, 625–632. [CrossRef]
59. Kashani, A.H.; Uang, J.; Mert, M.; Rahhal, F.; Chan, C.; Avery, R.L.; Dugel, P.; Chen, S.; Lebkowski, J.; Clegg, D.O.; et al. Surgical Method for Implantation of a Biosynthetic Retinal Pigment Epithelium Monolayer for Geographic Atrophy: Experience from a Phase 1/2a Study. *Ophthalmol. Retin.* **2020**, *4*, 264–273. [CrossRef]
60. da Cruz, L.; Fynes, K.; Georgiadis, O.; Kerby, J.; Luo, Y.H.; Ahmado, A.; Vernon, A.; Daniels, J.T.; Nommiste, B.; Hasan, S.M.; et al. Phase 1 clinical study of an embryonic stem cell-derived retinal pigment epithelium patch in age-related macular degeneration. *Nat. Biotechnol.* **2018**, *36*, 328–337. [CrossRef] [PubMed]
61. Zhao, C.; Wang, Q.; Temple, S. Stem cell therapies for retinal diseases: Recapitulating development to replace degenerated cells. *Development* **2017**, *144*, 1368–1381. [CrossRef]
62. Zhu, D.; Deng, X.; Spee, C.; Sonoda, S.; Hsieh, C.L.; Barron, E.; Pera, M.; Hinton, D.R. Polarized secretion of PEDF from human embryonic stem cell-derived RPE promotes retinal progenitor cell survival. *Investig. Ophthalmol. Vis. Sci.* **2011**, *52*, 1573–1585. [CrossRef]
63. Radtke, N.D.; Aramant, R.B.; Seiler, M.J.; Petry, H.M.; Pidwell, D. Vision change after sheet transplant of fetal retina with retinal pigment epithelium to a patient with retinitis pigmentosa. *Arch. Ophthalmol.* **2004**, *122*, 1159–1165. [CrossRef]
64. Aramant, R.B.; Seiler, M.J. Progress in retinal sheet transplantation. *Prog. Retin Eye Res.* **2004**, *23*, 475–494. [CrossRef]
65. Cordero, A.; West, E.L.; Pearson, R.A.; Duran, Y.; Carvalho, L.S.; Chu, C.J.; Naeem, A.; Blackford, S.J.I.; Georgiadis, A.; Lakowski, J.; et al. Photoreceptor precursors derived from three-dimensional embryonic stem cell cultures integrate and mature within adult degenerate retina. *Nat. Biotechnol.* **2013**, *31*, 741–747. [CrossRef]
66. Klassen, H.J.; Ng, T.F.; Kurimoto, Y.; Kirov, I.; Shatos, M.; Coffey, P.; Young, M.J. Multipotent retinal progenitors express developmental markers, differentiate into retinal neurons, and preserve light-mediated behavior. *Investig. Ophthalmol. Vis. Sci.* **2004**, *45*, 4167–4173. [CrossRef] [PubMed]
67. Lamba, D.A.; Gust, J.; Reh, T.A. Transplantation of Human Embryonic Stem Cell-Derived Photoreceptors Restores Some Visual Function in Crx-Deficient Mice. *Cell Stem Cell* **2009**, *4*, 73–79. [CrossRef]
68. Tucker, B.A.; Park, I.H.; Qi, S.D.; Klassen, H.J.; Jiang, C.; Yao, J.; Redenti, S.; Daley, G.Q.; Young, M.J. Transplantation of adult mouse iPS cell-derived photoreceptor precursors restores retinal structure and function in degenerative mice. *PLoS ONE* **2011**, *6*, e18992. [CrossRef]
69. Homma, K.; Okamoto, S.; Mandai, M.; Gotoh, N.; Rajasimha, H.K.; Chang, Y.S.; Chen, S.; Li, W.; Cogliati, T.; Swaroop, A.; et al. Developing rods transplanted into the degenerating retina of Crx-knockout mice exhibit neural activity similar to native photoreceptors. *Stem Cells* **2013**, *31*, 1149–1159. [CrossRef]
70. Santos-Ferreira, T.; Völkner, M.; Borsch, O.; Haas, J.; Cimalla, P.; Vasudevan, P.; Carmeliet, P.; Corbeil, D.; Michalakis, S.; Koch, E.; et al. Stem Cell-Derived Photoreceptor Transplants Differentially Integrate Into Mouse Models of Cone-Rod Dystrophy. *Investig. Ophthalmol. Vis. Sci.* **2016**, *57*, 3509–3520. [CrossRef] [PubMed]
71. Singh, M.; Aslam, S.; Duncan, I.; Cramer, A.; Barnard, A.; MacLaren, R. Cell fusion following photoreceptor transplantation into the non-degenerate retina. *Investig. Ophthalmol. Vis. Sci.* **2014**, *55*, 3989.
72. Ortin-Martinez, A.; Tsai, E.L.; Nickerson, P.E.; Bergeret, M.; Lu, Y.; Smiley, S.; Comanita, L.; Wallace, V.A. A Reinterpretation of Cell Transplantation: GFP Transfer From Donor to Host Photoreceptors. *Stem Cells* **2017**, *35*, 932–939. [CrossRef] [PubMed]
73. Siqueira, R.C.; Messias, A.; Messias, K.; Arcieri, R.S.; Ruiz, M.A.; Souza, N.F.; Martins, L.C.; Jorge, R. Quality of life in patients with retinitis pigmentosa submitted to intravitreal use of bone marrow-derived stem cells (Reticell -clinical trial). *Stem Cell Res. Ther.* **2015**, *6*, 29. [CrossRef] [PubMed]
74. Terrell, D.; Comander, J. Current Stem-Cell Approaches for the treatment of inherited retinal degenerations. *Semin. Ophthalmol.* **2019**, *34*, 287–292. [CrossRef]
75. Zheng, A.; Li, Y.; Tsang, S.H. Personalized therapeutic strategies for patients with retinitis pigmentosa. *Expert Opin. Biol. Ther.* **2015**, *15*, 391–402. [CrossRef]

76. Cai, B.; Sun, S.; Li, Z.; Zhang, X.; Ke, Y.; Yang, J.; Li, X. Application of CRISPR/Cas9 technologies combined with iPSCs in the study and treatment of retinal degenerative diseases. *Hum. Genet.* **2018**, *137*, 679–688. [CrossRef] [PubMed]
77. Burnight, E.R.; Wiley, L.A.; Mullins, R.F.; Stone, E.M.; Tucker, B.A. Gene therapy using stem cells. *Cold Spring Harb. Perspect. Med.* **2014**, *5*, a017434. [CrossRef]
78. Chuang, K.; Fields, M.A.; Del Priore, L.V. Potential of Gene Editing and Induced Pluripotent Stem Cells (iPSCs) in Treatment of Retinal Diseases. *Yale J. Biol. Med.* **2017**, *90*, 635–642.
79. Liao, H.K.; Hatanaka, F.; Araoka, T.; Reddy, P.; Wu, M.Z.; Sui, Y.; Yamauchi, T.; Sakurai, M.; O'Keefe, D.D.; Núñez-Delicado, E.; et al. In Vivo Target Gene Activation via CRISPR/Cas9-Mediated Trans-epigenetic Modulation. *Cell* **2017**, *171*, 1495–1507. [CrossRef]
80. Santiago, C.P.; Keuthan, C.J.; Boye, S.L.; Boye, S.E.; Imam, A.A.; Ash, J.D. A Drug-Tunable Gene Therapy for Broad-Spectrum Protection against Retinal Degeneration. *Mol. Ther.* **2018**, *26*, 2407–2417. [CrossRef]
81. Cereso, N.; Pequignot, M.O.; Robert, L.; Becker, F.; De Luca, V.; Nabholz, N.; Rigau, V.; De Vos, J.; Hamel, C.P.; Kalatzis, V. Proof of concept for AAV2/5-mediated gene therapy in iPSC-derived retinal pigment epithelium of a choroideremia patient. *Mol. Ther. Methods Clin. Dev.* **2014**, *1*, 14011. [CrossRef]
82. Burnight, E.R.; Wiley, L.A.; Drack, A.V.; Braun, T.A.; Anfinson, K.R.; Kaalberg, E.E.; Halder, J.A.; Affatigato, L.M.; Mullins, R.F.; Stone, E.M.; et al. CEP290 gene transfer rescues Leber congenital amaurosis cellular phenotype. *Gene Ther.* **2014**, *21*, 662–672. [CrossRef] [PubMed]
83. Bassuk, A.G.; Zheng, A.; Li, Y.; Tsang, S.H.; Mahajan, V.B. Precision Medicine: Genetic Repair of Retinitis Pigmentosa in Patient-Derived Stem Cells. *Sci. Rep.* **2016**, *6*, 19969. [CrossRef]
84. Garita-Hernandez, M.; Lampič, M.; Chaffiol, A.; Guibbal, L.; Routet, F.; Santos-Ferreira, T.; Gasparini, S.; Borsch, O.; Gagliardi, G.; Reichman, S.; et al. Restoration of visual function by transplantation of optogenetically engineered photoreceptors. *Nat. Commun.* **2019**, *10*, 4524. [CrossRef]
85. Drori, T.; Chapman, J. Diagnosis and classification of neuromyelitis optica (Devic's syndrome). *Autoimmun Rev.* **2014**, *13*, 531–533. [CrossRef] [PubMed]
86. Mallick, J.; Devi, L.; Malik, P.K.; Mallick, J. Update on Normal Tension Glaucoma. *J. Ophthalmic Vis. Res.* **2016**, *11*, 204–208. [CrossRef] [PubMed]
87. Kauper, K.; McGovern, C.; Sherman, S.; Heatherton, P.; Rapoza, R.; Stabila, P.; Dean, B.; Lee, A.; Borges, S.; Bouchard, B.; et al. Two-year intraocular delivery of ciliary neurotrophic factor by encapsulated cell technology implants in patients with chronic retinal degenerative diseases. *Investig. Ophthalmol. Vis. Sci.* **2012**, *53*, 7484–7491. [CrossRef]
88. Birch, D.G.; Weleber, R.G.; Duncan, J.L.; Jaffe, G.J.; Tao, W. Ciliary Neurotrophic Factor Retinitis Pigmentosa Study Groups. Randomized trial of ciliary neurotrophic factor delivered by encapsulated cell intraocular implants for retinitis pigmentosa. *Am. J. Ophthalmol.* **2013**, *156*, 283–292. [CrossRef]
89. Levison, S.W.; Ducceschi, M.H.; Young, G.M.; Wood, T.L. Acute exposure to CNTF in vivo induces multiple components of reactive gliosis. *Exp. Neurol.* **1996**, *141*, 256–268. [CrossRef]
90. Amore, G.; Romagnoli, M.; Carbonelli, M.; Barboni, P.; Carelli, V.; La Morgia, C. Therapeutic Options in Hereditary Optic Neuropathies. *Drugs* **2021**, *81*, 57–86. [CrossRef] [PubMed]
91. Zhao, T.; Li, Y.; Tang, L.; Li, Y.; Fan, F.; Jiang, B. Protective effects of human umbilical cord blood stem cell intravitreal transplantation against optic nerve injury in rats. *Graefes Arch. Clin. Exp. Ophthalmol.* **2011**, *249*, 1021–1028. [CrossRef]
92. Lopez Sanchez, M.I.; Crowston, J.G.; Mackey, D.A.; Trounce, I.A. Emerging Mitochondrial Therapeutic Targets in Optic Neuropathies. *Pharmacol. Ther.* **2016**, *165*, 132–152. [CrossRef]
93. Usategui-Martín, R.; Puertas-Neyra, K.; García-Gutiérrez, M.T.; Fuentes, M.; Pastor, J.C.; Fernandez-Bueno, I. Human Mesenchymal Stem Cell Secretome Exhibits a Neuroprotective Effect over In Vitro Retinal Photoreceptor Degeneration. *Mol. Ther. Methods Clin. Dev.* **2020**, *17*, 1155–1166. [CrossRef] [PubMed]
94. Labrador-Velandia, S.; Alonso-Alonso, M.L.; Di Lauro, S.; García-Gutierrez, M.T.; Srivastava, G.K.; Pastor, J.C.; Fernandez-Bueno, I. Mesenchymal stem cells provide paracrine neuroprotective resources that delay degeneration of co-cultured organotypic neuroretinal cultures. *Exp. Eye Res.* **2019**, *185*, 107671. [CrossRef]
95. Weiss, J.N.; Levy, S. Stem Cell Ophthalmology Treatment Study (SCOTS): Bone marrow derived stem cells in the treatment of Dominant Optic Atrophy. *Stem Cell Investig.* **2019**, *6*, 41. [CrossRef]
96. Nascimento-Dos-Santos, G.; Teixeira-Pinheiro, L.C.; da Silva-Júnior, A.J.; Carvalho, L.R.P.; Mesentier-Louro, L.A.; Hauswirth, W.W.; Mendez-Otero, R.; Santiago, M.F.; Petrs-Silva, H. Effects of a combinatorial treatment with gene and cell therapy on retinal ganglion cell survival and axonal outgrowth after optic nerve injury. *Gene Ther.* **2020**, *27*, 27–39. [CrossRef]
97. Huang, H.; Kolibabka, M.; Eshwaran, R.; Chatterjee, A.; Schlotterer, A.; Willer, H.; Bieback, K.; Hammes, H.P.; Feng, Y. Intravitreal injection of mesenchymal stem cells evokes retinal vascular damage in rats. *FASEB J.* **2019**, *33*, 14668–14679. [CrossRef] [PubMed]
98. Labrador Velandia, S.; Di Lauro, S.; Alonso-Alonso, M.L.; Tabera Bartolome, S.; Srivastava, G.K.; Pastor, J.C.; Fernandez-Bueno, I. Biocompatibility of intravitreal injection of human mesenchymal stem cells in immunocompetent rabbits. *Graefes Arch. Clin. Exp. Ophthalmol.* **2018**, *256*, 125–134. [CrossRef] [PubMed]
99. Park, S.S.; Bauer, G.; Abedi, M.; Pontow, S.; Panorgias, A.; Jonnal, R.; Zawadzki, R.J.; Werner, J.S.; Nolta, J. Intravitreal autologous bone marrow CD34+ cell therapy for ischemic and degenerative retinal disorders: Preliminary phase 1 clinical trial findings. *Investig. Ophthalmol Vis. Sci.* **2014**, *56*, 81–89. [CrossRef]

100. Gu, X.; Yu, X.; Zhao, C.; Duan, P.; Zhao, T.; Liu, Y.; Li, S.; Yang, Z.; Li, Y.; Qian, C.; et al. Efficacy and Safety of Autologous Bone Marrow Mesenchymal Stem Cell Transplantation in Patients with Diabetic Retinopathy. *Cell Physiol. Biochem.* **2018**, *49*, 40–52. [CrossRef]
101. China. Shanghai General Hospital, Shanghai Jiao Tong University School of Medicine. Role of the Serum Exosomal miRNA in Diabetic Retinopathy (DR). Available online: https://clinicaltrials.gov/ct2/show/NCT03264976 (accessed on 2 May 2021).
102. Castanheira, P.; Torquetti, L.; Nehemy, M.B.; Goes, A.M. Retinal incorporation and differentiation of mesenchymal stem cells intravitreally injected in the injured retina of rats. *Arq. Bras. Oftalmol.* **2008**, *71*, 644–650. [CrossRef]
103. van Zeeburg, E.J.; Maaijwee, K.J.; Missotten, T.O.; Heimann, H.; van Meurs, J.C. A free retinal pigment epithelium-choroid graft in patients with exudative age-related macular degeneration: Results up to 7 years. *Am. J. Ophthalmol.* **2012**, *153*, 120–127. [CrossRef]
104. Ma, Z.; Han, L.; Wang, C.; Dou, H.; Hu, Y.; Feng, X.; Xu, Y.; Wang, Z.; Yin, Z.; Liu, Y. Autologous transplantation of retinal pigment epithelium-Bruch's membrane complex for hemorrhagic age-related macular degeneration. *Investig. Ophthalmol Vis. Sci.* **2009**, *50*, 2975–2981. [CrossRef]
105. Jung, Y.H.; Phillips, M.J.; Lee, J.; Xie, R.; Ludwig, A.L.; Chen, G.; Zheng, Q.; Kim, T.J.; Zhang, H.; Barney, P.; et al. 3D Microstructured Scaffolds to Support Photoreceptor Polarization and Maturation. *Adv. Mater.* **2018**, *30*, e1803550. [CrossRef] [PubMed]
106. Boyd, A.S.; Higashi, Y.; Wood, K.J. Transplanting stem cells: Potential targets for immune attack. Modulating the immune response against embryonic stem cell transplantation. *Adv. Drug Deliv. Rev.* **2005**, *57*, 1944–1969. [CrossRef] [PubMed]
107. Drukker, M.; Katz, G.; Urbach, A.; Schuldiner, M.; Markel, G.; Itskovitz-Eldor, J.; Reubinoff, B.; Mandelboim, O.; Benvenisty, N. Characterization of the expression of MHC proteins in human embryonic stem cells. *Proc. Natl. Acad. Sci. USA* **2002**, *99*, 9864–9869. [CrossRef]
108. Araki, R.; Uda, M.; Hoki, Y.; Sunayama, M.; Nakamura, M.; Ando, S.; Sugiura, M.; Ideno, H.; Shimada, A.; Nifuji, A.; et al. Negligible immunogenicity of terminally differentiated cells derived from induced pluripotent or embryonic stem cells. *Nature* **2013**, *494*, 100–104. [CrossRef]
109. Sugita, S.; Iwasaki, Y.; Makabe, K.; Kamao, H.; Mandai, M.; Shiina, T.; Ogasawara, K.; Hirami, Y.; Kurimoto, Y.; Takahashi, M. Successful Transplantation of Retinal Pigment Epithelial Cells from MHC Homozygote iPSCs in MHC-Matched Models. *Stem Cell Rep.* **2016**, *7*, 635–648. [CrossRef] [PubMed]
110. Umekage, M.; Sato, Y.; Takasu, N. Overview: An iPS cell stock at CiRA. *Inflamm. Regen.* **2019**, *39*, 17. [CrossRef]
111. Sugita, S.; Mandai, M.; Hirami, Y.; Takagi, S.; Maeda, T.; Fujihara, M.; Matsuzaki, M.; Yamamoto, M.; Iseki, K.; Hayashi, N.; et al. HLA-Matched Allogeneic iPS Cells-Derived RPE Transplantation for Macular Degeneration. *J. Clin. Med.* **2020**, *9*, 2217. [CrossRef]
112. Hazra, S.; Stepps, V.; Bhatwadekar, A.D.; Caballero, S.; Boulton, M.E.; Higgins, P.J.; Nikonova, E.V.; Pepine, C.J.; Thut, C.; Finney, E.M.; et al. Enhancing the function of CD34(+) cells by targeting plasminogen activator inhibitor-1. *PLoS ONE* **2013**, *8*, e79067. [CrossRef]
113. Ueki, Y.; Wilken, M.S.; Cox, K.E.; Chipman, L.; Jorstad, N.; Sternhagen, K.; Simic, M.; Ullom, K.; Nakafuku, M.; Reh, T.A. Transgenic expression of the proneural transcription factor Ascl1 in Müller glia stimulates retinal regeneration in young mice. *Proc. Natl. Acad. Sci. USA* **2015**, *112*, 13717–13722. [CrossRef]
114. Mesentier-Louro, L.A.; Teixeira-Pinheiro, L.C.; Gubert, F.; Vasques, J.F.; Silva-Junior, A.J.; Chimeli-Ormonde, L.; Nascimento-Dos-Santo, G.; Mendez-Otero, R.; Santiago, M.F. Long-term neuronal survival, regeneration, and transient target reconnection after optic nerve crush and mesenchymal stem cell transplantation. *Stem Cell Res. Ther.* **2019**, *10*, 121. [CrossRef]
115. Barber, A.; Farmer, K.; Martin, K.R.; Smith, P.D. Retinal regeneration mechanisms linked to multiple cancer molecules: A therapeutic conundrum. *Prog. Retin. Eye Res.* **2017**, *56*, 19–31. [CrossRef] [PubMed]
116. Mead, B.; Tomarev, S. Bone Marrow-Derived Mesenchymal Stem Cells-Derived Exosomes Promote Survival of Retinal Ganglion Cells Through miRNA-Dependent Mechanisms. *Stem Cells Transl. Med.* **2017**, *6*, 1273–1285. [CrossRef] [PubMed]
117. Gramlich, O.W.; Brown, A.J.; Godwin, C.R.; Chimenti, M.S.; Boland, L.K.; Ankrum, J.A.; Kardon, R.H. Systemic Mesenchymal Stem Cell Treatment Mitigates Structural and Functional Retinal Ganglion Cell Degeneration in a Mouse Model of Multiple Sclerosis. *Transl. Vis. Sci. Technol.* **2020**, *9*, 16. [CrossRef] [PubMed]

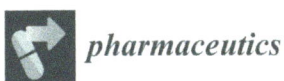 *pharmaceutics*

Review

Significance of Crosslinking Approaches in the Development of Next Generation Hydrogels for Corneal Tissue Engineering

Promita Bhattacharjee [1,2] and Mark Ahearne [1,2,*]

1. Trinity Centre for Biomedical Engineering, Trinity Biomedical Sciences Institute, Trinity College Dublin, University of Dublin, D02 R590 Dublin, Ireland; promitabhatt@gmail.com
2. Department of Mechanical, Manufacturing and Biomedical Engineering, School of Engineering, Trinity College Dublin, University of Dublin, D02 R590 Dublin, Ireland
* Correspondence: ahearnm@tcd.ie; Tel.: +353-0-1896-2359

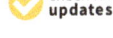

Citation: Bhattacharjee, P.; Ahearne, M. Significance of Crosslinking Approaches in the Development of Next Generation Hydrogels for Corneal Tissue Engineering. *Pharmaceutics* 2021, 13, 319. https://doi.org/10.3390/pharmaceutics13030319

Academic Editors: Dimitrios A. Lamprou and Yolanda Diebold

Received: 21 December 2020
Accepted: 24 February 2021
Published: 28 February 2021

Publisher's Note: MDPI stays neutral with regard to jurisdictional claims in published maps and institutional affiliations.

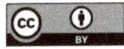

Copyright: © 2021 by the authors. Licensee MDPI, Basel, Switzerland. This article is an open access article distributed under the terms and conditions of the Creative Commons Attribution (CC BY) license (https://creativecommons.org/licenses/by/4.0/).

Abstract: Medical conditions such as trachoma, keratoconus and Fuchs endothelial dystrophy can damage the cornea, leading to visual deterioration and blindness and necessitating a cornea transplant. Due to the shortage of donor corneas, hydrogels have been investigated as potential corneal replacements. A key factor that influences the physical and biochemical properties of these hydrogels is how they are crosslinked. In this paper, an overview is provided of different crosslinking techniques and crosslinking chemical additives that have been applied to hydrogels for the purposes of corneal tissue engineering, drug delivery or corneal repair. Factors that influence the success of a crosslinker are considered that include material composition, dosage, fabrication method, immunogenicity and toxicity. Different crosslinking techniques that have been used to develop injectable hydrogels for corneal regeneration are summarized. The limitations and future prospects of crosslinking strategies for use in corneal tissue engineering are discussed. It is demonstrated that the choice of crosslinking technique has a significant influence on the biocompatibility, mechanical properties and chemical structure of hydrogels that may be suitable for corneal tissue engineering and regenerative applications.

Keywords: cornea; hydrogel; keratoplasty; scaffold; tissue engineering; collagen

1. Introduction

The cornea is the outermost transparent layer of the anterior eye consisting of five distinct layers: Epithelium, Bowman's layer, Stroma, Descemets membrane and Endothelium. Damage to any of these layers can result in a loss of vision. More than 10 million people worldwide suffer from corneal related blindness due to disease or injury [1]. Corneal blindness can result from infection, inflammation, trauma, dystrophies and degenerative medical conditions. Partial or full corneal transplantation (keratoplasty) is often the only viable treatment to regain vision. However, some of the problems associated with keratoplasties include immunological rejection (around 18%) [2] and donor shortages [3,4].

An alternative to traditional keratoplasty is to develop an artificial cornea or keratoprosthesis. This approach has the advantage of overcoming the donor supply problems associated with keratoplasties. However, current keratoprostheses have a number of limitations including an increased risk of glaucoma, inflammation and abnormal tissue growth [5]. Amniotic membrane (AM) obtained from the inner wall of the fetal placenta has been used for ocular surface reconstruction [6,7]. The AM promotes re-epithelialization of the corneal surface, reduces inflammation and inhibits vascularization [8]. However, using AM to reconstruct the ocular surface has drawbacks, including reduced transparency [9], poor mechanical strength [10] and varying tissue quality between donors [11].

To overcome these problems, tissue engineering approaches have been under investigation to fabricate whole corneas or specific layers of the cornea that are suitable for transplantation. These may be generated using decellularized xenogenic tissues [12–15] or natural or synthetic polymers [16–19], as a scaffold to support cells in a three-dimensional construct. To engineer a functional corneal equivalent, constructs should ideally mimic the native cornea, both structurally and functionally. Tissue engineered corneas need to exhibit three functional characteristics: protection, light transmission, and refraction [20]. To fulfill these characteristics, constructs should support the development of a functional corneal epithelium by supporting proliferation and migration of cells from the limbus. This newly formed epithelium should protect the intra-ocular contents from pathogenic invasion. The mechanical stiffness and strength of the constructs should be equivalent to the native cornea. Ideally, the constructs should mimic the nanoscale fibrillar structure of the corneal stroma to achieve a high degree of transparency (>90%). To prevent the formation of an optical haze, the construct's swelling ratio should be similar to the native cornea. Engineered corneal equivalents should also have a high water content to allow nutrient diffusion through the tissue, enhance cell survival and replicate the cornea's viscoelastic characteristics.

Hydrogels are water-swollen polymers that have been under investigation as scaffolds to engineer corneal tissue for many reasons including their high water content, biocompatibility, transparency and permeability (Figure 1). While many hydrogels tend not to be suturable, some can adhere directly to tissue when gelation occurs in vivo, avoiding the need for sutures [21]. Hydrogels can also be used to deliver drugs to the eye to support tissue regeneration and inhibit inflammation. They offer many advantages over colloidal [22,23] and polymeric [24] drug delivery systems including a high water content that assists in preserving the activity of bio-pharmaceuticals such as peptides, proteins or nucleic acids [25,26]. Temperature-responsive and in situ chemically crosslinked hydrogels can be administered by minimally invasive methods [27–29]. While hydrogels have been shown to support the formation of the functional epithelium [30], many have poor mechanical strength and rigidity compared to native corneas [31], they can undergo rapid degradation in vivo and they often lack signaling molecules normally resident in the extracellular matrix that are necessary to control cell behavior.

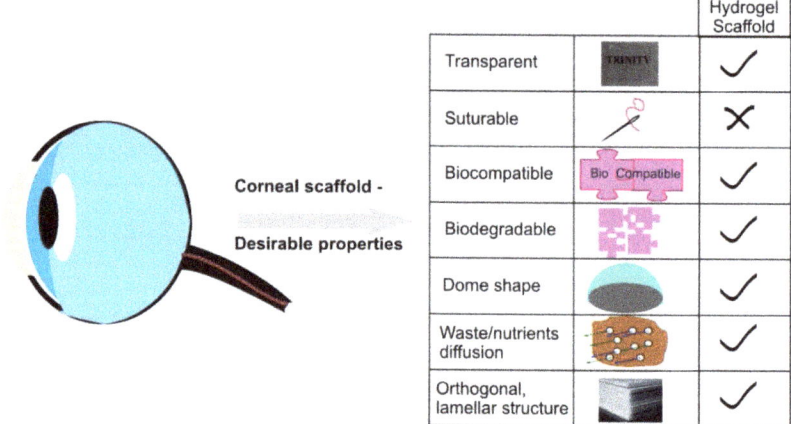

Figure 1. Schematic representation of desirable properties that hydrogels should possess for corneal tissue engineering.

To assist in improving the mechanical and degradation characteristics of hydrogels, the application of exogenous small molecules, i.e., crosslinkers [28] has been investigated. Crosslinking agents have been introduced to functionally modify the mechanical, biological and degradation properties of various biomaterials depending on their compositional and structural features [32]. It is important to select a suitable crosslinker for specific tissue applications that allows the possibility to tune the hydrogels micro/macro-structure and physico-chemical, biological and mechanical properties.

While many different types of crosslinkers have been investigated for controlling the properties of hydrogels for corneal tissue engineering and regeneration, these have not been previously compared in any detail. Here, we report on the recent investigations involving the functional modification of hydrogels using different crosslinking reagents. This paper reviews different crosslinking approaches that have been employed to fabricate several standard and innovative hydrogels for corneal regeneration. The basic mechanisms of each crosslinking method are described and examples are used to illustrate each of the approaches. Several studies are highlighted that have undertaken comparative analyses of different crosslinking reagents. The development of injectable hydrogels and the impact of different crosslinking initiators on the characteristics of hydrogels are discussed. The benefits, limitations and future prospects of these crosslinkers used for corneal regeneration are outlined.

2. Crosslinking in Hydrogel Fabrication for Corneal Regeneration

Recently, there has been much progress in fabricating mechanically stable biomimetic scaffolds and hydrogels by incorporating different crosslinking mechanisms. Crosslinking is an important parameter in the fabrication of hydrogels that can result in enhanced biomechanical properties by developing inter-molecular network linkages. Among the different major functional groups (hydroxyl, methyl, carbonyl, carboxyl, amino, phosphate, and sulfhydryl) of a polymer chain, any two functional groups can couple covalently or non-covalently through crosslinking. These types of bonds (especially covalent bonding) regulate the protein activity, stability and complex structural assembly within fabricated biomaterials [29]. Ideally, crosslinking agents should be capable of improving mechanical strength and stiffness, must be non-toxic, enhance enzymatic resistance, effectively influence cross-talk between cells and material, and retain shape memory [33]. The specific chemical and structural properties of a hydrogel have a significant impact on the crosslinking mechanism. These crosslinking mechanisms can be classified into two groups: physical involving non-covalent bonding or chemical involving covalent bonding (Figure 2A). For hydrogels, physical crosslinking is accompanied by chemical crosslinking since physical crosslinking alone would be insufficient to maintain the integrity of the hydrogel. Specific examples of crosslinking techniques are shown (Figure 2B).

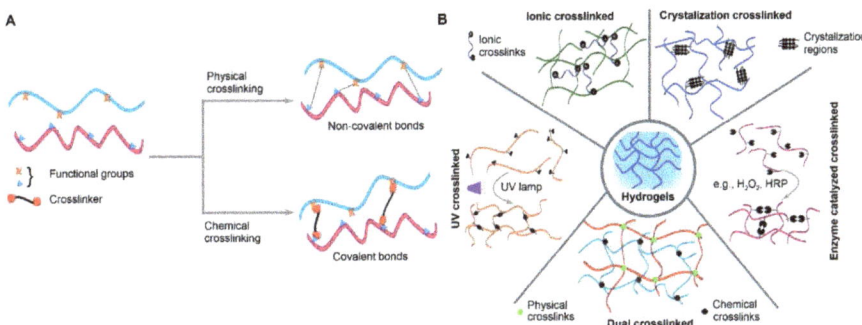

Figure 2. Representation showing (**A**) the effect of physical and chemical crosslinking on the type of bonds formed and (**B**) several examples of different crosslinking techniques.

2.1. Dehydrothermal Treatment (DHT)

During DHT, the hydrogel is exposed to an elevated temperature under vacuum. Intermolecular crosslinking is initiated via esterification or amide formation when water molecules are evacuated at a high temperature [34]. Carboxyl and amine groups situated in adjacent proximity of protein backbone become covalently coupled. One advantage of this mechanism is that it results in sterilization of the materials, hence, removing the need for further sterilization steps later in the process as well as reducing the potential immunogenic response to the material after implantation [35,36].

An ophthalmic drug delivery system was developed using biodegradable cationized gelatin hydrogels loaded with an epidermal growth factor [37]. These hydrogels were fabricated by air-drying and DHT crosslinking. Corneal epithelial defects in rabbits were created to study the potential of this hydrogel for wound repair. A controlled release of epidermal growth factor was reported from hydrogels that led to accelerated wound healing. In a separate comparative study, DHT crosslinked gelatin hydrogel sheets and atelocollagen sheets with human corneal endothelial cells were compared, where gelatin hydrogels displayed better transparency, permeability and elasticity [38]. ZO-1 bonding between cells and Na^+/K^+-ATPase indicated that the crosslinked gelatin supported the formation of a functional endothelium. In another study, collagen scaffolds were crosslinked using either UV irradiation or DHT [39]. Both treatments led to increased tensile strength but also the fragmentation of the collagen molecules structure. There was no significant difference between the two mechanisms. German et al. demonstrated that they could engineer a cornea by culturing human epithelial cells on DHT crosslinked collagen hydrogels containing fibroblasts [40]. A promising result was reported with the formation of 4–5 layers of regenerated corneal epithelium as well as basement membrane components after 3 days of culture. While DHT does not induce any potential toxic effects, controlling the degree of the crosslinking remains a challenge to be addressed [41].

2.2. Ultra-Violet (UV) Irradiation

UV mediated crosslinking is an easy, robust and non-toxic procedure when two characteristic phenomena take place simultaneously: crosslinking and UV-induced denaturation. The combination of these two phenomena improves the mechanical properties and degradation resistance of collagen based scaffolds [42]. Protein molecules can be covalently coupled via UV light with aromatic residues such as tyrosine and phenylalanine. UV light also creates covalent bonds between polypeptide chains, important cell recognition sites situated in the proteins backbone, without involving the acidic and basic side chains [43].

UV crosslinking has been used to modify collagen based biomaterials and tissues. For example, the Young's modulus of collagen-based hydrogels has been shown to significantly increase after UV mediated crosslinking between riboflavin and collagen without hindering the growth of human corneal fibroblasts [44,45]. The final modulus of the hydrogel was dependent on the UV exposure time. UV crosslinking also enhances enzymatic resistance in collagen hydrogels [46]. Incorporation of glucose into the hydrogel can help to lower collagen fragmentation during the UV crosslinking process [47]. Therefore, this technique could potentially be used for in vitro stabilization of collagen hydrogels [48]. UV crosslinking is also a promising technique to treat degenerative diseases such as keratoconus that directly affects the corneal stroma. In this process, photosensitive riboflavin is crosslinked with corneal collagen through UV irradiation [49].

In addition to collagen, silk fibroin has also been crosslinked via UV irradiation. A highly transparent silk fibroin-based hydrogel has been developed using photo-crosslinking between riboflavin and silk fibroin. This hydrogel was examined for corneal reshaping through photo-lithography to provide visual acuity. Excellent adherence between the hydrogel and ocular surface makes this approach very promising for corneal regeneration [50]. Silk fibroin based matrices also positively influence corneal stromal cell behavior when the riboflavin content and UV exposure are optimized. Riboflavin crosslinked silk fibroin matrices supported cellular adhesion, proliferation, ECM formation, and keratocyte-associated gene expression [51].

An injectable, photocurable and biocompatible gelatin-based thiol-acrylate hydrogel with tunable mechanical properties has been used for corneal regeneration in rabbit model [52]. This hydrogel supported epithelial wound coverage in less than three days.

The study also demonstrated the non-toxic effect of UV irradiation on the cornea as well as the posterior segment of the eye [52]. Semi-synthetic gelatin methacrylate (GelMA) is a popular biomaterial in tissue engineering due to its adjustable physical properties, biocompatibility and ability to be used in 3D bioprinting. In the presence of a photoinitiator, GelMA hydrogels can be easily fabricated through free radical polymerization. To generate GelMA hydrogels suitable for corneal endothelium formation and transplantation, physical networks were formed in the solution prior to UV crosslinking by incubating a pre-polymer solution at 4 °C for 1 h [53]. The hydrogels displayed excellent in vitro biocompatibility with corneal endothelial cells and had favorable biodegradation kinetics and high cellular viability in a rabbit model following transplantation.

In addition to natural polymer-based hydrogels, UV crosslinking can be used to produce stable hydrogels from synthetic polymers. Transparent, UV crosslinked polyethylene glycol (PEG)-diacrylate and PEG-diacrylamide hydrogels have been successfully manufactured and tested as corneal replacements in rabbit studies [54]. Although PEG-diacrylate hydrogels resulted in corneal inflammation and ulceration that led to corneal haze, PEG-diacrylamide hydrogels showed more promise. UV crosslinked PEG-diacrylamide hydrogels did not show any inflammation up to 6 months after implantation and appeared healthy and transparent. UV mediated photo-crosslinking is only effective for transparent and thin scaffolds that allow the light to penetrate the structure. For this reason, this crosslinking technique is generally acceptable and has fewer limitations for its applications with a comparatively thin tissue like the cornea.

2.3. Crosslinking Using Chemical Additives

Crosslinking using chemical additives accelerates the modification of the polymeric backbone and leads to a higher degree of crosslinking. For this reason, these crosslinkers are widely accepted for tissue engineering and regenerative medicine applications. The most commonly used crosslinking additives are glutaraldehyde (GA), 1,4-butanediol di glycidyl ether (BDDGE), genipin and 1-ethyl-3-[3-dimethylaminopropyl] carbodiimide hydrochloride (EDC). Examples of hydrogels crosslinked using chemical additives and that have been used for corneal regeneration are shown in Table 1.

2.3.1. Glutaraldehyde (GA)

Bi-functional crosslinking agent, GA induces covalent linkages between the aldehyde groups of GA with the amine groups of lysine or hydroxylysine residues of the polypeptide chains. This mechanism contributes to increased degradation resistivity of the protein molecules. GA is one of the most commonly used crosslinking agents due to its fast reaction time, firm stabilization, low cost and easy availability [55]. The main limitation of using GA is its cytotoxicity and the immune response it elicits in the body [56]. Unbound free aldehyde groups are mainly responsible for the toxic effect of GA crosslinked scaffolds. Vigorous washing of the crosslinked scaffold using glycine solution helps to eliminate unbound aldehyde groups reducing the scaffold's toxicity. Several studies that have used GA crosslinked hydrogels for corneal regeneration [41,57–67] are summarized in Table 1. These studies show that researchers are trying to obtain a stable crosslinker by varying the concentration of GA. However, due to the toxicity of GA, alternative chemical agents had to be explored.

2.3.2. 1,4-Butanediol Diglycidyl Ether (BDDGE)

The application of BDDGE as a crosslinking agent is limited in the field of corneal tissue engineering (Table 1). BDDGE is more commonly used to efficiently stabilize collagen dermal filler [68]. The crosslinking reactivity of BDDGE with a biopolymer depends on environmental conditions such as pH and temperature. Through hydroxyl group linkage, BDDGE is also able to covalently bond with the macromolecular substrate. The crosslinking mechanism depends on the reactivity of the epoxide groups situated on the ends of the molecules. In alkaline conditions, amine groups can open up the epoxide ring, forming strong ether bonds and secondary amide bonding [68]. One example of a BDDGE crosslinked hydrogels that have been used as a bioactive corneal stromal substitute are hydroxypropyl chitosan–gelatin-chondroitin sulfate hydrogels. These hydrogels were highly transparent, retained a high water content, were permeable and showed good biocompatibility [69]. In another study, Koh et al. reported that BDDGE cross-linking of collagen hydrogels resulted in a slow gelation time [70]. The bi-functional BDDGE cross-linking exhibited through secondary amine bond formation via epoxide ring opening by amine groups of collagens under basic pH conditions. This phenomenon facilitates slower gelation and enables drug molecule encapsulation within the collagen matrix for therapeutic application.

2.3.3. Genipin

Genipin is a green colored chemical derived from gardenia fruits that enables protein macromolecules to be easily crosslinked via intra- and inter-molecular linkages. This crosslinking mechanism undergoes the following two steps. First, a nucleophilic substitution takes place at C_3 carbon atom of genipin. This leads to the immediate formation of an intermediate aldehyde group. Next, a heterocyclic compound is formed due to the reaction between the aldehyde group and secondary amine. Subsequently, the substitution of ester groups takes place on the protein backbone via secondary amide bridging and leads to nucleophilic substitution [71]. Consequently, a heterocyclic compound (bluish-green in color) is formed due to the reaction between genipin and protein amine groups via oxygen-radical-induced polymerization [72].

Genipin is widely used for tissue engineering applications due to its low toxicity and negligible immunogenicity [73]. Genipin's cytotoxicity appears to be highly dose dependent but time independent. To eliminate the toxic effect and undesired immunogenic reaction, a 0.5 mM concentration of genipin is recommended for most tissue engineering application [74]. Further dose optimization may still be required for specific applications. Table 1, elaborates on the studies that use genipin crosslinking in developing hydrogels for corneal tissue engineering [75–77].

2.3.4. Ethyl-3-[3-dimethylaminopropyl] Carbodiimide Hydrochloride (EDC) and N-hydroxy-succinimide (NHS)

EDC, a zero-length crosslinking agent, commonly conjugates carboxyl or phosphate groups to primary amines through a covalent linkage. EDC forms an active O-urea that subsequently couples with the amino groups through an amide bridging [78]. As a result, a water soluble sub-product, iso-urea, is formed that can be easily eliminated by washing. This crosslinking mechanism is significantly pH dependent and the reactivity is higher with improved efficiency in an acidic environment (in presence of 2-(N-morpholino)ethanesulfonic acid (MES) buffer solution) compared to alkaline environments [79]. Conjugation of water soluble NHS, or its analog sulfo-NHS, in EDC enhances the efficiency of the crosslinking reaction as well as its stability. NHS esters are formed due to direct coupling between EDC/NHS and carboxyls. These NHS esters are more stable than the O-acyl-isourea intermediates and positively assist in proficient coupling of primary amines at physiological pH [80]. When using EDC for crosslinking, unreacted free groups of EDC do not remain in the material. This consequently means that the final product is not affected by EDC toxicity [81]. EDC mediated crosslinking generally utilizes cell reactive carboxylate anions (on glutamate or aspartate residues) or primary amino groups (on lysine residues), which are the major cell binding motif sites of many biomaterials for forming hydrogels, such as collagen or silk fibroin. As a result, there is a shortage of available cell binding motif sites after crosslinking [82]. To address this issue, more investigation is required to optimize the concentration of EDC for fabricating hydrogels with improved cellular reactivity, without altering surface chemistry or biomechanics. A significant improvement in mechanical integrity and stability along with cellular biocompatibility has been recorded for collagen-based scaffolds when the concentration of EDC was significantly reduced [83]. The standard concentration (100%) of carbodiimide is 11.5 mg/ml and was diluted progressively down to 0.1%. This reduction resulted in an almost 4-fold increment in the amount of free amine groups without altering the mechanics or stability in water of the resultant scaffolds. This 10-fold reduction in carbodiimide crosslinking demonstrated in near native-like cell attachment to collagen scaffolds.

From analyzing Table 1 it is found that EDC/NHS has been commonly used as a crosslinker for developing hydrogels for corneal regeneration [41,59,84–90]. There are considerable variations in the concentration of EDC/NHS used in the reported articles. Almost all reported articles (8 out of 10) performed in vivo evaluations of EDC/NHS crosslinked hydrogels supported by in vitro studies using corneal specific cells.

2.4. Other Approaches

Several alternative crosslinking chemicals and approaches have been evaluated to improve the mechanical properties and stability of hydrogels for corneal tissue engineering [85,86,91–101] (Table 1). These hydrogels are made using a variety of biomaterials. For example, several studies have used novel crosslinkers on collagen hydrogels. Generation 2 polypropylenimine octaamine dendrimers have successfully crosslinked collagen hydrogels with high degree of transparency and good mechanical properties for corneal regeneration [91]. The biocompatibility of these hydrogels, in respect of cellular adhesion and proliferation, was evaluated with human corneal epithelial cells and the crosslinker showed no toxicity [91].

Table 1. Complete details of the different crosslinkers used in corneal regeneration to synthesize corneal hydrogels identified in this review.

Paper	Biomaterial	Crosslinkers	Fabrication Method	Cell Study	In Vivo Study
		Glutaraldehyde (GA)			
[57]	Gelatin	10% GA at 4 °C for 14 h	Lyophilization	-	Pigmented rabbits
[58]	Collagen I + chondroitin sulphate	GA conc. (0.02, 0.04, 0.06 and 0.08%)	Air-lifted and maintained at air-liquid interfaces	Keratocytes ± corneal epithelial and endothelial cells	-
[67]	Collagen + poly(ethylene oxide dialdehyde)	GA	Air drying and argon plasma surface modification	Human epithelial cells	-
[59]	Hyaluronic acid	100 mM GA at 25 °C for 2 days	Solution casting and air-drying	Corneal endothelial cells	-
[60]	Hyaluronic acid	100 mM GA at 25 °C for 2 days	Solution casting and air-drying	-	New Zealand white rabbits
[41]	Gelatin	50 mM GA at 25 °C for 80 min	Solution casting and air-drying	Rat iris pigment epithelial cells	New Zealand white rabbits
[61]	Collagen, copolymers of collagen and TERP	0.22% GA at room temperature for 7 days	Air drying	-	Adult laboratory beagles
[62]	Amniotic membrane	0.1% GA and hyperdried	Far infrared rays and microwaves	-	Three eyes of three patients
[63]	Hyaluronic acid + itaconic acid + PEGDE	GA under acidic pH	Air drying	Human corneal epithelial cell line	New Zealand white rabbits
[64]	Amniotic membrane (AM)	0.05 mmol GA per mg AM	Air drying	Limbal epithelial cells	-
[65]	Canine AM + atelocollagen	0.1% GA	Air drying	Canine corneal epithelial cells	-
[66]	Carboxymethyl chitosan + poloxamer	1% GA for 1 h at 50 °C	Air drying	Human corneal epithelial cells	-

Table 1. Cont.

Paper	Biomaterial	Crosslinkers	Fabrication Method	Cell Study	In Vivo Study
\multicolumn{6}{c}{1,4-Butanediol diglycidyl ether (BDDGE)}				
[69]	Chitosan + gelatin + chondroitin sulfate	0.5% BDDGE	Lyophilization	Human and rabbit keratocytes	-
[70]	Porcine collagen type I	BDDGE at pH 11	Air drying	Human corneal epithelial and rodent DRG cell	-
\multicolumn{6}{c}{Genipin (GP)}				
[75]	Chitosan + collagen, cellulose or elastin	GP (40 µL)	Air drying	Human corneal epithelial cells	-
[76]	Chitosan	0.5–5.0 mM GP	Lyophilization	Human corneal epithelial cells	-
[77]	Carboxymethyl chitosan + poloxamer	02–0.8% GP	Lyophilization	-	New Zealand rabbits (ex vivo)
\multicolumn{6}{c}{Ethyl-3-[3-dimethylaminopropyl] carbodiimide hydrochloride (EDC) & N-hydroxy-succinimide (NHS)}				
[87]	Amniotic membranes (AM)	0–0.25 mmol EDC per mg AM EDC:NHS molar ratios = 5:1	Immersion	Limbal epithelial cells	New Zealand white rabbits
[41]	Gelatin	50 mM EDC	Solution casting and air-drying	Rat iris pigment epithelial cells	New Zealand white rabbits
[88]	Hyaluronic acid	10 mM EDC at 25 °C for 2 days	Lyophilization	Corneal endothelia	New Zealand white rabbits
[89]	Hyaluronic acid	10 mM EDC	Lyophilization	Corneal endothelia	New Zealand white rabbits
[90]	Collagen I + gelatin (Col/Gel)	EDC:NHS:(Col/Gel) = 1:1:12 for 4 h	Lyophilization	Human mesenchymal stem cells	-
\multicolumn{6}{c}{Other crosslinkers}				
[91]	Type I collagen	Generation 2 polypropyleneimine octaamine dendrimers	Chemical crosslinking	Human corneal epithelial cells	-
[92,93]	PEG and PAAc double network hydrogel	50% acrylic acid 1% v/v with respect to hydroxyl-2-methyl propiophenone and triethylene glycol dimethacrylate	Two-step sequential network formation technique	Primary corneal epithelial and fibroblast cells	New Zealand Red rabbits
[94]	Collagen coupled PEG/PAAc	1% triethylene glycol dimethacrylate for 24 h at room temperature	UV- free radical polymerization	Rabbit corneal cell line	New Zealand Red rabbits
[85]	PEG-stabilized collagen + chitosan	Hybrid cross-linking system comprising of a long-range bi-functional cross-linker	Chemical crosslinking	Human corneal epithelial cells, and DRG	Yucatan porcine cornea and rat subcutaneous
[86]	Collagen–phosphorylcholine	PEG diacrylate initiated by ammonium persulphate or 0.5% Irgacure 2959	Photopolymerization	Human corneal epithelial cell line and DRG	Mini-pigs and New Zealand white rabbits

Table 1. Cont.

Paper	Biomaterial	Crosslinkers	Fabrication Method	Cell Study	In Vivo Study
[95]	Neoglycopolymer—recombinant collagen III	Carbohydrate-functionalized norbornenes	Tandem ring-open metathesis polymerization hydrogenation	Human corneal epithelial cells	-
[96]	Hydroxypropyl chitosan (HPCTS)	Sodium alginate dialdehyde (20 mg/mL) mixed equal volume with HPCTS	Self-cross-linking process of chitosan and oxidized alginate	Corneal endothelial cells	New Zealand rabbits
[97]	Collagen I-Immobilized PEG	1% Triethylene glycol dimethacrylate and poly(2-hydroxyethyl methacrylate)	UV-initiated free radical polymerization	Human corneal epithelial cells	-
[98]	Chitosan + PEG	Diepoxy-PEG:cystamine (4:1 molar ratio)	Casting and chemical crosslinking for 24 h at 25 °C	Sheep endothelial cell	Ovine eyes (ex vivo)
[99]	Poly(2-hydroxyethyl methacrylate)	N, N'-methylenebis 0.5% acrylamide	Polymerization and molding processes	Rabbit corneal stromal cells	New Zealand rabbits
[100]	Levofloxacin loaded glycol chitosan	4-arm polyethylene glycol with aldehyde end groups (4-arm PEG-CHO)	Chemical crosslinking	L-929 cells	-
[101]	GelCORE bioadhesive hydrogels	Photocrosslinking with visible light (450 to 550 nm)	Lyophilization, chemical and photo-crosslinking	Corneal fibroblast cells	New Zealand white rabbits

New crosslinkers have also been used to crosslink collagen with other biomaterials. A hybrid cross-linking system was developed using a long-range bi-functional cross-linker PEG-dibutyraldehyde (PEG-DBA) and short-range amide-type cross-linkers (EDC and NHS) to crosslink collagen–chitosan composite hydrogels [85]. The hydrogels exhibited excellent optical clarity (superior to human eye bank corneas), suturability, permeability to albumin and glucose, and significantly higher mechanical strength and elasticity, an increase of 100% and 20%, respectively, when compared to its non-hybrid counterpart. These hydrogels showed excellent biocompatibility both in vitro, using dorsal root ganglia (DRG) and human corneal epithelial cells, and in vivo using rat subcutaneous and pig cornea implants. The hydrogels supported host–graft integration with successful regeneration of corneal stroma, nerve and epithelium after 12 months implantation in pigs.

A bio-interactive collagen-phospholipid corneal substitute was developed from interpenetrating polymeric networks, utilizing EDC/NHS crosslinked porcine atelocollagen, and PEG-diacrylate crosslinked 2-methacryloyloxyethyl phosphorylcholine (MPC) [86]. Fabricated hydrogels showed increased mechanical strength along with enhanced stability against collagenase and UV degradation and improved in vitro biocompatibility with DRG and human corneal epithelial cells. A 12 months in vivo study of hydrogels into mini pig demonstrated regeneration ability of corneal stroma, epithelium, tear film and sensory nerves.

Chitosan and chitosan composites are also commonly used biomaterials for corneal tissue engineering. In addition to using standard crosslinking chemicals like GA, several different approaches have been explored to crosslinking chitosan. For example, an in situ formed biodegradable hydrogel was fabricated involving the water-soluble derivative of chitosan, hydroxypropyl chitosan, and sodium alginate dialdehyde for corneal endothelial regeneration [96]. Periodate oxidized alginate rapidly cross-links hydroxypropyl chitosan due to the formation of Schiff's base between the available amino groups and aldehyde. The fabricated hydrogels were biocompatible with corneal endothelial cells, biodegradable and were evaluated as a potential scaffolds for in vivo endothelium regeneration in New Zealand rabbits.

A new post crosslinking mechanism via epoxy–amine chemistry was introduced to fabricate ultrathin (thickness in hydrated condition 50μm) chitosan–PEG hydrogel for corneal tissue regeneration [98]. The resultant hydrogel showed desirable optical transparency, biodegradability, comparable mechanical property with cornea to support a suitable mechano-responsive environment for corneal endothelial cell and supported adhesion and proliferation of sheep's corneal endothelial cells. Ex vivo trials on ovine eyes showed that the hydrogels exhibited excellent properties for physical manipulation and implantation, which made them a potential scaffold for minimally invasive surgical procedures, such as Descemet's Stripping Endothelial Keratoplasty (DSEK).

Porous chitosan hydrogel sheets were developed and evaluated as a potential ophthalmic delivery substrate for levofloxacin [100]. Hydrogel sheets were fabricated spontaneously under mild conditions when a 4-arm polyethylene glycol crosslinker was mixed with aldehyde end groups (4-arm PEGCHO) and glycol chitosan (GC) at various ratios. Upon decreasing the concentration of 4-arm PEGCHO and GC, the swelling ratio of fabricated hydrogels was increased. Biocompatibility assays reported that the hydrogels were non-toxic and exhibited an excellent cytocompatibility with L929 cells.

In addition to collagen and chitosan, there has also been considerable interest in the development of PEG based hydrogels for corneal engineering. A two-step sequential network formation approach was employed to fabricate interpenetrating hydrogels by using poly(2-hydroxyethyl methacrylate) and triethylene glycol dimethacrylate (1% v/v) as a crosslinker inside collagen immobilized PEG hydrogels [97]. Fabricated hydrogels were non-toxic and supported adhesion and proliferation of corneal epithelial cells.

UV-initiated free radical polymerization, using a two-step sequential network formation technique was used to fabricate PEG/poly(acrylic acid) (PEG/PAA) hydrogels for corneal tissue engineering [92]. Both in vitro (using primary corneal epithelial and fibroblast cells) [92] and preliminary in vivo (New Zealand Red rabbits) [93] studies were carried out to assess the biocompatibility of the fabricated hydrogel. A similar UV-initiated free radical polymerization and crosslinking network technique was used to fabricate collagen-coupled PEG/PAA hydrogels that support corneal epithelial wound healing [94]. The bioactive surface of the hydrogels showed promising results for epithelial wound closure. In vivo results conducted on rabbits demonstrated that the implanted hydrogel supported the migration of corneal epithelial cells, although the morphology and migration rate of cells were different from normal.

A mechanically and structurally efficient artificial cornea using poly(2-hydroxyethyl methacrylate) was fabricated involving a T-style design of a keratoprosthetics [99]. N,N'-methylenebis (acrylamide) (0.5 %) was used as a crosslinker. The porous skirt was altered with hyaluronic acid and cationized gelatin, and the bottom of the optical column was coated with poly(ethylene glycol). In vitro (rabbit corneal stromal cells) and in vivo (New Zealand rabbits) analysis demonstrated that the artificial cornea was a potential corneal substitute and could be suitable for patients with corneal opacity and massive limbal stem cell deficiency.

A saturated neoglycopolymer was developed by tandem ring opening metathesis polymerization-hydrogenation of carbohydrate-functionalized norbornenes and examined as a promising crosslinking agent for corneal tissue engineering [95]. The resultant neoglycopolymer hydrogels were superior with respect to stability, enzymatic resistivity and permeability, compared to clinically tested control materials (recombinant human collagen type III (RHC III) crosslinked using EDC/NHS) as well as demonstrating biocompatibility in vitro with human corneal epithelial cells.

Recently a transparent, highly biocompatible, cost-effective, bio-adhesive hydrogel, using gelatin methacryloyl (GelMA) prepolymer with ~80% methacryloyl functionalization degree (GelCORE) were fabricated utilizing photo-crosslinking with visible light (450 to 550 nm) for 60 seconds [101]. The physical properties of fabricated hydrogel can be finely adjusted by altering the photo crosslinking time and concentration of pre-polymer. In situ photo-polymerization of GelCORE improved the adhesion between the hydrogel and tissue. In vitro and in vivo (rabbit model) evaluation demonstrated that the bio-adhesive hydrogel is highly biocompatible with corneal fibroblast, efficiently enclosing stromal defects in rabbit and promoting stromal regeneration and re-epithelialization.

2.5. Comparative Studies

A number of studies have compared different crosslinking reagents (Table 2) and their effectiveness at modifying physical properties, chemical structure, mechanical characteristics and biological effects [41,59,60,91,102,103].

Table 2. Works identified in this review focusing on the comparison of different crosslinkers used to develop corneal hydrogels.

Paper	Biomaterial	Crosslinkers & Concentration	Results
[91]	Type I collagen	Generation 2 polypropyleneimine octaamine dendrimers: EDC: molar ratio 1:1 GA: 0.02%.	Dendrimer-crosslinked gel had no cellular toxicity and higher glucose permeability than natural human cornea and more transparent than GA/EDC crosslinked gels
[59]	Hyaluronic acid (HA)	EDC:100 mM GA:100 mM	EDC-HA was more transparent, smoother surface, faster degradation and lower toxicity than GA-HA
[60]	Hyaluronic acid (HA)	EDC:100 mM GA:100 mM	EDC-HA gel had no adverse inflammatory reaction GA-HA gel induced significant inflammatory cell infiltration and foreign body reaction observed
[41]	Gelatin	EDC:50 mM GA:50 mM	EDC-gelatin was biocompatible without causing toxicity GA-gelatin showed significant inflammatory reaction
[102]	Chitosan	10 mM GA 10 mM Genipin (GP)	GP crosslinked implants were more biocompatible without providing significant intraocular inflammation
[103]	Recombinant human atelocollagen type III	EDC: 0.3 ME (Molar equivalent) CMC: 2.0 ME.	CMC crosslinked samples had comparable properties to EDC crosslinked hydrogels

In one study, collagen solutions (2–4%) were crosslinked with EDC, GA or polypropyleneimine-octa-amine dendrimers [91]. The multi-functional dendrimers were introduced after the activation of the carboxylic acid groups of glutamic and aspartic acid residues in collagen. The dendrimer crosslinked collagen hydrogels exhibited significantly higher optical transparency than EDC and GA crosslinked hydrogels as well as higher glucose permeability compared to human corneas. Adhesion and proliferation of human corneal epithelial cells were supported by dendrimer crosslinked collagen hydrogels without inducing cellular toxicity.

The crosslinking kinetics and properties of recombinant human atelocollagen type III hydrogels were examined using two different crosslinking agents: (i) sterically bulky carbodiimide, N-cyclohexyl-N'-(2-morpholinethyl) carbodiimide metho-p-toluenesulfonate (CMC) and (ii) EDC [103]. The major advantage of CMC crosslinking was that it supported crosslinking at room temperature (25 °C), while EDC crosslinking process was too fast to control at room temperature. Therefore, it is required to be executed at lower temperatures. CMC crosslinked hydrogels were significantly stiffer and exhibited higher collagenase resistivity compared to EDC crosslinked hydrogels. Comparable biocompatibility, in vitro (human corneal epithelial and endothelial cells, DRGs from chick embryos) and in vivo (mouse model), was demonstrated for both crosslinked hydrogels [103].

Another comparative analysis was conducted between EDC and GA to identify the more appropriate crosslinker for hyaluronic acid (HA) hydrogels. These hydrogels were developed as cell delivery vehicles for corneal endothelial cell therapy [59]. Water uptake capacity and enzymatic degradability were significantly decreased for HA hydrogels crosslinked with GA. EDC crosslinked HA hydrogels had a faster degradation rate and smoother surfaces. Lower cytotoxicity for the corneal endothelial cell was also recorded for EDC crosslinked HA hydrogels compared with GA crosslinked HA hydrogels. This study identified EDC as a better option for HA crosslinking. Comparative in vivo evaluation in rabbits for 24 weeks was also carried out to examine the ocular biocompatibility of the HA hydrogels crosslinked with EDC and GA [60]. EDC crosslinked HA hydrogels supported better ocular biocompatibility than GA crosslinked HA hydrogels. No significant inflammatory cell infiltration or foreign body reaction was observed after implantation for non-cross-linked or EDC cross-linked HA hydrogels, whereas adverse inflammatory reaction was quite prominent for GA crosslinked HA hydrogel.

Similar comparative studies between EDC and GA were carried out using gelatin [41]. In vitro analysis using primary rat iris pigment epithelial cells demonstrated that the cells cultured on EDC crosslinked gelatin hydrogels showed lower lactate dehydrogenase activity, cytotoxicity, and interleukin-1β and tumor necrosis factor-α levels compared to cells cultured on GA cross-linked gelatin hydrogels. In vivo analysis in rabbit model also reported better biocompatibility, less toxicity and fewer adverse effects for EDC cross-linked gelatin hydrogels compared to GA.

In vivo ocular biocompatibility of genipin and GA crosslinked chitosan hydrogel were compared in rabbits [102]. Genipin crosslinked implanted hydrogels showed no signs of ocular inflammation in the anterior chamber of the eye, enhanced the preservation of corneal endothelial cell density as well as supported better anti-inflammatory activities, when compared with non crosslinked and GA-crosslinked chitosan hydrogels.

3. Crosslinking Strategies for Injectable Hydrogel

Injectable hydrogels are hydrogels that form after injection into the body and have been used for drug delivery, tissue defects repair and as cell delivery vehicles [104]. In the eye, injectable hydrogels have been examined as a substitute for vitreous humor and more recently, for corneal defect repair [104]. Figure 3 represents such an idealized future situation where hydrogel precursors, loaded with stem cells and bioactive molecules, can be injected and form a hydrogel with desirable characteristics in vivo. The composition and quantity of bioactive molecules could be easily varied depending on the clinical requirements and could even be made patient specific. Injectable hydrogels demonstrate more potential than pre-formed hydrogels for the delivery of a therapeutic payload [105–107]. The most important properties that affect swelling, drug release rate and oxygen permeability of the hydrogels are the molecular weight of a polymer between two crosslink points and the mesh size. The gelation, crosslinking and the application of injectable hydrogels for corneal regeneration will be discussed here.

3.1. Gelation and Formulation

Injectable hydrogels are composed of synthetic or naturally derived hydrophilic polymers that are able to crosslink in situ following a variety of mechanisms [108]. The Food and Drug Administration, USA (FDA) has approved several synthetic polymers including polyvinyl alcohol (PVA), PEG, PAA, poly(N-isoproylacrylamine) (PNIPAAm) and Pluronic F-127. These polymers are able to crosslink hydrophilic co-polymers or homopolymers and effectively develop block co-polymers with other polymers [104]. Several naturally derived polymers such as polysaccharides (alginate, chitosan, hyaluronic acid and dextran) and proteins (collagen and gelatin) have also been used to develop injectable hydrogels for ophthalmic applications [104]. These hydrogels use covalent crosslinking, the Diels–Alder reaction, enzyme reactions to effect in situ Michael addition, Schiff base formation and click chemistry to form stable hydrogels [104]. Crosslinking of injectable hydrogels is often initiated by altering physico-chemical parameters such as temperature, pH, ionic strength, the glucose concentration or mechanical stress. These physico-chemical parameters induce phase separation and structural alteration of polymer chains to develop a crosslinked network [109]. Stimuli responsive polymers such as thermo-responsive PEG, PNIPAAm and Pluronic F-127 or pH-responsive polyacrylic acid (PAAc) and chitosan, can be easily formed by crosslinking an injected hydrogel network [104].

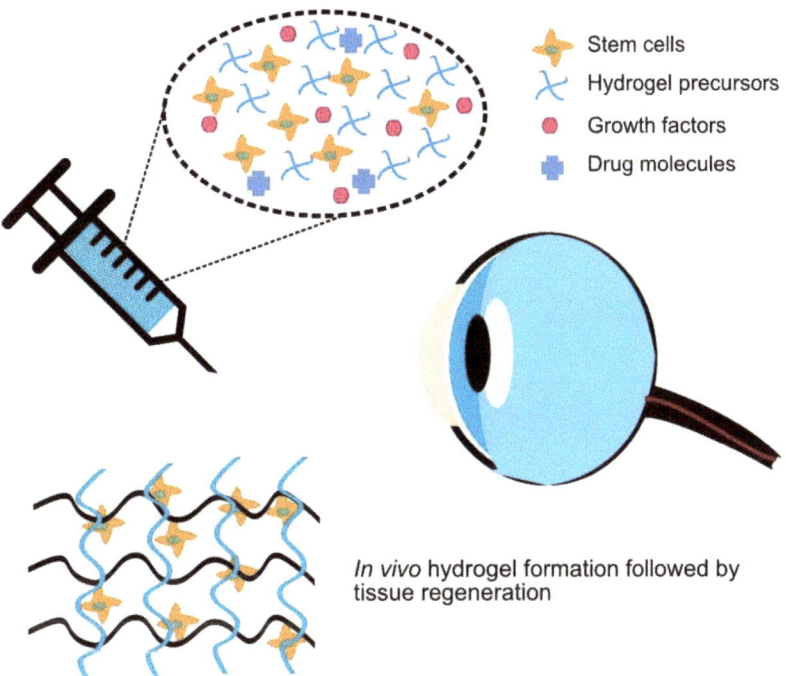

Figure 3. Schematic representing the potential different components of an injectable hydrogel to be used for corneal repair.

3.2. The Injectable Hydrogels in Treatment

In situ forming hydrogels are an efficient way to repair corneal wounds and defects by delivering drugs and cells to the damaged region of the cornea [110]. To examine the effectiveness of induced pluripotent stem cells (iPSCs) in bioengineered cornea for corneal regeneration, a thermo-responsive injectable amphiphatic carboxymethylhexanoyl chitosan (CHC) nanoscale hydrogel was synthesized [111]. This hydrogel supported increased cell viability and gene expression associated with stem cells. In vivo experiments involved administrating the injectable iPSCs laden CHC hydrogel in a defect site of the rat cornea. CHC hydrogels improved regeneration of damaged cornea by down regulating oxidative stress that led to the restoration of the corneal epithelial thickness. Therefore, CHC hydrogels are a potential scaffold for stem cell delivery to improve corneal wound healing [111].

A PEG based injectable hydrogel was developed by incorporating Tyr-Arg-Gly-AspSer (YRGDS) peptides [112]. Keratocytes encapsulated in these hydrogels maintained their viability over 4 weeks and displayed genetic and morphological characteristics associated with healthy, functional keratocytes. However, further advancement in the development of PEG based hydrogels as a cell based therapeutic approach for keratoconus treatment is required as it failed to restore the keratocyte phenotype completely.

A novel LiQD cornea has recently been developed as an alternative to donated corneas for transplantation [113]. This cell-free hydrogel liquid was synthesized using short collagen-like peptides combined with PEG and blended with fibrinogen. In vitro and in vivo analysis demonstrated that this self-assembled LiQD cornea is biocompatible, non-toxic and significantly reduced the risk of immune rejection associated with xenogeneic materials. LiQD cornea is also capable of undergoing rapid in situ gelation and may serve as a potential material for corneal regeneration.

An in situ, rapidly formed, PEG-based doxycycline laden transparent hydrogel was successfully fabricated through thiol reactions and was examined for corneal wound healing applications [114]. This hydrogel exhibited a prolonged release of doxycycline (up to 7 days) and was able to resist the structural deformation under shearing force. Remarkably, a decline in the production of matrix metalloproteinase-9 (MMP-9) was shown through immunofluorescence and histology analysis. This result supported better corneal healing for these hydrogels. Thus, PEG-based homo-polymers and co-polymers are an attractive choice for corneal repair.

An injectable hydrogel utilizing the thermo-responsive co-polymer of poly(lactic-co-glycolic acid) (PLGA) and PEG was synthesized through sol-gel transition at temperatures ranging between 5 and 60 °C [115]. In vitro biocompatibility tests showed that these hydrogels supported proliferation and migration of epithelial cells. In vivo (rabbit model) results of implanted hydrogels demonstrated that keratocytes retain a natural morphology appearance and there was desirable healing of corneal wounds [115].

There is limited availability of FDA approved injectable hydrogels for commercial use and they have only been used to prompt the healing process post ocular surgery. Ongoing investigations are aiming to use injectable hydrogels as a delivery vehicle of drugs and cells for corneal regeneration. They are also trying to overcome the complications associated with stem cell research. It may take several years before injectable hydrogels are clinically available as a delivery vehicle of cells and drugs for corneal repair and regeneration.

4. Impact of Crosslinkers on Hydrogel Characteristics

The type and duration of crosslinking affects the physical properties and biological compatibility of many hydrogels. For example, an increase in crosslinking will increase degradation resistance for most hydrogels. Similarly, hydrogel formation may often need to take place with cells and/or proteins present, thus necessitating the crosslinking process to be cytocompatibility. Thus, it is desirable to control the crosslinking process. An overview of the effect of different crosslinking actions on hydrogel properties is shown below (Figure 4).

4.1. Mechanical Characteristics

The mechanical characteristics of hydrogels are dependent on the type and magnitude of crosslinking that has been applied to them. In general, the use of chemical crosslinking reagents results in stable hydrogels with better mechanical properties while other methods such as photo-crosslinking can provide better cytocompatibility since no additional chemical agents are required. The mechanical properties of hydrogels are often described as viscoelastic, where they exhibit both viscous and elastic characteristics [116,117]. This results in time dependent deformation behaviors such as creep, relaxation and time dependent recovery. The viscoelastic characteristics of hydrogels tend to be dependent on the degree and density of crosslinking. Alternatively, many studies describe the behavior of hydrogels as being elastic with similar properties to rubber. The correct description of the hydrogel mechanical characteristics depends on the material composition and type of crosslinking. The crosslinks that improve mechanical strength also increase viscosity, reduces solubility and reduce glass transition temperature (T_g).

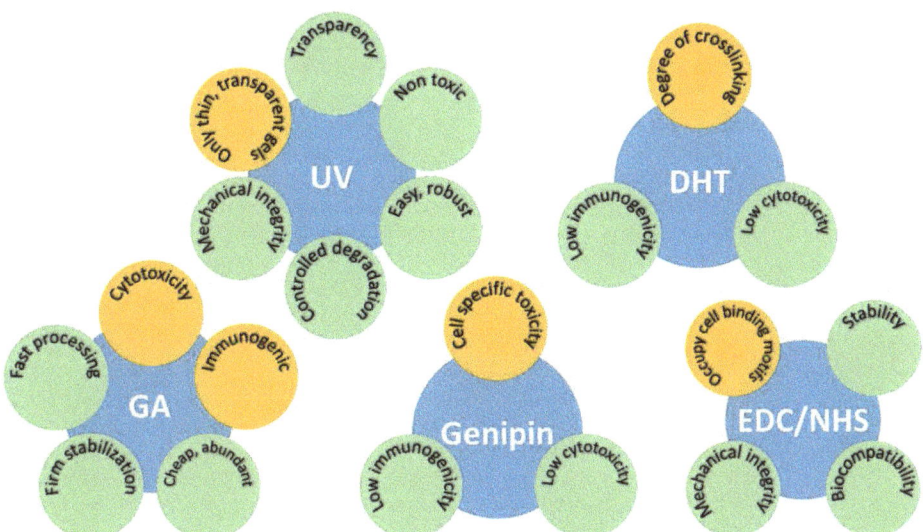

Figure 4. Schematic representation summarizing the pros (green) and cons (orange) of commonly used crosslinking techniques and chemical additives in terms of their impact on hydrogel characteristics.

At the macro-scale, the mechanical properties of hydrogels affect their stability, strength and stiffness while at the micro-scale mechanical properties can affect how the hydrogels interact with cells and affect cell signaling, proliferation, migration, and differentiation [118,119]. Hydrogel stiffness can be adjusted by tuning the crosslinker density, crosslinking time and the type of precursors used [120].

Both UV and DHT initiated crosslinking have been shown to improve the tensile strength of collagen based hydrogels although they led to fragmentation of the collagens basic structure [39,44]. Another limitation with photo-crosslinking is the inability of light to penetrate deep into a material, although this is less of a problem for thin, transparent hydrogels [54]. Photo-crosslinking can be used to finely control mechanical properties of hydrogels by adjusting the time of exposure and light intensity [101].

2 polypropylenimine octaamine dendrimers have been shown to produce transparent collagen hydrogels with good mechanical properties [91]. Interestingly, a hybrid approach of using a long-range bi-functional crosslinker (PEG-DBA) and short-range amide-type crosslinkers (EDC and NHS) was able to produce a collagen-chitosan hydrogel that was transparent, had good mechanical properties and could be sutured [85].

4.2. Degradation and Structural Properties

Chemical crosslinking produces covalently bonded hydrogels. These covalent bonds between the polymeric chains can be broken down by photo-catalytic cleaving, ester or enzymatic hydrolysis [121]. To provide adequate support as a scaffold, the hydrogels should degrade at a rate that matches new tissue formation so there is no loss of strength or function. To do this, chemical crosslinking parameters can be tailored as required by varying crosslinking time, crosslinker concentration and precursors [122]. Interestingly, degradation, which is a chemical process, alters the physical surroundings of cells and in turn can affect how those cells behave [123].

Hydrogel mesh size impacts solute transmission through the structure [124]. Particles that are larger than the effective pore size in the mesh will thus be excluded. A hydrogel with an asymmetric mesh size can provide bio-separation, that is a high solute flux, as well as selective cell capture and encapsulation [125]. Mesh size can also affect the hydrogel degradation rate. Hydrogels with a high crosslinking density, generally achievable through the use of chemical crosslinkers, reduces mesh size and slows down degradation [126]. The reduced mesh size also slows down the transport of larger molecules, like enzymes, thus limiting access of the enzymes to degradation sites [121]. However, the reduction of molecular diffusion due to smaller mesh size can pose a problem for nutrients transfer, which may be required for the survival of encapsulated cells.

Aimetti et al. [127] developed a hydrogel that degrades via surface erosion. A human neutrophil elastase (HNE) sensitive peptide was used as a crosslinker in PEG hydrogels, via thiol–ene photopolymerization. The high crosslinking density resulted in a reduced mesh structure, limiting HNE diffusion into the hydrogel. Thus, degradation gradually occurred via surface erosion and through this process, a protein entrapped physically in the hydrogel was released.

To mimic natural, soft tissues and their multi-scale, hierarchical structure, an ideal hydrogel for tissue engineering would need to be anisotropic and have a highly ordered architecture [128]. Hydrogel structural hierarchy is an important consideration in designing innovative hydrogels [129]. While physical methods such as plastic compress [130,131] and magnetic fields [132,133] can be used to organize the structure of some hydrogels, controlled crosslinking procedures may be adopted to develop hydrogels with specific architectures. For example, interpenetrating polymer network hydrogels, allow hydrogels to be formed that contains a desirable structural hierarchy by varying the ratio of the different polymers [134].

In addition to affecting the hydrogels mechanical characteristics, UV initiated crosslinking can also improve the degradation resistance of collagen hydrogels to different enzymes [46]. UV crosslinking of GelMA hydrogels has been shown to reduce the rate of degradation [53]. Crosslinking gelatin using DHT has also been able to achieve controlled release of hydrogel embedded bioactive molecules [37]. Use of GA also increases degradation resistance of gelatin [55]. Similarly, combined use of EDC and NHS produced crosslinked atelocollagen hydrogels that were stable against collagenase and UV degradation [86].

4.3. Toxicity and Biocompatibility

Crosslinkers have an important role in modulating chemical and mechanical features of hydrogels so that they lead to a desirable cell response [135]. Changes in the hydrogel properties after crosslinking can affect the behavior and activity of cells in contact with the material. Ideally, a crosslinker must be able to improve mechanical properties while maintaining the biocompatibility of the scaffold and without generating any toxic biproduct [136].

UV crosslinking is not only able to produce a biocompatible hydrogel with no toxic residuals [53], but UV irradiation has also been safely used on the cornea and posterior segment of the eye [52]. However, the wavelength and intensity of UV light need to be considered as over-exposure to UV or too low a wavelength can result in apoptosis.

In spite of its toxicity, GA is one of the mostly used crosslinkers that has been studied by many research groups for tissue engineering application [137]. Many studies reported that GA leaching undergoes simultaneously with scaffold degradation and results in cytotoxicity. Hence, GA residues can be harmful to the cells over long periods [138]. In contrast, genipin is less cytotoxic and still maintains a strong crosslinking ability. Safety issues regarding the use of genipin are still a concern as cellular behavior has been shown to vary significantly after crosslinking depending on the cell type [102]. Genipin can promote the differentiation of neurite cells and accelerate dose dependent neurite outgrowth [139]. However, immediate apoptosis was demonstrated with liver and dermal cells after genipin crosslinking. The concentration of genipin should be optimized for tissue specific studies using different cell types [135].

An alternative to GA and genipin crosslinking, EDC/NHS efficiently crosslinks amino acid based biomaterials with favorable cellular performance [90]. EDC/NHS results in fewer crosslinks compared to GA but it does not present itself in the final product, thus reducing the potential for toxicity [135,140]. However, EDC/NHS crosslinking occupies integrin binding sites in the same carboxylic chain of biopolymers, which are pivotal for integrin-mediated cell interactions [80]. Therefore, there is a requirement to try to conserve the active cell binding sites during crosslinking without altering the chemistry of biomaterial. The use of EDC-NHS creates stable and mechanically strong hydrogels with collagen [83]. An EDC concentration of 0.1% for collagen is recommended to maintain biocompatibility while still improving strength. When applied to hyaluronic acid hydrogels EDC led to lower cytotoxicity but faster degradation and a reduced water uptake compared to GA [59].

5. Challenges and Future Perspective

There are several challenges that need to be addressed before crosslinked hydrogels and scaffolds are more commonly used on patients for corneal tissue engineering. Sterilization of the biomaterials can cause some difficulties since most natural and synthetic polymers undergo degradation during radiation, heat or chemical sterilization processes [141]. These issues are made worse when bioactive molecules, proteins and drugs are incorporated into the polymer matrix [142]. In addition, some hydrogel polymers have a specific shelf life after which there is a reduced ability to form crosslinks. Chemical crosslinking agents support the fabrication of hydrogels with well-defined characteristics that may hinder the availability and stability of biopharmaceuticals. Physical crosslinking may be better at conserving the stability of incorporated biopharmaceuticals, but it is more difficult to control the release of drugs and the degradation kinetics of these hydrogels.

Optimization of crosslinking is required to successfully control the release of drugs or bioactive molecules from hydrogels. For drugs that are chemically bound to the hydrogel, these can be released via degradation. However, controlling the degradation kinetics after encapsulating drug molecules is challenging. The degradation rate of drug loaded hydrogels and their drug release profiles may vary from patient to patient depending on many factors including age, sex and health of the patients [141]. Rapid degradation of the hydrogel may accelerate the release of drugs, while inhibiting degradation may lead to incomplete drug release.

Another challenge is how best to control the spatial distribution of cells throughout a hydrogel. One approach to doing this is to employ 3D bioprinting to engineer constructs with a high degree of precision. Most hydrogels used for 3D bioprinting (called bioinks) utilize UVA light to generate crosslinks and form a stable hydrogel. This technology has the potential to assist clinicians and researchers to produce innovative constructs to address corneal donor shortages. In addition, 3D bioprinting could be used to incorporate drugs or biological reagents into the hydrogels. Recently a number of groups have started exploring the application of 3D bioprinting for corneal tissue engineering [143–146].

6. Conclusions

This review has explored different crosslinking mechanisms that are used to fabricate hydrogels for corneal regeneration. While there is not one ideal crosslinker with all the desirable properties for fabricating hydrogels for corneal regeneration, many of the crosslinking techniques described here are beneficial in controlling the mechanical behavior of hydrogels without adversely affecting their biocompatibility. Overall, variations in the type of hydrogel material selected and the crosslinking dosage significantly affect the properties of the resultant scaffold. Detailed studies that focus on the optimization of crosslinker concentration, cytocompatibility and biocompatibility are necessary to understand the advantages and limitations of each crosslinking approach.

Author Contributions: Writing—original draft preparation, P.B.; writing—review and editing, P.B. and M.A.; funding acquisition, M.A. All authors have read and agreed to the published version of the manuscript.

Funding: The research leading to these results has received funding from the European Research Council (ERC) under the European Union's Horizon 2020 research and innovation program (EYEREGEN-637460) and Science Foundation Ireland (15/ERC/3269).

Institutional Review Board Statement: Not applicable.

Informed Consent Statement: Not applicable.

Data Availability Statement: The data presented in this study are available on request from the corresponding author.

Conflicts of Interest: The authors declare no conflict of interest.

References

1. Whitcher, J.P.; Srinivasan, M.; Upadhyay, M.P. Corneal blindness: A global perspective. *Bull. World Health Organ.* **2001**, *79*, 214–221. [PubMed]
2. Thompson, R.W.; Price, M.O.; Bowers, P.J.; Price, F.W. Long-term graft survival after penetrating keratoplasty. *Ophthalmology* **2003**, *110*, 1396–1402. [CrossRef]
3. Shimazaki, J.; Shinozaki, N.; Shimmura, S.; Holland, E.J.; Tsubota, K. Efficacy and Safety of International Donor Sharing: A Single-Center, Case-Controlled Study on Corneal Transplantation. *Transplantation* **2004**, *78*, 216–220. [CrossRef]
4. Cao, K.Y.; Dorrepaal, S.J.; Seamone, C.; Slomovic, A.R. Demographics of corneal transplantation in Canada in 2004. *Can. J. Ophthalmol.* **2006**, *41*, 688–692. [CrossRef] [PubMed]
5. Salvador-Culla, B.; Kolovou, P.E. Keratoprosthesis: A Review of Recent Advances in the Field. *J. Funct. Biomater.* **2016**, *7*, 13. [CrossRef]
6. Dua, H.S.; Gomes, J.A.; King, A.J.; Maharajan, V. The amniotic membrane in ophthalmology. *Surv. Ophthalmol.* **2004**, *49*, 51–77. [CrossRef]
7. Shimazaki, J.; Shinozaki, N.; Tsubota, K. Transplantation of amniotic membrane and limbal autograft for patients with recurrent pterygium associated with symblepharon. *Br. J. Ophthalmol.* **1998**, *82*, 235–240. [CrossRef] [PubMed]
8. Tseng, S.C.; Espana, E.M.; Kawakita, T.; Di Pascuale, M.A.; Li, W.; He, H.; Liu, T.-S.; Cho, T.-H.; Gao, Y.-Y.; Yeh, L.-K.; et al. How Does Amniotic Membrane Work? *Ocul. Surf.* **2004**, *2*, 177–187. [CrossRef]
9. Connon, C.J.; Doutch, J.; Chen, B.; Hopkinson, A.; Mehta, J.S.; Nakamura, T.; Kinoshita, S.; Meek, K.M. The variation in transparency of amniotic membrane used in ocular surface regeneration. *Br. J. Ophthalmol.* **2009**, *94*, 1057–1061. [CrossRef]
10. Shortt, A.J.; Secker, G.A.; Rajan, M.S.; Meligonis, G.; Dart, J.K.; Tuft, S.J.; Daniels, J.T. Ex Vivo Expansion and Transplantation of Limbal Epithelial Stem Cells. *Ophthalmology* **2008**, *115*, 1989–1997. [CrossRef]
11. Dua, H.S.; Rahman, I.; Miri, A.; Said, D.G. Variations in amniotic membrane: Relevance for clinical applications. *Br. J. Ophthalmol.* **2010**, *94*, 963–964. [CrossRef]
12. Wilson, S.L.; Sidney, L.E.; Dunphy, S.E.; Rose, J.B.; Hopkinson, A. Keeping an Eye on Decellularized Corneas: A Review of Methods, Characterization and Applications. *J. Funct. Biomater.* **2013**, *4*, 114–161. [CrossRef]
13. Lynch, A.P.; Ahearne, M. Strategies for developing decellularized corneal scaffolds. *Exp. Eye Res.* **2013**, *108*, 42–47. [CrossRef]
14. Lynch, A.P.; Wilson, S.L.; Ahearne, M. Dextran Preserves Native Corneal Structure during Decellularization. *Tissue Eng. Part C Methods* **2016**, *22*, 561–572. [CrossRef] [PubMed]
15. Yin, H.; Qiu, P.; Wu, F.; Zhang, W.; Teng, W.; Qin, Z.; Li, C.; Zhou, J.; Fang, Z.; Tang, Q.; et al. Construction of a Corneal Stromal Equivalent with SMILE-Derived Lenticules and Fibrin Glue. *Sci. Rep.* **2016**, *6*, 33848. [CrossRef] [PubMed]
16. Ahearne, M.; Fernández-Pérez, J.; Masterton, S.; Madden, P.W.; Bhattacharjee, P. Designing Scaffolds for Corneal Regeneration. *Adv. Funct. Mater.* **2020**, *30*, 10. [CrossRef]
17. Fernández-Pérez, J.; Kador, K.E.; Lynch, A.P.; Ahearne, M. Characterization of extracellular matrix modified poly(ε-caprolactone) electrospun scaffolds with differing fiber orientations for corneal stroma regeneration. *Mater. Sci. Eng. C* **2020**, *108*, 110415. [CrossRef] [PubMed]
18. Xu, W.; Wang, Z.; Liu, Y.; Wang, L.; Jiang, Z.; Li, T.; Zhang, W.; Liang, Y. Carboxymethyl chitosan/gelatin/hyaluronic acid blended-membranes as epithelia transplanting scaffold for corneal wound healing. *Carbohydr. Polym.* **2018**, *192*, 240–250. [CrossRef]
19. Wu, Z.; Kong, B.; Liu, R.; Sun, W.; Mi, S. Engineering of Corneal Tissue through an Aligned PVA/Collagen Composite Nanofibrous Electrospun Scaffold. *Nanomaterials* **2018**, *8*, 124. [CrossRef]
20. Ruberti, J.W.; Zieske, J.D. Prelude to corneal tissue engineering—Gaining control of collagen organization. *Prog. Retin. Eye Res.* **2008**, *27*, 549–577. [CrossRef]
21. Zhao, Y.; Fan, J.; Bai, S. Biocompatibility of injectable hydrogel from decellularized human adipose tissue in vitro and in vivo. *J. Biomed. Mater. Res. Part B Appl. Biomater.* **2019**, *107*, 1684–1694. [CrossRef]
22. Pollinger, K.; Hennig, R.; Ohlmann, A.; Fuchshofer, R.; Wenzel, R.; Breunig, M.; Tessmar, J.; Tamm, E.R.; Goepferich, A. Ligand-functionalized nanoparticles target endothelial cells in retinal capillaries after systemic application. *Proc. Natl. Acad. Sci. USA* **2013**, *110*, 6115–6120. [CrossRef]

23. Luschmann, C.; Tessmar, J.; Schoeberl, S.; Strauss, O.; Framme, C.; Luschmann, K.; Goepferich, A. Developing an in situ nanosuspension: A novel approach towards the efficient administration of poorly soluble drugs at the anterior eye. *Eur. J. Pharm. Sci.* **2013**, *50*, 385–392. [CrossRef]
24. Lee, S.S.; Hughes, P.; Ross, A.D.; Robinson, M.R. Biodegradable Implants for Sustained Drug Release in the Eye. *Pharm. Res.* **2010**, *27*, 2043–2053. [CrossRef]
25. Lin, C.-C.; Anseth, K.S. PEG Hydrogels for the Controlled Release of Biomolecules in Regenerative Medicine. *Pharm. Res.* **2009**, *26*, 631–643. [CrossRef]
26. Vermonden, T.; Censi, R.; Hennink, W.E. Hydrogels for Protein Delivery. *Chem. Rev.* **2012**, *112*, 2853–2888. [CrossRef]
27. Van Tomme, S.R.; Storm, G.; Hennink, W.E. In situ gelling hydrogels for pharmaceutical and biomedical applications. *Int. J. Pharm.* **2008**, *355*, 1–18. [CrossRef]
28. Oryan, A.; Kamali, A.; Moshiri, A.; Baharvand, H.; Daemi, H. Chemical crosslinking of biopolymeric scaffolds: Current knowledge and future directions of crosslinked engineered bone scaffolds. *Int. J. Biol. Macromol.* **2018**, *107*, 678–688. [CrossRef]
29. Reddy, N.; Reddy, R.; Jiang, Q. Crosslinking biopolymers for biomedical applications. *Trends Biotechnol.* **2015**, *33*, 362–369. [CrossRef]
30. Atyabi, F.; Bakhshandeh, H.; Soleimani, M.; Hosseini, S.S.; Hashemi, H.; Shabani, I.; Shafiee, A.; Nejad, A.H.B.; Erfan, M.; Dinarvand, R. Poly (ε-caprolactone) nanofibrous ring surrounding a polyvinyl alcohol hydrogel for the development of a biocompatible two-part artificial cornea. *Int. J. Nanomed.* **2011**, *6*, 1509–1515. [CrossRef]
31. Ahearne, M.; Liu, K.-K.; El Haj, A.J.; Then, K.Y.; Rauz, S.; Yang, Y. Online Monitoring of the Mechanical Behavior of Collagen Hydrogels: Influence of Corneal Fibroblasts on Elastic Modulus. *Tissue Eng. Part C Methods* **2010**, *16*, 319–327. [CrossRef]
32. Gostynska, N.; Krishnakumar, G.S.; Campodoni, E.; Panseri, S.; Montesi, M.; Sprio, S.; Kon, E.; Marcacci, M.; Tampieri, A.; Sandri, M. 3D porous collagen scaffolds reinforced by glycation with ribose for tissue engineering application. *Biomed. Mater.* **2017**, *12*, 055002. [CrossRef]
33. Ruini, F.; Tonda-Turo, C.; Chiono, V.; Ciardelli, G. Chitosan membranes for tissue engineering: Comparison of different crosslinkers. *Biomed. Mater.* **2015**, *10*, 65002. [CrossRef]
34. Haugh, M.G.; Jaasma, M.J.; O'Brien, F.J. The effect of dehydrothermal treatment on the mechanical and structural properties of collagen-GAG scaffolds. *J. Biomed. Mater. Res. Part A* **2009**, *89*, 363–369. [CrossRef]
35. Gomes, S.; Rodrigues, G.; Martins, G.; Henriques, C.; Silva, J. In vitro evaluation of crosslinked electrospun fish gelatin scaffolds. *Mater. Sci. Eng. C* **2013**, *33*, 1219–1227. [CrossRef]
36. Ratanavaraporn, J.; Rangkupan, R.; Jeeratawatchai, H.; Kanokpanont, S.; Damrongsakkul, S. Influences of physical and chemical crosslinking techniques on electrospun type A and B gelatin fiber mats. *Int. J. Biol. Macromol.* **2010**, *47*, 431–438. [CrossRef]
37. Hori, K.; Sotozono, C.; Hamuro, J.; Yamasaki, K.; Kimura, Y.; Ozeki, M.; Tabata, Y.; Kinoshita, S. Controlled-release of epidermal growth factor from cationized gelatin hydrogel enhances corneal epithelial wound healing. *J. Control. Release* **2007**, *118*, 169–176. [CrossRef]
38. Watanabe, R.; Hayashi, R.; Kimura, Y.; Tanaka, Y.; Kageyama, T.; Hara, S.; Tabata, Y.; Nishida, K. A Novel Gelatin Hydrogel Carrier Sheet for Corneal Endothelial Transplantation. *Tissue Eng. Part A* **2011**, *17*, 2213–2219. [CrossRef]
39. Weadock, K.S.; Miller, E.J.; Bellincampi, L.D.; Zawadsky, J.P.; Dunn, M.G. Physical crosslinking of collagen fibers: Comparison of ultraviolet irradiation and dehydrothermal treatment. *J. Biomed. Mater. Res.* **1995**, *29*, 1373–1379. [CrossRef]
40. Germain, L.; Auger, F.A.; Grandbois, E.; Guignard, R.; Giasson, M.; Boisjoly, H.; Guérin, S.L. Reconstructed Human Cornea Produced in vitro by Tissue Engineering. *Pathobiology* **1999**, *67*, 140–147. [CrossRef]
41. Lai, J.-Y. Biocompatibility of chemically cross-linked gelatin hydrogels for ophthalmic use. *J. Mater. Sci. Mater. Med.* **2010**, *21*, 1899–1911. [CrossRef]
42. Lew, D.-H.; Liu, P.H.-T.; Orgill, D.P. Optimization of UV cross-linking density for durable and nontoxic collagen GAG dermal substitute. *J. Biomed. Mater. Res. Part B Appl. Biomater.* **2007**, *82*, 51–56. [CrossRef] [PubMed]
43. Davidenko, N.; Bax, D.V.; Schuster, C.F.; Farndale, R.W.; Hamaia, S.W.; Best, S.M.; Cameron, R.E. Optimisation of UV irradiation as a binding site conserving method for crosslinking collagen-based scaffolds. *J. Mater. Sci. Mater. Med.* **2016**, *27*, 1–17. [CrossRef]
44. Ahearne, M.; Yang, Y.; Then, K.Y.; Liu, K.-K. Non-destructive mechanical characterisation of UVA/riboflavin crosslinked collagen hydrogels. *Br. J. Ophthalmol.* **2007**, *92*, 268–271. [CrossRef]
45. Ahearne, M.; Coyle, A. Application of UVA-riboflavin crosslinking to enhance the mechanical properties of extracellular matrix derived hydrogels. *J. Mech. Behav. Biomed. Mater.* **2016**, *54*, 259–267. [CrossRef]
46. Heo, J.; Koh, R.H.; Shim, W.; Kim, H.D.; Yim, H.-G.; Hwang, N.S. Riboflavin-induced photo-crosslinking of collagen hydrogel and its application in meniscus tissue engineering. *Drug Deliv. Transl. Res.* **2015**, *6*, 148–158. [CrossRef] [PubMed]
47. Ohan, M.P.; Dunn, M.G. Glucose stabilizes collagen sterilized with gamma irradiation. *J. Biomed. Mater. Res. Part A* **2003**, *67*, 1188–1195. [CrossRef]
48. Mi, S.; Khutoryanskiy, V.V.; Jones, R.R.; Zhu, X.; Hamley, I.W.; Connon, C.J. Photochemical cross-linking of plastically compressed collagen gel produces an optimal scaffold for corneal tissue engineering. *J. Biomed. Mater. Res. Part A* **2011**, *99*, 1–8. [CrossRef] [PubMed]
49. Wollensak, G.; Spoerl, E.; Seiler, T. Riboflavin/ultraviolet-a–induced collagen crosslinking for the treatment of keratoconus. *Am. J. Ophthalmol.* **2003**, *135*, 620–627. [CrossRef]

50. Applegate, M.B.; Partlow, B.P.; Coburn, J.; Marelli, B.; Pirie, C.; Pineda, R.; Kaplan, D.L.; Omenetto, F.G. Photocrosslink-ing of silk fibroin using riboflavin for ocular prostheses. *Adv. Mater.* **2016**, *28*, 2417–2420.
51. Bhattacharjee, P.; Fernández-Pérez, J.; Ahearne, M. Potential for combined delivery of riboflavin and all-trans retinoic acid, from silk fibroin for corneal bioengineering. *Mater. Sci. Eng. C* **2019**, *105*, 110093. [CrossRef]
52. Li, L.; Lu, C.; Wang, L.; Chen, M.; White, J.F.; Hao, X.; McLean, K.M.; Chen, H.; Hughes, T.C. Gelatin-Based Photocurable Hydrogels for Corneal Wound Repair. *ACS Appl. Mater. Interfaces* **2018**, *10*, 13283–13292. [CrossRef]
53. Rizwan, M.; Peh, G.S.; Ang, H.-P.; Lwin, N.C.; Adnan, K.; Mehta, J.S.; Tan, W.S.; Yim, E.K. Sequentially-crosslinked bioactive hydrogels as nano-patterned substrates with customizable stiffness and degradation for corneal tissue engineering applications. *Biomaterials* **2017**, *120*, 139–154. [CrossRef] [PubMed]
54. Hartmann, L.; Watanabe, K.; Zheng, L.L.; Kim, C.-Y.; Beck, S.E.; Huie, P.; Noolandi, J.; Cochran, J.R.; Ta, C.N.; Frank, C.W. Toward the development of an artificial cornea: Improved stability of interpenetrating polymer networks. *J. Biomed. Mater. Res. Part B Appl. Biomater.* **2011**, *98*, 8–17. [CrossRef]
55. Bigi, A.; Cojazzi, G.; Panzavolta, S.; Rubini, K.; Roveri, N. Mechanical and thermal properties of gelatin films at different degrees of glutaraldehyde crosslinking. *Biomaterials* **2001**, *22*, 763–768. [CrossRef]
56. Bigi, A.; Cojazzi, G.; Panzavolta, S.; Roveri, N.; Rubini, K. Stabilization of gelatin films by crosslinking with genipin. *Biomaterials* **2002**, *23*, 4827–4832. [CrossRef]
57. Yang, C.-F.; Yasukawa, T.; Kimura, H.; Miyamoto, H.; Honda, Y.; Tabata, Y.; Ikada, Y.; Ogura, Y. Experimental Corneal Neovascularization by Basic Fibroblast Growth Factor Incorporated into Gelatin Hydrogel. *Ophthalmic Res.* **2000**, *32*, 19–24. [CrossRef] [PubMed]
58. Doillon, C.J.; Watsky, M.A.; Hakim, M.; Wang, J.; Munger, R.; Laycock, N.; Osborne, R.; Griffith, M. A collagen-based scaf-fold for a tissue engineered human cornea: Physical and physiological properties. *Int. J. Artif. Organs* **2003**, *26*, 764–773. [CrossRef]
59. Lu, P.-L.; Lai, J.-Y.; Ma, D.H.-K.; Hsiue, G.-H. Carbodiimide cross-linked hyaluronic acid hydrogels as cell sheet delivery vehicles: Characterization and interaction with corneal endothelial cells. *J. Biomater. Sci. Polym. Ed.* **2008**, *19*, 1–18. [CrossRef]
60. Lai, J.-Y.; Ma, D.H.-K.; Cheng, H.-Y.; Sun, C.-C.; Huang, S.-J.; Li, Y.-T.; Hsiue, G.-H. Ocular Biocompatibility of Carbodiimide Cross-Linked Hyaluronic Acid Hydrogels for Cell Sheet Delivery Carriers. *J. Biomater. Sci. Polym. Ed.* **2010**, *21*, 359–376. [CrossRef] [PubMed]
61. Bentley, E.; Murphy, C.J.; Li, F.; Carlsson, D.J.; Griffith, M. Biosynthetic Corneal Substitute Implantation in Dogs. *Cornea* **2010**, *29*, 910–916. [CrossRef]
62. Kitagawa, K.; Okabe, M.; Yanagisawa, S.; Zhang, X.-Y.; Nikaido, T.; Hayashi, A. Use of a hyperdried cross-linked amniotic membrane as initial therapy for corneal perforations. *Jpn. J. Ophthalmol.* **2011**, *55*, 16–21. [CrossRef] [PubMed]
63. Calles, J.; Tártara, L.; López-García, A.; Diebold, Y.; Palma, S.; Vallés, E. Novel bioadhesive hyaluronan–itaconic acid crosslinked films for ocular therapy. *Int. J. Pharm.* **2013**, *455*, 48–56. [CrossRef] [PubMed]
64. Lai, J.-Y.; Ma, D.H.-K. Glutaraldehyde cross-linking of amniotic membranes affects their nanofibrous structures and limbal epithelial cell culture characteristics. *Int. J. Nanomed.* **2013**, *8*, 4157–4168. [CrossRef] [PubMed]
65. Nam, E.; Fujita, N.; Morita, M.; Tsuzuki, K.; Lin, H.Y.; Chung, C.S.; Nakagawa, T.; Nishimura, R. Comparison of the canine corneal epithelial cell sheets cultivated from limbal stem cells on canine amniotic membrane, atelocollagen gel, and temperature-responsive culture dish. *Veter Ophthalmol.* **2014**, *18*, 317–325. [CrossRef] [PubMed]
66. Yu, S.; Zhang, X.; Tan, G.; Tian, L.; Liu, D.; Liu, Y.; Yang, X.; Pan, W. A novel pH-induced thermosensitive hydrogel composed of carboxymethyl chitosan and poloxamer cross-linked by glutaraldehyde for ophthalmic drug delivery. *Carbohydr. Polym.* **2017**, *155*, 208–217. [CrossRef]
67. Rafat, M.; Griffith, M.; Hakim, M.; Muzakare, L.; Li, F.; Khulbe, K.; Matsuura, T. Plasma surface modification and characterization of collagen-based artificial cornea for enhanced epithelialization. *J. Appl. Polym. Sci.* **2007**, *106*, 2056–2064. [CrossRef]
68. Nicoletti, A.; Fiorini, M.; Paolillo, J.; Dolcini, L.; Sandri, M.; Pressato, D. Effects of different crosslinking conditions on the chemical–physical properties of a novel bio-inspired composite scaffold stabilised with 1,4-butanediol diglycidyl ether (BDDGE). *J. Mater. Sci. Mater. Med.* **2012**, *24*, 17–35. [CrossRef] [PubMed]
69. Wang, S.; Liu, W.; Han, B.; Yang, L. Study on a hydroxypropyl chitosan–gelatin based scaffold for corneal stroma tissue engineering. *Appl. Surf. Sci.* **2009**, *255*, 8701–8705. [CrossRef]
70. Koh, L.B.; Islam, M.M.; Mitra, D.; Noel, C.W.; Merrett, K.; Odorcic, S.; Fagerholm, P.; Jackson, W.B.; Liedberg, B.; Phopase, J.; et al. Epoxy Cross-Linked Collagen and Collagen-Laminin Peptide Hydrogels as Corneal Substitutes. *J. Funct. Biomater.* **2013**, *4*, 162–177. [CrossRef] [PubMed]
71. Butler, M.F.; Ng, Y.-F.; Pudney, P.D.A. Mechanism and kinetics of the crosslinking reaction between biopolymers containing primary amine groups and genipin. *J. Polym. Sci. Part A Polym. Chem.* **2003**, *41*, 3941–3953. [CrossRef]
72. Tonda-Turo, C.; Gentile, P.; Saracino, S.; Chiono, V.; Nandagiri, V.; Muzio, G.; Canuto, R.; Ciardelli, G. Comparative analysis of gelatin scaffolds crosslinked by genipin and silane coupling agent. *Int. J. Biol. Macromol.* **2011**, *49*, 700–706. [CrossRef]
73. Madhavan, K.; Belchenko, D.; Motta, A.; Tan, W. Evaluation of composition and crosslinking effects on collagen-based composite constructs. *Acta Biomater.* **2010**, *6*, 1413–1422. [CrossRef]
74. Fessel, G.; Cadby, J.; Wunderli, S.; van Weeren, R.; Snedeker, J.G. Dose- and time-dependent effects of genipin crosslinking on cell viability and tissue mechanics—Toward clinical application for tendon repair. *Acta Biomater.* **2014**, *10*, 1897–1906. [CrossRef] [PubMed]

75. Grolik, M.; Szczubiałka, K.; Wowra, B.; Dobrowolski, D.; Orzechowska-Wylęgała, B.; Wylęgała, E.; Nowakowska, M. Hydrogel membranes based on genipin-cross-linked chitosan blends for corneal epithelium tissue engineering. *J. Mater. Sci. Mater. Med.* **2012**, *23*, 1991–2000. [CrossRef] [PubMed]
76. Li, Y.-H.; Cheng, C.-Y.; Wang, N.-K.; Tan, H.-Y.; Tsai, Y.-J.; Hsiao, C.-H.; Ma, D.H.-K.; Yeh, L.-K. Characterization of the modified chitosan membrane cross-linked with genipin for the cultured corneal epithelial cells. *Colloids Surf. B Biointerfaces* **2015**, *126*, 237–244. [CrossRef] [PubMed]
77. Yu, Y.; Feng, R.; Li, J.; Wang, Y.; Song, Y.; Tan, G.; Liu, D.; Liu, W.; Yang, X.; Pan, H.; et al. A hybrid genipin-crosslinked dual-sensitive hydrogel/nanostructured lipid carrier ocular drug delivery platform. *Asian J. Pharm. Sci.* **2019**, *14*, 423–434. [CrossRef]
78. Nam, K.; Kimura, T.; Kishida, A. Controlling Coupling Reaction of EDC and NHS for Preparation of Collagen Gels Using Ethanol/Water Co-Solvents. *Macromol. Biosci.* **2008**, *8*, 32–37. [CrossRef] [PubMed]
79. Cammarata, C.R.; Hughes, M.E.; Ofner, C.M. Carbodiimide Induced Cross-Linking, Ligand Addition, and Degradation in Gelatin. *Mol. Pharm.* **2015**, *12*, 783–793. [CrossRef]
80. Bax, D.V.; Davidenko, N.; Gullberg, D.; Hamaia, S.W.; Farndale, R.W.; Best, S.M.; Cameron, R.E. Fundamental insight into the effect of carbodiimide crosslinking on cellular recognition of collagen-based scaffolds. *Acta Biomater.* **2017**, *49*, 218–234. [CrossRef] [PubMed]
81. Damink, L.O.; Dijkstra, P.J.; Van Luyn, M.; Van Wachem, P.; Nieuwenhuis, P.; Feijen, J. Cross-linking of dermal sheep collagen using a water-soluble carbodiimide. *Biomaterials* **1996**, *17*, 765–773. [CrossRef]
82. Pieper, J.; Hafmans, T.; Veerkamp, J.; Van Kuppevelt, T. Development of tailor-made collagen–glycosaminoglycan matrices: EDC/NHS crosslinking, and ultrastructural aspects. *Biomaterials* **2000**, *21*, 581–593. [CrossRef]
83. Davidenko, N.; Schuster, C.; Bax, D.; Raynal, N.; Farndale, R.; Best, S.; Cameron, R. Control of crosslinking for tailoring collagen-based scaffolds stability and mechanics. *Acta Biomater.* **2015**, *25*, 131–142. [CrossRef]
84. Liu, W.; Merrett, K.; Griffith, M.; Fagerholm, P.; Dravida, S.; Heyne, B.; Scaiano, J.C.; Watsky, M.A.; Shinozaki, N.; Lagali, N.; et al. Recombinant human collagen for tissue engineered corneal substitutes. *Biomaterials* **2008**, *29*, 1147–1158. [CrossRef] [PubMed]
85. Rafat, M.; Li, F.; Fagerholm, P.; Lagali, N.S.; Watsky, M.A.; Munger, R.; Matsuura, T.; Griffith, M. PEG-stabilized carbodiimide crosslinked collagen–chitosan hydrogels for corneal tissue engineering. *Biomaterials* **2008**, *29*, 3960–3972. [CrossRef]
86. Liu, W.; Deng, C.; McLaughlin, C.R.; Fagerholm, P.; Lagali, N.S.; Heyne, B.; Scaiano, J.C.; Watsky, M.A.; Kato, Y.; Munger, R.; et al. Collagen–phosphorylcholine interpenetrating network hydrogels as corneal substitutes. *Biomaterials* **2009**, *30*, 1551–1559. [CrossRef] [PubMed]
87. Ma, D.H.-K.; Lai, J.-Y.; Cheng, H.-Y.; Tsai, C.-C.; Yeh, L.-K. Carbodiimide cross-linked amniotic membranes for cultivation of limbal epithelial cells. *Biomaterials* **2010**, *31*, 6647–6658. [CrossRef]
88. Lai, J.-Y. Hyaluronic acid concentration-mediated changes in structure and function of porous carriers for corneal endothelial cell sheet delivery. *Mater. Sci. Eng. C* **2016**, *59*, 411–419. [CrossRef]
89. Lai, J.Y.; Cheng, H.Y.; Ma, D.H.K. Investigation of overrun-processed porous hyaluronic acid carriers in corneal endo-thelial tissue engineering. *PLoS ONE* **2015**, *10*, e0136067. [CrossRef]
90. Goodarzi, H.; Jadidi, K.; Pourmotabed, S.; Sharifi, E.; Aghamollaei, H. Preparation and in vitro characterization of cross-linked collagen–gelatin hydrogel using EDC/NHS for corneal tissue engineering applications. *Int. J. Biol. Macromol.* **2019**, *126*, 620–632. [CrossRef]
91. Duan, X.; Sheardown, H. Dendrimer crosslinked collagen as a corneal tissue engineering scaffold: Mechanical properties and corneal epithelial cell interactions. *Biomaterials* **2006**, *27*, 4608–4617. [CrossRef]
92. Myung, D.; Koh, W.; Bakri, A.; Zhang, F.; Marshall, A.; Ko, J.; Noolandi, J.; Carrasco, M.; Cochran, J.R.; Frank, C.W.; et al. Design and fabrication of an artificial cornea based on a photolithographically patterned hydrogel construct. *Biomed. Microdevices* **2007**, *9*, 911–922. [CrossRef]
93. Farooqui, N.; Myung, D.; Koh, W.; Masek, R.; Dalal, M.; Carrasco, M.R.; Noolandi, J.; Frank, C.W.; Ta, C.N. Histological processing of ph-sensitive hydrogels used in corneal implant applications. *J. Histotechnol.* **2007**, *30*, 157–163. [CrossRef]
94. Myung, D.; Farooqui, N.; Zheng, L.L.; Koh, W.; Gupta, S.; Bakri, A.; Noolandi, J.; Cochran, J.R.; Frank, C.W.; Ta, C.N. Bioactive interpenetrating polymer network hydrogels that support corneal epithelial wound healing. *J. Biomed. Mater. Res. Part A* **2009**, *90*, 70–81. [CrossRef]
95. Merrett, K.; Liu, W.; Mitra, D.; Camm, K.D.; McLaughlin, C.R.; Liu, Y.; Watsky, M.A.; Li, F.; Griffith, M.; Fogg, D.E. Synthetic neoglycopolymer-recombinant human collagen hybrids as biomimetic crosslinking agents in corneal tissue engineering. *Biomaterials* **2009**, *30*, 5403. [CrossRef]
96. Liang, Y.; Liu, W.; Han, B.; Yang, C.; Ma, Q.; Song, F.; Bi, Q. An in situ formed biodegradable hydrogel for reconstruction of the corneal endothelium. *Colloids Surf. B Biointerfaces* **2011**, *82*, 1–7. [CrossRef] [PubMed]
97. Park, S.; Nam, S.H.; Koh, W.-G. Preparation of collagen-immobilized poly(ethylene glycol)/poly(2-hydroxyethyl methacrylate) interpenetrating network hydrogels for potential application of artificial cornea. *J. Appl. Polym. Sci.* **2011**, *123*, 637–645. [CrossRef]
98. Ozcelik, B.; Brown, K.D.; Blencowe, A.; Daniell, M.; Stevens, G.W.; Qiao, G.G. Ultrathin chitosan–poly(ethylene glycol) hydrogel films for corneal tissue engineering. *Acta Biomater.* **2013**, *9*, 6594–6605. [CrossRef] [PubMed]
99. Xiang, J.; Sun, J.; Hong, J.; Wang, W.; Wei, A.; Le, Q.; Xu, J. T-style keratoprosthesis based on surface-modified poly (2-hydroxyethyl methacrylate) hydrogel for cornea repairs. *Mater. Sci. Eng. C* **2015**, *50*, 274–285. [CrossRef]

100. Lei, L.; Li, X.; Xiong, T.; Yu, J.; Yu, X.; Song, Z.; Li, X. Covalently Cross-Linked Chitosan Hydrogel Sheet for Topical Ophthalmic Delivery of Levofloxacin. *J. Biomed. Nanotechnol.* **2018**, *14*, 371–378. [CrossRef] [PubMed]
101. Sani, E.S.; Kheirkhah, A.; Rana, D.; Sun, Z.M.; Foulsham, W.; Sheikhi, A.; Khademhosseini, A.; Dana, R.; Annabi, N. Su-tureless repair of corneal injuries using naturally derived bioadhesive hydrogels. *Sci. Adv.* **2019**, *5*, eaav1281. [CrossRef]
102. Lai, J.-Y. Biocompatibility of Genipin and Glutaraldehyde Cross-Linked Chitosan Materials in the Anterior Chamber of the Eye. *Int. J. Mol. Sci.* **2012**, *13*, 10970–10985. [CrossRef]
103. Ahn, J.-I.; Kuffova, L.; Merrett, K.; Mitra, D.; Forrester, J.V.; Li, F.; Griffith, M. Crosslinked collagen hydrogels as corneal implants: Effects of sterically bulky vs. non-bulky carbodiimides as crosslinkers. *Acta Biomater.* **2013**, *9*, 7796–7805. [CrossRef] [PubMed]
104. Wang, K.; Han, Z. Injectable hydrogels for ophthalmic applications. *J. Control. Release* **2017**, *268*, 212–224. [CrossRef] [PubMed]
105. Overstreet, D.J.; Dutta, D.; Stabenfeldt, S.E.; Vernon, B.L. Injectable hydrogels. *J. Polym. Sci. Part B Polym. Phys.* **2012**, *50*, 881–903. [CrossRef]
106. Li, Y.L.; Rodrigues, J.; Tomas, H. Injectable and biodegradable hydrogels: Gelation, biodegradation and biomedical ap-plications. *Chem. Soc. Rev.* **2012**, *41*, 2193–2221. [CrossRef]
107. Yang, J.-A.; Yeom, J.; Hwang, B.W.; Hoffman, A.S.; Hahn, S.K. In situ-forming injectable hydrogels for regenerative medicine. *Prog. Polym. Sci.* **2014**, *39*, 1973–1986. [CrossRef]
108. Hoffman, A.S. Hydrogels for biomedical applications. *Adv. Drug Deliv. Rev.* **2002**, *54*, 3–12. [CrossRef]
109. Ulijn, R.V.; Bibi, N.; Jayawarna, V.; Thornton, P.D.; Todd, S.J.; Mart, R.J.; Smith, A.M.; Gough, J.E. Bioresponsive hydro-gels. *Mater. Today* **2007**, *10*, 40–48. [CrossRef]
110. Xinming, L.; Yingde, C.; Lloyd, A.W.; Mikhalovsky, S.V.; Sandeman, S.R.; Howel, C.A.; Liewen, L. Polymeric hydrogels for novel contact lens-based ophthalmic drug delivery systems: A review. *Contact Lens Anterior Eye* **2008**, *31*, 57–64. [CrossRef]
111. Chien, Y.; Liao, Y.W.; Liu, D.M.; Lin, H.L.; Chen, S.J.; Chen, H.L.; Peng, C.H.; Liang, C.M.; Mou, C.Y.; Chiou, H. Corneal repair by human corneal keratocyte-reprogrammed ipscs and amphiphatic carboxymethyl-hexanoyl chitosan hy-drogel. *Biomaterials* **2012**, *33*, 8003–8016. [CrossRef]
112. Garagorri, N.; Fermanian, S.; Thibault, R.; Ambrose, W.M.; Schein, O.D.; Chakravarti, S.; Elisseeff, J. Keratocyte behavior in three-dimensional photopolymerizable poly(ethylene glycol) hydrogels. *Acta Biomater.* **2008**, *4*, 1139–1147. [CrossRef] [PubMed]
113. McTiernan, C.D.; Simpson, F.C.; Haagdorens, M.; Samarawickrama, C.; Hunter, D.; Buznyk, O.; Fagerholm, P.; Ljunggren, M.K.; Lewis, P.; Pintelon, I.; et al. LiQD Cornea: Pro-regeneration collagen mimetics as patches and alternatives to corneal transplantation. *Sci. Adv.* **2020**, *6*, eaba2187. [CrossRef] [PubMed]
114. Anumolu, S.S.; DeSantis, A.S.; Menjoge, A.R.; Hahn, R.A.; Beloni, J.A.; Gordon, M.K.; Sinko, P.J. Doxycycline loaded poly(ethylene glycol) hydrogels for healing vesicant-induced ocular wounds. *Biomaterials* **2010**, *31*, 964–974. [CrossRef] [PubMed]
115. Pratoomsoot, C.; Tanioka, H.; Hori, K.; Kawasaki, S.; Kinoshita, S.; Tighe, P.J.; Dua, H.; Shakesheff, K.M.; Rose, F.R.A. A thermo-versible hydrogel as a biosynthetic bandage for corneal wound repair. *Biomaterials* **2008**, *29*, 272–281. [CrossRef] [PubMed]
116. Fanesi, G.; Abrami, M.; Zecchin, F.; Giassi, I.; Dal Ferro, E.; Boisen, A.; Grassi, G.; Bertoncin, P.; Grassi, M.; Marizza, P. Com-bined used of rheology and lf-nmr for the characterization of pvp-alginates gels containing liposomes. *Pharm. Res.* **2018**, *35*, 1–11. [CrossRef] [PubMed]
117. Ahearne, M.; Yang, Y.; El Haj, A.J.; Then, K.Y.; Liu, K.-K. Characterizing the viscoelastic properties of thin hydrogel-based constructs for tissue engineering applications. *J. R. Soc. Interface* **2005**, *2*, 455–463. [CrossRef]
118. Wen, J.H.; Vincent, L.G.; Fuhrmann, A.; Choi, Y.S.; Hribar, K.C.; Taylor-Weiner, H.; Chen, S.; Engler, A.J. Interplay of matrix stiffness and protein tethering in stem cell differentiation. *Nat. Mater.* **2014**, *13*, 979–987. [CrossRef]
119. Ahearne, M.; Wilson, S.L.; Liu, K.-K.; Rauz, S.; El Haj, A.J.; Yang, Y. Influence of cell and collagen concentration on the cell–matrix mechanical relationship in a corneal stroma wound healing model. *Exp. Eye Res.* **2010**, *91*, 584–591. [CrossRef]
120. Li, X.; Zhang, J.; Kawazoe, N.; Chen, G. Fabrication of highly crosslinked gelatin hydrogel and its influence on chondro-cyte proliferation and phenotype. *Polymers* **2017**, *9*, 309. [CrossRef]
121. Kharkar, P.M.; Kiick, K.L.; Kloxin, A.M. Designing degradable hydrogels for orthogonal control of cell microenviron-ments. *Chem. Soc. Rev.* **2013**, *42*, 7335–7372. [CrossRef]
122. Bryant, S.J.; Bender, R.J.; Durand, K.L.; Anseth, K.S. Encapsulating chondrocytes in degrading PEG hydrogels with high modulus: Engineering gel structural changes to facilitate cartilaginous tissue production. *Biotechnol. Bioeng.* **2004**, *86*, 747–755. [CrossRef] [PubMed]
123. Li, X.; Sun, Q.; Li, Q.; Kawazoe, N.; Chen, G. Functional hydrogels with tunable structures and properties for tissue engi-neering applications. *Front. Chem.* **2018**, *6*, 499. [CrossRef]
124. Richbourg, N.R.; Peppas, N.A. The swollen polymer network hypothesis: Quantitative models of hydrogel swelling, stiffness, and solute transport. *Prog. Polym. Sci.* **2020**, *105*, 101243. [CrossRef]
125. Dai, W.; Barbari, T. Hydrogel membranes with mesh size asymmetry based on the gradient crosslinking of poly(vinyl alcohol). *J. Membr. Sci.* **1999**, *156*, 67–79. [CrossRef]
126. Peppas, N.A.; Hilt, J.Z.; Khademhosseini, A.; Langer, R. Hydrogels in Biology and Medicine: From Molecular Principles to Bionanotechnology. *Adv. Mater.* **2006**, *18*, 1345–1360. [CrossRef]
127. Aimetti, A.A.; Machen, A.J.; Anseth, K.S. Poly(ethylene glycol) hydrogels formed by thiol-ene photopolymerization for enzyme-responsive protein delivery. *Biomaterials* **2009**, *30*, 6048–6054. [CrossRef]

128. Hu, W.; Wang, Z.; Xiao, Y.; Zhang, S.; Wang, J. Advances in crosslinking strategies of biomedical hydrogels. *Biomater. Sci.* **2019**, *7*, 843–855. [CrossRef] [PubMed]
129. Lu, S.; Lam, J.; Trachtenberg, J.E.; Lee, E.J.; Seyednejad, H.; van den Beucken, J.J.J.P.; Tabata, Y.; Wong, M.E.; Jansen, J.A.; Mikos, A.G.; et al. Dual growth factor delivery from bilayered, biodegradable hydrogel composites for spatially-guided osteochondral tissue repair. *Biomaterials* **2014**, *35*, 8829–8839. [CrossRef] [PubMed]
130. Hadjipanayi, E.; Ananta, M.; Binkowski, M.; Streeter, I.; Lu, Z.; Cui, Z.F.; Brown, R.A.; Mudera, V. Mechanisms of structure generation during plastic compression of nanofibrillar collagen hydrogel scaffolds: Towards engineering of collagen. *J. Tissue Eng. Regen. Med.* **2010**, *5*, 505–519. [CrossRef] [PubMed]
131. Cheema, U.; Brown, R.A. Rapid Fabrication of Living Tissue Models by Collagen Plastic Compression: Understanding Three-Dimensional Cell Matrix Repair In Vitro. *Adv. Wound Care* **2013**, *2*, 176–184. [CrossRef] [PubMed]
132. Torbet, J.; Ronzière, M.C. Magnetic alignment of collagen during self-assembly. *Biochem. J.* **1984**, *219*, 1057–1059. [CrossRef] [PubMed]
133. Torbet, J.; Malbouyres, M.; Builles, N.; Justin, V.; Roulet, M.; Damour, O.; Oldberg, A.; Ruggiero, F.; Hulmes, D.J. Orthogo-nal scaffold of magnetically aligned collagen lamellae for corneal stroma reconstruction. *Biomaterials* **2007**, *28*, 4268–4276. [CrossRef]
134. Panteli, P.A.; Patrickios, C.S. Multiply Interpenetrating Polymer Networks: Preparation, Mechanical Properties, and Applications. *Gels* **2019**, *5*, 36. [CrossRef]
135. Krishnakumar, G.S.; Sampath, S.; Muthusamy, S.; John, M.A. Importance of crosslinking strategies in designing smart biomaterials for bone tissue engineering: A systematic review. *Mater. Sci. Eng. C* **2019**, *96*, 941–954. [CrossRef]
136. Martínez, A.; Blanco, M.; Davidenko, N.; Cameron, R. Tailoring chitosan/collagen scaffolds for tissue engineering: Effect of composition and different crosslinking agents on scaffold properties. *Carbohydr. Polym.* **2015**, *132*, 606–619. [CrossRef]
137. Khor, E. Methods for the treatment of collagenous tissues for bioprostheses. *Biomaterials* **1997**, *18*, 95–105. [CrossRef]
138. Casali, D.M.; Yost, M.J.; Matthews, M.A. Eliminating glutaraldehyde from crosslinked collagen films using supercritical CO_2. *J. Biomed. Mater. Res. Part A* **2018**, *106*, 86–94. [CrossRef]
139. Yamazaki, M.; Chiba, K.; Mohri, T.; Hatanaka, H. Activation of the mitogen-activated protein kinase cascade through nitric oxide synthesis as a mechanism of neuritogenic effect of genipin in PC12h cells. *J. Neurochem.* **2008**, *79*, 45–54. [CrossRef] [PubMed]
140. Kim, B.-C.; Kim, H.-G.; Lee, S.-A.; Lim, S.; Park, E.-H.; Kim, S.-J.; Lim, C.-J. Genipin-induced apoptosis in hepatoma cells is mediated by reactive oxygen species/c-Jun NH2-terminal kinase-dependent activation of mitochondrial pathway. *Biochem. Pharmacol.* **2005**, *70*, 1398–1407. [CrossRef] [PubMed]
141. Kirchhof, S.; Goepferich, A.M.; Brandl, F.P. Hydrogels in ophthalmic applications. *Eur. J. Pharm. Biopharm.* **2015**, *95*, 227–238. [CrossRef] [PubMed]
142. Hammer, N.; Brandl, F.P.; Kirchhof, S.; Messmann, V.; Goepferich, A.M. Protein Compatibility of Selected Cross-linking Reactions for Hydrogels. *Macromol. Biosci.* **2015**, *15*, 405–413. [CrossRef]
143. Zhang, B.; Xue, Q.; Li, J.; Ma, L.; Yao, Y.; Ye, H.; Cui, Z.; Yang, H. 3d bioprinting for artificial cornea: Challenges and perspectives. *Med. Eng. Phys.* **2019**, *71*, 68–78. [CrossRef] [PubMed]
144. Sorkio, A.; Koch, L.; Koivusalo, L.; Deiwick, A.; Miettinen, S.; Chichkov, B.; Skottman, H. Human stem cell based corneal tissue mimicking structures using laser-assisted 3D bioprinting and functional bioinks. *Biomaterials* **2018**, *171*, 57–71. [CrossRef] [PubMed]
145. Isaacson, A.; Swioklo, S.; Connon, C.J. 3D bioprinting of a corneal stroma equivalent. *Exp. Eye Res.* **2018**, *173*, 188–193. [CrossRef] [PubMed]
146. Campos, D.F.D.; Rohde, M.; Ross, M.; Anvari, P.; Blaeser, A.; Vogt, M.; Panfil, C.; Yam, G.H.; Mehta, J.S.; Fischer, H.; et al. Corneal bioprinting utilizing collagen-based bioinks and primary human keratocytes. *J. Biomed. Mater. Res. Part A* **2019**, *107*, 1945–1953. [CrossRef] [PubMed]

Article

MPC Polymer Promotes Recovery from Dry Eye via Stabilization of the Ocular Surface

Noriaki Nagai [1,*], **Shunsuke Sakurai** [2], **Ryotaro Seiriki** [1], **Misa Minami** [1], **Mizuki Yamaguchi** [1], **Saori Deguchi** [1] and **Eiji Harata** [2]

1. Faculty of Pharmacy, Kindai University, 3-4-1 Kowakae, Higashi-Osaka, Osaka 577-8502, Japan; 1611610157u@kindai.ac.jp (R.S.); 2033420004w@kindai.ac.jp (M.M.); 2033420005s@kindai.ac.jp (M.Y.); 2045110002h@kindai.ac.jp (S.D.)
2. Life Science Products Division, NOF Corporation, Yebisu Garden Place Tower, 20-3 Ebisu 4-chome, Shibuya-ku, Tokyo 150-6019, Japan; shunsuke_sakurai@nof.co.jp (S.S.); eiji_harata@nof.co.jp (E.H.)
* Correspondence: nagai_n@phar.kindai.ac.jp; Tel.: +81-6-4307-3638

Abstract: The polymer that includes 2-methacryloyloxy ethyl phosphorylcholine (MPC) is well-known as an effectively hydrating multifunction agent. In this study, we prepared an MPC polymer (MPCP) using radical polymerization with co-monomers—MPC/Stearyl Methacrylate/N,N-dimethylacrylamide—and evaluated the MPCP's usefulness for dry eye treatment using a rabbit model treated with N-acetylcysteine. The MPCP particle size was 50–250 nm, and the form was similar to that of micelles. The MPCP viscosity (approximately 0.95 mPa·s) was 1.17-fold that of purified water, and a decrease in the transepithelial electrical resistance value (corneal damage) was not observed in the immortalized human corneal epithelial cell line HCE-T cell (HCE-T cell layer). The MPCP enhanced the water maintenance on the cornea, and the instillation of MPCP increased the lacrimal fluid volume and prolonged the tear film breakup time without an increase in total mucin contents in the lacrimal fluid of the normal rabbits. The therapeutic potential of the MPCP for dry eye was evaluated using an N-acetylcysteine-treated rabbit model, and, in our investigation, we found that MPCP enhanced the volume of lacrimal fluid and promoted an improvement in the tear film breakup levels. These findings regarding the creation and characteristics of a novel MPCP will provide relevant information for designing further studies to develop a treatment for dry eyes.

Keywords: MPC polymer; dry eye; ocular surface; lacrimal fluid; mucin

1. Introduction

Dry eye disease is a complex and multifactorial ocular disease, and tear film instability, visual disturbance, and discomfort are commonly observed, with potential damage to the ocular surface [1]. It was reported that dry eye disease has multiple causes, such as air pollution, medication, androgen deficiency, contact lens usage, and excessive computer use [2]. Inflammation and enhanced osmolarity on the ocular surface are also important factors in the onset of dry eye disease [3]. It has also been reported that oxidant stress and aging are other factors that contribute to dry eye disease [4]. The prevalence of dry eye disease is estimated at approximately 5–50% of the global adult population [5], and it is expected that the economic burden from the disease will increase as the population ages [6].

Current treatments for dry eye disease aim to prevent the objective signs and clinical symptoms of the disease and recover the quality of life of the patients. The main approved treatments are as follows: Mucosta® (rebamipide ophthalmic suspension 2%, Otsuka Pharmaceutical, Tokyo, Japan) and Diquas® (diquafosol ophthalmic solution 3%, Santen Pharmaceutical, Osaka, Japan) in Asia; Xiidra® (lifitegrast ophthalmic solution 5.0%, Shire, Lexington, KY, USA) and Restasis® (Cyclosporine ophthalmic emulsion 0.05%, Allergan,

Irvine, CA, USA) in North America; and Ikervis® (CsA cationic emulsion, Santen Pharmaceutical, Osaka, Japan) in Europe. In addition, Cequa™ (ananomicellar formulation of CsA 0.09%, Sun Pharmaceuticals, Mumbai, India) has been used in the US since 2018. Cequa™ enhances lacrimal fluid production in patients with dry eye disease. Overall, these medicines are used to stabilize the tear film and/or prevent the inflammation of the ocular surface [7].

The polymer including 2-methacryloyloxy ethyl phosphorylcholine (MPC) is well-known for being not only an antiadhesive and antithrombogenetic agent, but also a significant hydrating multifunction agent [8–10]. These characteristics are due to the polymer's phosphorylcholine group and the water structure surrounding the polar group. To date, soft contact lenses containing this MPC have been approved by the Food and Drug Administration (FDA) and Pharmaceuticals and Medical Devices Agency (PMDA). Hall et al. have reported that the dehydration of this soft contact lens is significantly less than that of other conventional lenses [11]. Eye drops, soft contact lens care products, oral care products, and cosmetics containing the MPC-BMA polymer have also been approved by the PMDA. Ayaki et al. reported that, after treatment with eye drops containing MPC polymer (MPC-BMA), cell viability rates were maintained at over 80%. Moreover, the conformation of proteins did not change, even when they were adsorbed on the surface or came into contact with the surface, and were similar to those of clinically approved artificial tear products [12]. In this way, the polymer including MPC, which is significantly hydrating and safe, could be used to improve the ocular surface and treat dry eye disease with the potential to be added to dry-eye drugs.

In this study, we prepared a novel MPC polymer using radical polymerization with co-monomers, MPC/stearyl methacrylate/N,N-dimethylacrylamide (MPCP), and evaluated the polymer's usefulness for dry eye treatment using a rabbit model treated with N-acetylcysteine.

2. Materials and Methods

2.1. Animals

Male adult rabbits (weight 2.58 ± 0.75 kg) were obtained from Shimizu Laboratory Supplies Co., Ltd. (Kyoto, Japan), and the protocol was approved by the Kindai University (KAPS-31-002, 1 April 2019). The experiments using the rabbits were performed according to the Association for Research in Vision and Ophthalmology (ARVO) and Kindai University guidelines. Thirty microliters of 0.1% MPCP were instilled in single applications at 14:00 h. For repeat applications, 0.1% MPCP (30 µL) was instilled once a day (14:00 h) for 5 days, and the measurement of the levels of lacrimal fluid, mucin, tear film breakup time (TBUT), ocular surface, and tear film breakup began at 16:00 h (single application) and 18:00 h (repetitive application). The dry eye model using rabbits was conducted via the instillation (30 µL) of 10% N-acetylcysteine six times per day (at 9:00, 11:00, 13:00, 15:00, 17:00, and 19:00 h). This protocol was performed following our previous report [13].

2.2. Chemicals

Dulbecco's modified Eagle's medium/Ham's F12, penicillin, streptomycin, and fetal bovine serum were provided from GIBCO (Tokyo, Japan). Cell Count Reagent SF was purchased from Nacalai Tesque, Inc. (Kyoto, Japan), and the Tear mucin assay ELISA kit was obtained from Cosmo Bio Co., Ltd. (Tokyo, Japan). Transwell-Clear™ (polyester filters, surface area 1.0 cm^2 and 0.4 µm pore size) and rat tail collagen type 1 were purchased from Costar (Cambridge, MA, USA) and Sigma (Tokyo, Japan), respectively. All other chemicals used were of the highest purity commercially available.

2.3. Preparation of MPCP

MPCP was obtained via radical polymerization with co-monomers, MPC/stearyl methacrylate/N,N-dimethylacrylamide, with a composition ratio of 50:5:45, and purified using the dialysis method. After polymerization, we measured the residual monomers and calculated that the conversion rate of this polymer in each monomer was >99%. We thus confirmed that the target polymer was obtained. In this study, we used MPCP diluted to a 1% aqueous solution with purified water. To confirm the MPCP concentration of the aqueous solution, we studied the residue upon drying. The structural formula of the MPCP is illustrated in Figure 1.

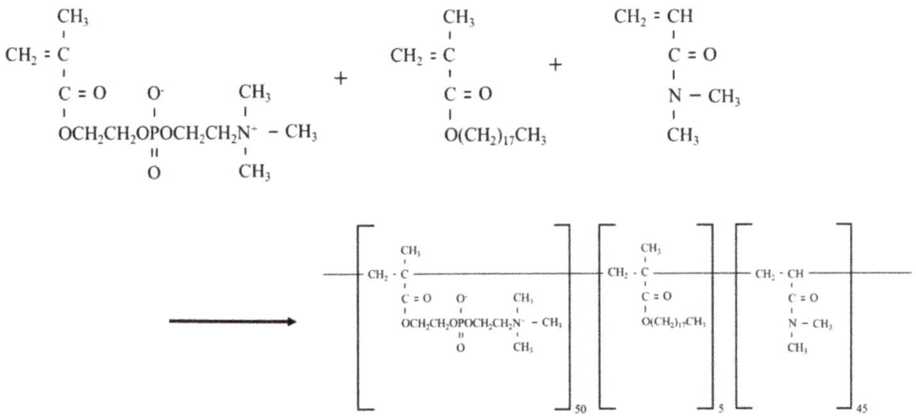

Figure 1. The structural formula for MPCP in this study. The MPCP based on MPC/stearyl methacrylate/N,N-dimethylacrylamide was prepared via radical polymerization. MPC—2-methacryloyloxy ethyl phosphorylcholine; MPCP—MPC polymer.

2.4. Measurement of Characteristics in MPCP

A NANOSIGHT LM10 (Quantum Design Japan, Tokyo, Japan) was used to measure the size and number of MPCP nanoparticles—the measurement was performed for 60 s at 405 nm. Atomic force microscopy (AFM) images were obtained via an A SPM-9700 (Shimadzu Corp., Kyoto, Japan), and AFM images were created by combining the phase and height images. The viscosity of MPCP was measured with an SV-1A at 10–40 °C (A&D Company, Limited, Tokyo, Japan) [14]. To confirm the wettability, defined as the tendency of one fluid to spread on or adhere to a solid surface, we performed contact angle measurements in 0.1% MPCP and 0.1% MPC-BMA aqueous solutions. In total, 1 µL of each of the 0.1% MPCP and 0.1% MPC-BMA aqueous solutions (or purified water as a control) was dropped onto a slide glass, and the contact angle was measured using a contact angle meter (DropMaster500, Kyowa Interface Science Co., Ltd., Saitama, Japan).

2.5. Cell Culture and Treatment

The immortalized human corneal epithelial cell line (HCE-T cell) used in this study were developed by Araki-Sasaki et al. [15]. The HCE-T cells were cultured in Dulbecco's modified Eagle's medium/Ham's F12 with heat-inactivated fetal bovine serum (5%), penicillin (1000 IU/mL), and streptomycin (0.1 mg/mL).

2.6. Measurement of Cell Adhesion

The MPCP treatment was carried out by seeding HCE-T cells (1×10^4 cells) in a culture medium containing 0.1% MPCP and incubating the medium for 12 h. Then, a Cell Count Reagent SF was added, and the absorbance (Abs) at 450 nm was measured according to the manufacturer's protocol. The Cell Count Reagent SF is based on the conversion of the reagent to formazan salts according to mitochondrial activity and, as a metabolic assay, is related to the cell number and its metabolic state and efficiency. Therefore, the cell number was also measured via counting under a microscope (Olympus Corporation, Tokyo, Japan), and the cell adhesion was evaluated using a combination of data on the cell number and Cell Count Reagent SF. The cell adhesion (%) was represented as the Abs ratio of the MPCP treatment and non-treatment [16].

2.7. Measurement of Cell Proliferation

The cell cultures were treated with MPCP 1 d after seeding (1×10^4 cells) by changing to a culture medium with 0.1% MPCP and incubating the medium for 24 h. Then, the Cell Count Reagent SF was added, and the Abs at 450 nm was measured according to the manufacturer's protocol. Cell proliferation (%) was recorded as the Abs ratio of the MPCP treatment and non-treatment [16]. The cell proliferation was also evaluated by a combination of the data on the cell number and Cell Count Reagent SF in this study.

2.8. Preparation of HCE-T Cell Layer Model

The cell layer models (multilayer) consisting of one cell (only HCE-T cells) were cultured by following our previous reports [17,18]. The HCE-T cells were seeded onto Transwell-Clear^{TM} (90,000 cells/cm^2) coated with rat tail collagen type 1 (71.5 µg/cm^2) and grown for seven days until the cells reached confluency. The HCE-T cells were then exposed to an air–liquid interface for two weeks with the culture medium containing the vehicle or 0.1% MPCP replaced every other day. In this process, 50 µL of the medium solution with or without MPCP was dropped onto the donor side twice a day (9:00 and 19:00 h) so that the donor would not dry completely. In this study, chopstick electrodes connected to an epithelial Volt–Ohm meter Millicell-ERS (Millipore Co., Bedford, MA, USA) were used to measure the transepithelial electrical resistance (TER) and followed the differentiation stages during cultivation.

2.9. Cell Toxicity of MPCP

Differentiated cells with TER values greater than 350 Ω·cm^2 were used for the cell toxicity analysis. The HCE-T cell layer model was treated with the vehicle and 0.1% MPCP, and the changes in TER values were measured for 60 min [17].

2.10. Measurement of Water Retention in the Cornea

The rabbits were euthanized by injecting a lethal dose of pentobarbital, and the corneas were carefully separated from other ocular tissues. The individual corneas were treated with the vehicle, 0.1% MPC-BMA, and 0.1% MPCP for 1 min. After that, the cornea was placed on a plastic cell, and the changes in the weight and number of MPCP particles were measured at 22 °C. In this study, the changes in weight were expressed as water retention in the cornea. Moreover, the samples (vehicle, MPC-BMA, and MPCP) on the cornea were collected by pipette, and the number of MPCP particles in the samples was measured with NANOSIGHT LM10, as described above.

2.11. Monitoring the Ocular Surface of Rabbits Instilled with MPCP

The ocular surface was monitored by using a dry eye monitor DR-1 (KOWA Co., LTD., Aichi, Japan), and the TBUT and changes in the ocular surface were monitored following our previous study [13]. Each rabbit treated with a fluorescein strip was allowed to blink several times to distribute the fluorescein. The time from the opening of the eyes to the appearance of the first dry spot in the central cornea was analyzed. The changes in tear film after blinking were monitored by the dry eye monitor DR-1. The TBUT and the tear film breakup level changes in the ocular surface were evaluated 2 h (16:00 h) and 4 h (18:00 h) after the application of the MPCP, respectively. The tear film breakup levels (area) were measured 2 s after the last blink using the Image J software (ver. 1.51, NIH, USA), and the measurement was performed three times; the mean was used as the value.

2.12. Lacrimal Fluid and Mucin Levels in Rabbits Instilled with MPCP

The volume of lacrimal fluid in rabbits instilled with MPCP was measured using Schirmer tear test strips (AYUMI Pharmaceutical Corporation, Tokyo, Japan), and the mucin was measured using a Tear mucin assay ELISA kit according to the manufacturer's instructions. Briefly, lacrimal fluid was collected with Schirmer tear test strips, and the Schirmer tear test strips were added into elution buffer of a tear mucin assay ELISA kit to extract the mucin. After that, the extracted mucin was measured by the Tear mucin assay ELISA kit, and a fluorescence microplate reader (Absorption/Emission = 336/383 nm) [13]. The mucin levels in the total lacrimal fluid volume of the eye are expressed as total mucin content (μg). The mucin concentration in lacrimal fluid (mg/mL) is estimated from the mucin level/lacrimal fluid volume.

2.13. Statistical Analysis

Differences between the mean values were analyzed with an ANOVA, followed by Student's t-test, and Dunnett's multiple comparisons test was used for the statistical analysis, where $p < 0.05$ was considered significant. The data are expressed as the mean ± standard error (S.E.).

3. Results

3.1. Design of the MPCP

Figure 1 shows the structural formula of the MPCP. We designed the MPCP structure based on three points: (1) the MPC, indicating the zwitterionic group, shows the hydrophilic part and gives hydrophilicity to MPCP; (2) stearyl methacrylate including the long-chain alkyl group shows its hydrophobic part and forms a hydrous polymer nano-sphere in an aqueous solution; (3) coupled with the acryl group as a highly reactive functional group, N,N-dimethylacrylamide accelerates the polymerization between MPC and stearyl methacrylate and strengthens the structure of polymer nano-sphere in an aqueous solution. Figure 2A,B shows the particle distribution and an AFM image of the MPCP. This polymer includes monomer forms similar to micelles (polymer nanosphere), with a hydrophilic outer-most layer and a hydrophobic inner-most layer in an aqueous solution, featuring a particle size of from 50 to 250 nm. In addition, the particle number was 349 ± 0.336 ($\times 10^8$ particles/mL). Figure 2C,D shows the viscosity of MPCP at 10–40 °C. The viscosity of MPCP was 1.17- and 0.92-fold that of the purified water and MPC-BMA reported previously (preexisting MPC polymer) [12], respectively, and the viscosity levels of MPCP were similar under 10–40 °C conditions. We also measured the hydrophilicity of MPCP and MPC-BMA. The contact angle using MPCP was 25.5 ± 1.3° (n = 3), the contact angle using MPC-BMA was 26.2 ± 2.0° (n = 3), and the control was 29.2 ± 0.4° (n = 3). These results indicate that the MPCP was slightly hydrophilic and had a higher wettability than the MPC-BMA and the control.

3.2. Changes in Cell Conditions in the Immortalized Human Corneal Epithelial Cell Line (HCE-T Cell) Treated with MPCP

Figure 3A,B shows the effects of MPCP treatment on cell adhesion and growth in the HCE-T cells. No significant differences were observed between the cell adhesion and growth of HCE-T cells treated with and without MPCP. Figure 3C shows the effect of MPCP treatment on the TER during the HCE-T cell layer model preparation. The TER values of HCE-T cells increased to over 380 Ω·cm² when we exposed them to an air–liquid interface for two weeks. The TER in the MPCP-treated HCE-T cells was similar to non-treated values before exposure to the air–liquid interface; however, during exposure to the air–liquid interface, the TER values in the MPCP-treated HCE-T cells were significantly higher than those found in the HCE-T cells without MPCP treatment. Figure 3D shows the cell toxicity caused by MPCP treatment. The cell toxicity caused by the MPCP was mild, since the decrease in TER in the MPCP-treated HCE-T cells was similar to that in the vehicle-treated HCE-T cells.

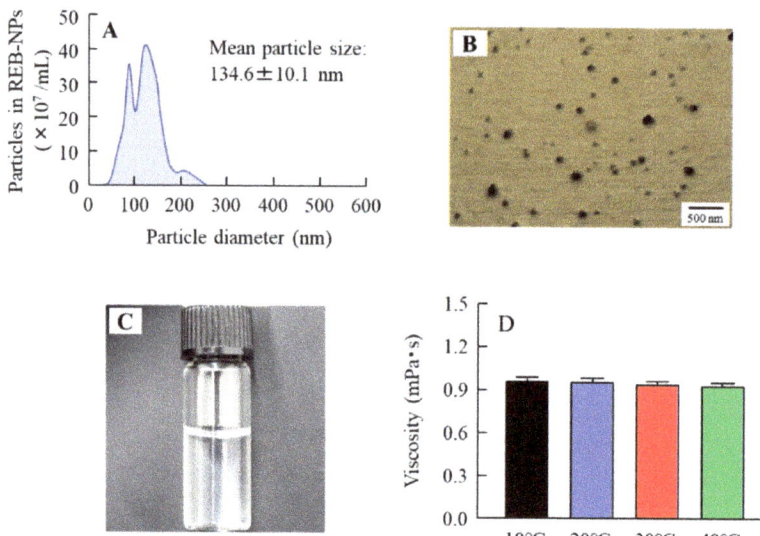

Figure 2. Particle size and viscosity of the MPCP. (**A,B**) Particle distribution (**A**) and atomic force microscopy (AFM) images (**B**) of MPCP. (**C**) Image of MPCP. (**D**) Changes in the viscosity of the MPCP at 10–40 °C. n = 8–10. The particle size of MPCP was 50–250 nm, and the viscosity of MPCP was 0.95 mPa·s at 20 °C. The temperature (10–40 °C) did not affect the viscosity.

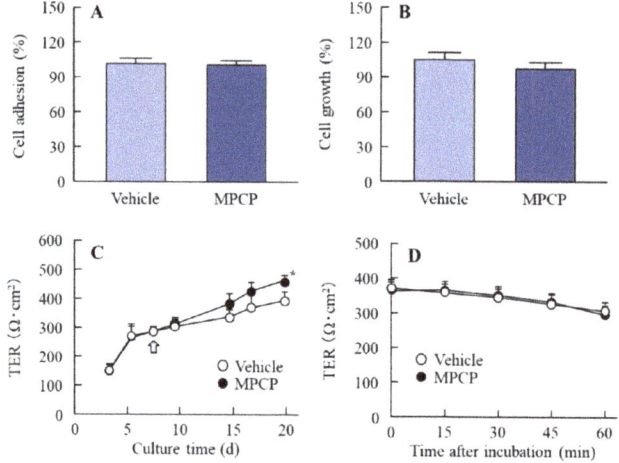

Figure 3. Corneal epithelial cell adhesion, growth, and stimulation of MPCP in the immortalized human corneal epithelial cell line (HCE-T cells). (**A**) Effect of MPCP on the adhesion of HCE-T cells. (**B**) Effect of MPCP on the growth of HCE-T cells. (**C**) Changes in transepithelial electrical resistance (TER) values during the formation of the HCE-T cell layer model treated with MPCP. The arrow indicates the beginning of the air–liquid interface. (**D**) Effect of MPCP on the TER values in the HCE-T cell layer model. n = 10–12. * $p < 0.05$ vs. the vehicle for each group. The treatment with MPCP did not affect the cell adhesion and growth of the HCE-T cells, and no stimulation was observed; however, the TER values in the HCE-T cell layer model were enhanced by the MPCP treatment.

3.3. Effect of MPCP on the Ocular Surface Stability in the Normal Model

As shown in Figure 3, the treatment with MPCP enhanced cell stability in the HCE-T cell layer model. We investigated whether the ocular surface stability in a normal rabbit was increased via the instillation of MPCP. The lacrimal fluid volume and TBUT were significantly increased via treatment with MPCP (Figure 4A,D); however, the mucin concentration in the lacrimal fluid decreased in the MPCP-instilled rabbits; for the total mucin levels in the lacrimal fluid, no difference between the vehicle- and MPCP-treated groups was found (Figure 4B,C). On the other hand, the lacrimal fluid volume (18.4 ± 1.9 µL, $n = 5$) and TBUT (24.1 ± 2.0 s, $n = 5$) in the rabbits instilled with MPC-BMA tended to increase, although both the lacrimal fluid volume and TBUT were significantly lower than those in the MPCP. Figure 5 shows the effects of MPCP on moisture retention in the excised rabbit cornea. The water content in the cornea instilled with the vehicle decreased with time and completely evaporated after 90 min. The MPCP instillation prolonged the time needed for water evaporation from the cornea and the number of MPCP nanoparticles to decrease on the cornea. Preexisting MPC-BMA prolonged the time needed for water maintenance in comparison with the vehicle, but this ability was significantly lower than that in MPCP.

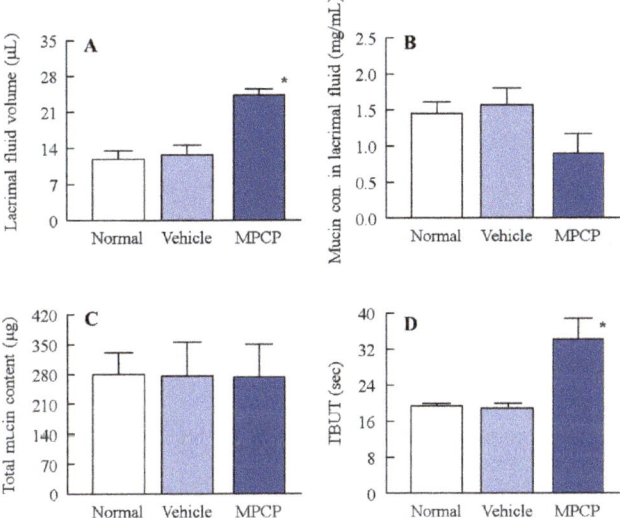

Figure 4. Effect of a single application of MPCP on lacrimal fluid volume, mucin levels, and tear film breakup time (TBUT) in normal rabbits. (**A,B**) Changes in lacrimal fluid volume (**A**) and mucin concentration in lacrimal fluid (**B**) after the application of MPCP. (**C**) Changes in total mucin levels in the lacrimal fluid after the application of MPCP. (**D**) Changes in the TBUT in rabbits instilled with the vehicle and MPCP. These measurements were performed 2 h after the instillation of MPCP (16:00). $n = 6$–8. * $p < 0.05$ vs. the vehicle for each group. Although the application of MPCP induced an increase in lacrimal fluid volume and TBUT in the rabbit eye, the total mucin contents in the rabbits instilled with MPCP were similar to those in the vehicle.

3.4. Therapeutic Potential of the MPCP for Dry Eye Disease

Next, we investigated the usefulness of MPCP as a therapy for dry eye using the N-acetylcysteine-treated rabbit model (Figure 6). The levels of lacrimal fluid and mucin decreased under treatment with N-acetylcysteine, with levels 0.8- and 0.67-fold greater than those of normal rabbits, respectively (Figure 6A,B). Both the lacrimal fluid volume and mucin levels were approximately 2.5-fold greater in comparison with the control group (non-instillation group) (Figure 6A,B). Figure 6C,D show the changes in the levels of tear film breakup in the N-acetylcysteine-treated dry eye model rabbits instilled with (or without) MPCP. Strong tear film breakup levels were observed and still persisted five days later. Repeat treatment with MPCP attenuated the tear film breakup levels five days post-N-acetylcysteine treatment, and the therapeutic effect of MPCP was significantly higher than that in MPC-BMA (tear film breakup levels at 5 days, 4.26 ± 1.09 mm², $n = 5$).

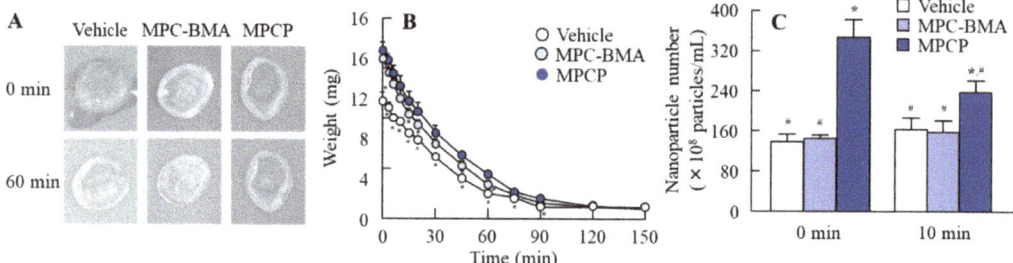

Figure 5. Changes in moisture retention in the cornea instilled with the vehicle, MPC-BMA, and MPCP. (**A**) Image of the cornea at 0 and 60 min after the instillation of MPCP. (**B**) Moisture retention curve in the extracted cornea instilled with the vehicle, MPC-BMA, and MPCP for 150 min. (**C**) the number of nanoparticles on the cornea at 10 min after the instillation of MPCP. Vehicle, vehicle-treated cornea. MPC-BMA, MPC-BMA-treated cornea. MPCP, MPCP-treated cornea. $n = 5$–7. * $p < 0.05$ vs. the vehicle for each group. # $p < 0.05$ vs. MPCP at 0 min. The water content in the cornea instilled with MPCP was higher than that found in the cornea instilled with the vehicle, and the time needed for water maintenance was prolonged in comparison with the vehicle and MPC-BMA. The number of MPCP particles on the cornea decreased after treatment.

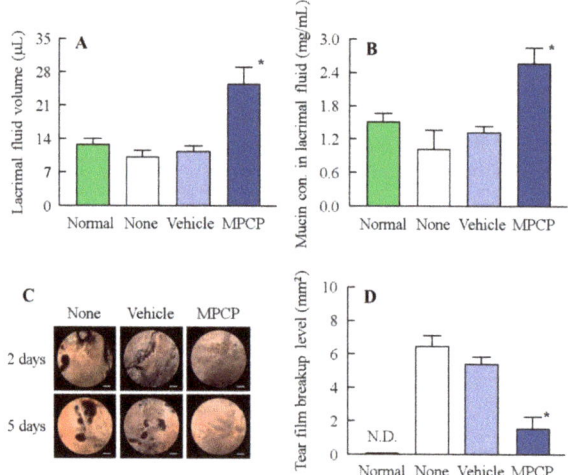

Figure 6. The therapeutic effect of the repetitive application of MPCP on dry eye in the N-acetylcysteine-treated rabbit model (dry eye model). (**A,B**) The effect of MPCP on the lacrimal fluid volume (**A**) and mucin levels (**B**) in the dry eye model. The mucin levels in the lacrimal fluid are expressed as the ratios of the mucin contents at the start of the experiment. (**C**) Images of the ocular surface in the dry eye model after repetitive applications of MPCP. The bar indicates 1 mm. The dark spots reflect the tear film breakup. (**D**) Effect of MPCP on tear film breakup levels in the dry eye model. Rabbits were instilled with MPCP at 14:00 h once a day for five days, and the experiments were performed at 18:00 h. This protocol was performed by following our previous reports [13]. $n = 9$–12. N.D., not detectable. * $p < 0.05$ vs. none for each group. The application of MPCP increased the volume of lacrimal fluid and normalized the decreased mucin levels in the dry eye model. The levels of tear film breakup were attenuated by the application of MPCP.

4. Discussion

In this study, we designed a novel MPCP that includes the zwitterionic group stearyl methacrylat, and the acryl group, and found that the MPCP has a high affinity for water and moisturizes the ocular surface in comparison with the MPC-BMA reported previously (preexisting MPC polymer) [12]. We also showed that the instillation of MPCP appears to provide a useful therapy for dry eye (Figure 7).

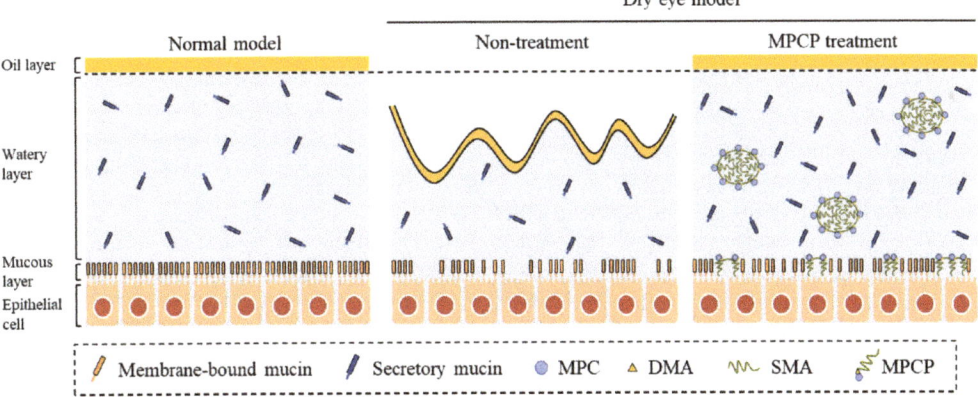

Figure 7. Schematic illustration for the amelioration of dry eye via the instillation of the MPCP. DMA—N,N-dimethylacrylamide; SMA—stearyl methacrylate.

First, we designed MPCP and evaluated its characteristics. MPC/stearyl methacrylate/N,N-dimethylacrylamide was used to prepare the MPCP in this study, and MPCP was purified using the dialysis method. The over-30-nm nanoparticles reported previously were not detected in the MPC-BMA [12]. In contrast with the results for MPC-BMA, this polymer (MPCP) included monomer forms similar to micelles (polymer nanosphere), with particle sizes of 50–250 nm (Figure 2A,B). The viscosity of MPCP was 0.92 fold that of MPC-BMA and was not different under 10–40 °C conditions (Figure 2D). On the other hand, the contact angle value of MPCP tended to decrease compared to that of the MPC-BMA. These results suggest that the MPCP has different physicochemical properties from preexisting MPC-BMP due to the formation of nanoparticles.

Next, we investigated the effects of MPCP on corneal epithelial cells using HCE-T cells. We previously reported that MPC-BMA does not affect the cell adhesion and growth of HCE-T cells, with little toxicity in HCE-T cells [19]. The MPCP did not affect the cell adhesion and growth of the HCE-T cells (Figure 3A,B), and no cell toxicity was observed (Figure 3D); however, we know that the barrier properties of the HCE-T cell layer model are very similar to those in rabbit corneas, and an increase in the barrier properties of the HCE-T cell layer model is expressed as an enhancement of the TER value [15,18]. To prepare the HCE-T cell layer model, the cells were exposed to air in order to increase the TER value, as this step was important to instill the medium solution to the cells twice a day (9:00 and 19:00 h), ensuring that the cell layer model would not dry completely. As a result, we demonstrated that the stabilization of the cell layer model increased via the instillation of a drop of MPCP to the therapeutic target. The MPCP enhanced the TER values of HCE-T cells during exposure to the air–liquid interface (Figure 3C). Taken together, the MPCP may attenuate the desiccation on the donor side, resulting in the enhancement of the TER value in the HCE-T cell layer model.

Further, we investigated the changes in the ocular surface in normal rabbits instilled with MPCP (Figure 4). The instillation of MPCP enhanced the lacrimal fluid volume and prolonged the TBUT (Figure 4A,D). These results show that the instillation of MPCP stabilized the ocular surface conditions; thus, the mucin level relates to the increase in lacrimal fluid and TBUT. The mucins composed of numerous sugar chains linked to an apomucin, which is a core protein, were heavy molecular glycoproteins, and 50–80% of their mass was comprised of carbohydrates. It was reported that mucin leads to the formation of a smooth spherical surface, offering good vision, the provision of a barrier for the ocular surface, lubrication of the ocular surface to facilitate smooth blinking, and maintenance of the lacrimal fluid on the ocular surface [20,21]. Moreover, the mucin layer spreads lacrimal fluid over the surface of the eye by decreasing the surface tension of the water content. In addition, the mucin can remove foreign materials and prevent damage and infections in the eye [22]; therefore, an increase in mucin may enhance the lacrimal fluid volume and TBUT. Based on previous studies, we also measured the mucin levels in the lacrimal fluid of normal rabbits instilled with MPCP. Against all expectations, the total mucin content in the lacrimal fluid of the MPCP-instilled rabbits was similar to that of the vehicle-instilled rabbits, and the concentration of lacrimal fluid of the MPCP-instilled rabbits was lower than that of the vehicle-instilled rabbits (Figure 4B,C). These results suggest that MPCP is not affected by mucin production, since the total mucin levels were similar in rabbits instilled with or without MPCP. On the other hand, the mucin levels may be diluted by the enhanced lacrimal fluid volume via MPCP instillation, resulting in an apparent reduction in the mucin concentration in lacrimal fluid. To understand this result, we investigated whether MPCP enhanced the moisture retention in the excised rabbit cornea, and the results showed that the MPCP instillation prolonged the time needed for water evaporation from the cornea (Figure 5A,B). Although the preexisting MPC-BMA [12] also prolonged the time needed for water maintenance in comparison with the vehicle, this ability was significantly lower than that in MPCP. These results suggest that the preexisting MPC-BMA and MPCP exert similar effects. However, the MPCP has a strong ability to retain water on the cornea in comparison with MPC-BMA, and this high water affinity may enhance the lacrimal fluid volume and TBUT in normal rabbits. Moreover, this water affinity on the cornea may be enhanced by the formulation of hydrous polymer nano-spheres and polymerization of the MPC, since the time needed for water maintenance was prolonged in comparison with the MPC-BMA.

We found that the number of MPCP nanoparticles decreased on the cornea after treatment (Figure 5C). The MPCP may bind to the cornea, resulting in a decrease in forms like micelles in the solution. Further studies are needed to demonstrate the binding of MPCP on the cornea.

It is important to elucidate the therapeutic effect of MPCP in a dry eye model. The N-acetylcysteine, a reducing agent and mucolytic [23], acts on corneal and conjunctival epithelial cells and decreases mucin production and retention. Further, the instillation of 20% N-acetylcysteine caused a decrease in the mucin layer in the conjunctiva and cornea, desquamation of conjunctival and corneal epithelial cells, elimination of microvilli [24], and decreased thickness of the tear fluid layer [25]. Because of these actions, a rabbit model treated with N-acetylcysteine is widely applied as a mucin-reduced model and may be useful for evaluating the therapeutic effect of the MPC polymer for dry eye. Therefore, we treated a rabbit model with N-acetylcysteine and measured the effect of MPCP on the ocular surface. First, we attempted to measure the tear film break-up time (as in Figure 4D). However, the tear film in the N-acetylcysteine-treated rabbit model was broken 1–2 s after the last blink, so that the TBUT could not be detected. Therefore, we measured the break up level to evaluate the therapeutic effect of the repetitive application of MPCP (Figure 6). The instillation of N-acetylcysteine decreased the lacrimal fluid volume and tear film breakup level (Figure 6). The instillation of MPCP significantly increased both the lacrimal fluid volume and tear film breakup level in comparison with the vehicle and MPC-BMA (Figure 6A,C,D). In this study, we showed that the MPCP has a strong ability to retain water on the cornea in comparison with MPC-BMA (Figure 5). The in vitro study illustrated in Figure 5 supports the in vivo study shown in Figure 6. In contrast with the results of the normal rabbits (Figure 4), the mucin levels were found to be approximately 2.5-fold greater when compared with the control (non-instillation group) (Figure 6B).

Urashima et al. reported that N-acetylcysteine reduces the mucin-like substances in the cornea and conjunctiva and that the mucin levels are enhanced by positive feedback during the healing process [26]. Therefore, mucin production in rabbits instilled with MPCP may be overexpressed, since MPCP accelerates the normalization of the ocular surface in the dry eye model by keeping the tear film on the cornea. Taken together, we hypothesized that the MPCP would show a high affinity for lacrimal fluid on the cornea after instillation and prolonged moisture retention in the rabbit cornea, resulting in an acceleration of the improvement in tear film breakup levels. In addition, normalization of the ocular surface conditions may induce high mucin production in dry eye models.

In this study, rabbit body weight did not change with the repetitive application of MPCP over 30 d (once a day), although it remains important to assess the systemic parameters and pharmakokinetics in the rabbit model. In addition, further studies are needed to apply the MPCP as dry eye drops. In future work, we intend to measure the therapeutic effect under a combination of MPCP and commercially available eye drops, such as Mucosta®, Diquas®, Xiidra® Restasis®, and Ikervis®, in a rabbit model treated with N-acetylcysteine.

5. Conclusions

In this study, we prepared a novel MPCP using MPC/stearyl methacrylate/N,N-dimethylacrylamide (50:5:45) and demonstrated that this MPCP provides high water affinity in comparison with the preexisting MPC polymer. The instillation of the MPCP prolonged the retention of lacrimal fluid in the eye and enhanced the TBUT in the rabbits. In addition, the MPCP accelerated the normalizing of the ocular surface in the dry eye model by keeping the tear film on the cornea. Moreover, the therapeutic effect of MPCP was significantly higher than that of the MPC-BMA reported previously [12]. Thus, this MPCP may provide an effective therapeutic treatment for dry eye.

Author Contributions: conceptualization, N.N. and S.S.; data curation, R.S., M.M., M.Y., and S.D.; formal analysis, R.S., M.M., M.Y., and S.D.; funding acquisition, N.N.; investigation, S.S., R.S., M.M., M.Y., and E.H.; methodology, N.N., S.S., and E.H.; supervision, N.N. and E.H.; visualization, N.N. and S.S.; writing—original draft, N.N. and S.S.; writing—review and editing, N.N. and S.S. All authors have read and agreed to the published version of the manuscript.

Funding: This research received no external funding.

Institutional Review Board Statement: The protocol was conducted according to the guidelines of the Association for Research in Vision and Ophthalmology (ARVO) and Kindai University, and approved by the Kindai University (KAPS-31-002, 1 April 2019).

Informed Consent Statement: Not applicable.

Data Availability Statement: Not applicable.

Conflicts of Interest: Shunsuke Sakurai and Eiji Harata work for the NOF Corporation. The authors report no other conflict of interest in this work.

References

1. Craig, J.P.; Nichols, K.K.; Akpek, E.K.; Caffery, B.; Dua, H.S.; Joo, C.K.; Liu, Z.; Nelson, J.D.; Nichols, J.J.; Tsubota, K.; et al. TFOS DEWS II Definition and Classification Report. *Ocul. Surf.* **2017**, *15*, 276–283. [CrossRef] [PubMed]
2. Marshall, L.L.; Roach, J.M. Treatment of dry eye disease. *Consult. Pharm.* **2016**, *31*, 96–106. [CrossRef] [PubMed]
3. Lemp, M.A. The definition and classification of dry eye disease: Report of the definition and classification subcommittee of the international dry eye Work Shop. *Ocul. Surf.* **2007**, *5*, 75–92.
4. Ogenesis of dry eye. *Inflamm. Regen.* **2007**, *27*, 559–564.
5. Stapleton, F.; Alves, M.; Bunya, V.Y.; Jalbert, I.; Lekhanont, K.; Malet, F.; Na, K.S.; Schaumberg, D.; Uchino, M.; Vehof, J.; et al. TFOS DEWS II epidemiology report. *Ocul. Surf.* **2017**, *15*, 334–365. [CrossRef] [PubMed]
6. Stapleton, F.; Garrett, Q.; Chan, C.; Craig, J.P. The epidemiology of dry eye diseas. In *Dry Eye: A Practical Approach, Essentials in Ophthalmology*; Chan, C., Ed.; Springer: Berlin/Heidelberg, Germany, 2015.
7. Nebbioso, M.; Fameli, V.; Gharbiya, M.; Sacchetti, M.; Zicari, A.M.; Lambiase, A. Investigational drugs in dry eye disease. *Expert Opin. Investig. Drugs* **2016**, *25*, 1437–1446. [CrossRef] [PubMed]

8. Ishihara, K.; Takai, M. Bioinspired interface for nanobiodevices based on phospholipid polymer chemistry. *J. R. Soc. Interface* **2009**, *6*, S279–S291. [CrossRef]
9. Ishihara, K. Bioinspired phospholipid polymer biomaterials for making high performance artificial organs. *Sci. Technol. Adv. Mater.* **2000**, *1*, 131–138. [CrossRef]
10. Ishihara, K. New polymeric biomaterials–phospholipid polymers with a biocompatible surface. *Front. Med. Biol. Eng.* **2000**, *10*, 83–95. [CrossRef]
11. Hall, B.; Janes, S.; Young, G.; Coleman, S. The on-eye dehydration of proclear compatibles lenses. *CLAO J.* **1999**, *25*, 233–237.
12. Ayaki, M.; Iwasawa, A.; Niwano, Y. Cytotoxicity assays of new artificial tears containing 2-methacryloyloxyehtyl phospholylcholine polymer for ocular surface cells. *Jpn. J. Ophthalmol.* **2011**, *55*, 541–546. [CrossRef]
13. Nagai, N.; Ishii, M.; Seiriki, R.; Ogata, F.; Otake, H.; Nakazawa, Y.; Okamoto, N.; Kanai, K.; Kawasaki, N. Novel sustained-release drug delivery system for dry eye therapy by rebamipide nanoparticles. *Pharmaceutics* **2020**, *12*, E155. [CrossRef] [PubMed]
14. Nagai, N.; Isaka, T.; Deguchi, S.; Minami, M.; Yamaguchi, M.; Otake, H.; Okamoto, N.; Nakazawa, Y. In situ gelling systems using pluronic F127 enhance corneal permeability of indomethacin nanocrystals. *Int. J. Mol. Sci.* **2020**, *21*, 7083. [CrossRef] [PubMed]
15. Araki-Sasaki, K.; Ohashi, Y.; Sasabe, T.; Hayashi, K.; Watanabe, H.; Tano, Y.; Handa, H. An SV40-immortalized human corneal epithelial cell line and its characterization. *Investig. Ophthalmol. Vis. Sci.* **1995**, *36*, 614–621.
16. Nagai, N.; Fukuoka, Y.; Ishii, M.; Otake, H.; Yamamoto, T.; Taga, A.; Okamoto, N.; Shimomura, Y. Instillation of sericin enhances corneal wound healing through the erk pathway in rat debrided corneal epithelium. *Int. J. Mol. Sci.* **2018**, *19*, 1123. [CrossRef]
17. Nagai, N.; Ogata, F.; Otake, H.; Nakazawa, Y.; Kawasaki, N. Energy-dependent endocytosis is responsible for drug transcorneal penetration following the instillation of ophthalmic formulations containing indomethacin nanoparticles. *Int. J. Nanomed.* **2019**, *14*, 1213–1227. [CrossRef]
18. Toropainen, E.; Ranta, V.P.; Talvitie, A.; Suhonen, P.; Urtti, A. Culture model of human corneal epithelium for prediction of ocular drug absorption. *Investig. Ophthalmol. Vis. Sci.* **2001**, *42*, 2942–2948.
19. Minami, M.; Yamaguchi, M.; Yamasaki, Y.; Otake, H.; Sakurai, S.; Harata, E.; Nagai, N. Effect of MPC polymer on corneal toxicity and corneal drug permeation of benzalkonium chloride in corneal epithelial cells. *J. Eye* **2020**, *37*, 1309–1314.
20. Gipson, I.K.; Hori, Y.; Argueso, P. Character of ocular surface mucins and their alteration in dry eye disease. *Ocul. Surf.* **2004**, *2*, 131–148. [CrossRef]
21. Gipson, I.K.; Argueso, P. Role of mucins in the function of the corneal and conjunctival epithelia. *Int. Rev. Cytol.* **2003**, *231*, 1–49.
22. Rose, M.C. Mucins:structure, function, and role in pulmonary diseases. *Am. J. Physiol.* **1992**, *263*, L413–L492. [PubMed]
23. Sheffner, A.L.; Medler, E.M.; Jacobs, L.W.; Sarett, H.P. The in vitro reduction in viscosity of human tracheobronchial secretions by acetylcysteine. *Am. Rev. Respir. Dis.* **1964**, *90*, 721–729. [PubMed]
24. Thermes, F.; Molon-Noblot, S.; Grove, J. Effects of acetylcysteine on rabbit conjunctival and corneal surfaces. *Investig. Ophthalmol. Vis. Sci.* **1991**, *32*, 2958–2963. [PubMed]
25. Anderton, P.; Tragoulias, S. Mucous contribution to rat tear-film thickness measured with a microelectrode technique. In *Lacrimal Gland, Tear Film, and Dry Eye Syndrome 2*; Plenum Press: New York, NY, USA, 1998; pp. 247–252.
26. Urashima, H.; Okamoto, T.; Takeji, Y.; Shinohara, H.; Fujisawa, S. Rebamipide increases the amount of mucin-like substances on the conjunctiva and cornea in the N-acetylcysteine-treated in vivo model. *Cornea* **2004**, *23*, 613–619. [CrossRef]

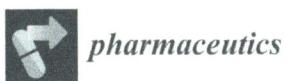

Review

Current Insights into 3D Bioprinting: An Advanced Approach for Eye Tissue Regeneration

Sandra Ruiz-Alonso [1,2,3,†], Ilia Villate-Beitia [1,2,3,†], Idoia Gallego [1,2,3], Markel Lafuente-Merchan [1,2,3], Gustavo Puras [1,2,3], Laura Saenz-del-Burgo [1,2,3,*] and José Luis Pedraz [1,2,3,*]

1. NanoBioCel Research Group, Laboratory of Pharmacy and Pharmaceutical Technology, Department of Pharmacy and Food Science, Faculty of Pharmacy, University of the Basque Country (UPV/EHU), Paseo de la Universidad 7, 01006 Vitoria-Gasteiz, Spain; sandra.ruiz@ehu.eus (S.R.-A.); aneilia.villate@ehu.eus (I.V.-B.); idoia.gallego@ehu.eus (I.G.); mlafuente004@ikasle.ehu.eus (M.L.-M.); gustavo.puras@ehu.eus (G.P.)
2. Networking Research Centre of Bioengineering, Biomaterials and Nanomedicine (CIBER-BBN), Institute of Health Carlos III, 28029 Madrid, Spain
3. Bioaraba, NanoBioCel Research Group, 01009 Vitoria-Gasteiz, Spain
* Correspondence: laura.saenzdelburgo@ehu.eusl (L.S.-d.-B.); joseluis.pedraz@ehu.eus (J.L.P.); Tel.: +(34)-945014542 (L.S.-d.-B.); +(34)-945013691 (J.L.P.)
† These authors contributed equally to this work.

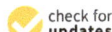

Citation: Ruiz-Alonso, S.; Villate-Beitia, I.; Gallego, I.; Lafuente-Merchan, M.; Puras, G.; Saenz-del-Burgo, L.; Pedraz, J.L. Current Insights into 3D Bioprinting: An Advanced Approach for Eye Tissue Regeneration. *Pharmaceutics* **2021**, *13*, 308. https://doi.org/10.3390/pharmaceutics13030308

Academic Editors: Yolanda Diebold and Laura García-Posadas

Received: 11 January 2021
Accepted: 19 February 2021
Published: 26 February 2021

Publisher's Note: MDPI stays neutral with regard to jurisdictional claims in published maps and institutional affiliations.

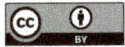

Copyright: © 2021 by the authors. Licensee MDPI, Basel, Switzerland. This article is an open access article distributed under the terms and conditions of the Creative Commons Attribution (CC BY) license (https://creativecommons.org/licenses/by/4.0/).

Abstract: Three-dimensional (3D) printing is a game changer technology that holds great promise for a wide variety of biomedical applications, including ophthalmology. Through this emerging technique, specific eye tissues can be custom-fabricated in a flexible and automated way, incorporating different cell types and biomaterials in precise anatomical 3D geometries. However, and despite the great progress and possibilities generated in recent years, there are still challenges to overcome that jeopardize its clinical application in regular practice. The main goal of this review is to provide an in-depth understanding of the current status and implementation of 3D bioprinting technology in the ophthalmology field in order to manufacture relevant tissues such as cornea, retina and conjunctiva. Special attention is paid to the description of the most commonly employed bioprinting methods, and the most relevant eye tissue engineering studies performed by 3D bioprinting technology at preclinical level. In addition, other relevant issues related to use of 3D bioprinting for ocular drug delivery, as well as both ethical and regulatory aspects, are analyzed. Through this review, we aim to raise awareness among the research community and report recent advances and future directions in order to apply this advanced therapy in the eye tissue regeneration field.

Keywords: 3D bioprinting; cornea; retina; ophthalmology; tissue regeneration

1. Introduction

The development of new revolutionary technologies during recent years, such as the use of Big Data, virtual reality systems and three-dimensional (3D) bioprinting, has created great expectations in the scientific community, not only regarding the improvement of the quality of life in patients affected by devastating pathologies, but also in terms of saving health-care associated resources [1–3]. In this regard, 3D bioprinting is an emerging manufacturing technology which holds great promise for a wide variety of biomedical applications, including drug testing, pathophysiological studies and regenerative medicine [4]. Specific benefits of such a technology would include the development of more targeted and personalized therapeutic approaches, as well as the possibility of obtaining functional models of tissues and organs for research purposes, increased reproducibility and higher capacity for drug lab testing studies, etc. In addition, for regenerative medicine applications, key advantages include automated tissue fabrication and the flexibility of incorporating many different materials and cell types in precise anatomical 3D geometries [4]. Consequently, the interest and investment in this promising technology has dramatically increased during the last five years [5] and, in fact, there is a clear exponential tendency regarding the number of published papers in the last decade (Figure 1A).

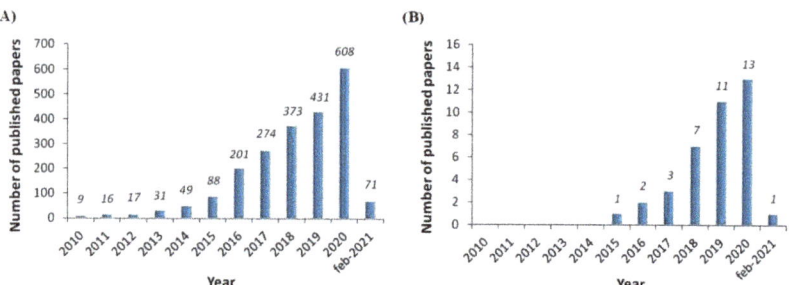

Figure 1. Histogram showing the timeline of publications (number per year), from the PubMed website, using the key "3D bioprinting" (**A**), and "eye/ocular/cornea/retina 3D bioprinting" (**B**) (updated to 2 February 2021).

From a conceptual standpoint, 3D bioprinting refers to the "additive manufacturing" process based on a layer-by-layer approach with the deposition of bio-inks in a precise spatial arrangement [6], which makes it a suitable technology for obtaining highly complex structures similar to the original tissues of the eye [7]. The bio-ink is composed of structural components or biomaterials, crosslinkers, functional elements and living cells. Compared to non-biological printing, which has been proved suitable for the manufacturing of medical devices and patient-tailored prosthetics for more than 30 years [8], 3D bioprinting involves additional challenges and requires the multidisciplinary integration of different technological and medical fields. These complexities refer mainly to the selection of biocompatible materials, cell types, biomechanical cues and the overcoming of technical difficulties due to the sensitivities of living cells [9]. By using different materials and designs, the structural, physicochemical and mechanical properties of the bio-printed structure can be adjusted [10]. In general terms, the fundamental aspects that need to be taken into account for an appropriate selection of biomaterials include their printability, biocompatibility, degradation kinetics and byproducts, structural and mechanical properties, and biomimicry. Nowadays, for eye tissue regeneration applications, the most commonly used biomaterials in bio-inks are based on naturally derived polymers such as collagen, gelatin, alginate or hyaluronic acid [11], whose similarity to human extracellular matrix (ECM) and inherent bioactivity represent a relevant advantage [9]. Additional to the selection of suitable biomaterials, the target tissue determines the type of cells that need to be used in the bio-ink. In most cases, the tissues of the eye are made up of more than one cell type. For this reason, many of the approaches made to date incorporate more than one cell type or contemplate, as future steps, the incorporation of more cell types in the obtained scaffolds.

In 3D bioprinting, the three major techniques include inkjet bioprinting, based on the deposition of bio-ink droplets, laser-assisted bioprinting, based on laser stimulation, and extrusion bioprinting, which uses mechanical force to deposit a continuous flow of bio-ink, each presenting specific features [4]. The choice of the most suitable approach depends on the specific application of interest, since each 3D printing technique holds its own peculiarities and these result in different outcomes [12–17] (Figure 2).

Some success has been demonstrated in early attempts to recreate complex tissue structures, and latest research evidences significant improvement in terms of effectiveness, resolution, accuracy and manufacturing speed of this customizable technique. All of this suggests, from a technical point of view, that the fabrication of biocompatible and functionalized full bio-printed organs will be possible in the near future [18]. In this regard, the success of 3D bioprinting for tissues and organs also depends on the target organ or tissue. For instance, for structurally simple tissues such as skin, 3D bioprinting is close to becoming a clinically relevant method for producing skin grafts and is already being used in the cosmetic industry [4]. On the other hand, for more complex organs such as the heart, it becomes more challenging to precisely reproduce its diverse functionality and heterogeneous composition, so is still far from clinical translation [4].

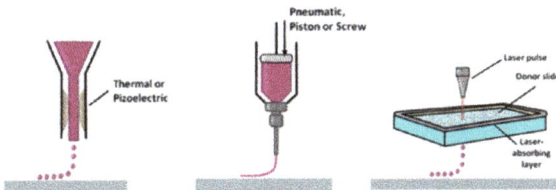

3D bioprinting method	Inkjet	Extrusion	Laser-assisted
Actuator	Temperature / voltage	Pressure	Laser
Bioink viscosity	Low (1 – 15 mPa/s)	High (30 – 6 · 10^7 mPa/s)	Wide range (1 – 300 mPa/s)
Mechanical and structural integrity	Low	High	Low
Print speed	Fast	Slow	Medium
Resolution	High (0.5 – 50 μm)	Moderate (≈200μm)	High (≈1μm)
Cell viability	70 – 90 %	45 – 98 %	>95%
Cost	Low	Medium	High

Figure 2. Major three-dimensional bioprinting techniques and their specific features.

The field of ophthalmological applications of 3D bioprinting is also gaining interest due to the specific features of the eye (Figure 1B). In addition, its anatomical disposition provides easy access for surgery and implantation in both the inner layer and overall in the anterior chamber. Furthermore, the privileged immune condition of the eye coupled with the disposition of multiple diagnostic tools, turn it into an attractive organ for the application of 3D bioprinting technology, reducing the lack of organ donors along with the problems associated with rejection of transplanted grafts due to inappropriate immune response [19]. Some of the ophthalmological applications are the development of 3D bioprinting of anatomically realistic ocular models to enhance both education and clinical practice, providing better training opportunities, or the design of cost-effective personalized approaches by manufacturing specific ocular structures to treat serious eye diseases that affect more than 30% of the world's population [20]. Depending on the specific eye disease to be treated, different ocular structures can be 3D bio-printed taking into account each disease's specific structural and functional complexities.

As known, the eye is a complex, isolated, highly evolved organ with different and specifically organized tissue structures, which embrace, from an anatomical point of view, "simple" cell multilayer structures such as the cornea and more complex structures enclosing central nervous system cells, such as the retina. However, it is noteworthy that each eye tissue possesses its complexities when implementing 3D bioprinting. In this regard, the cornea represents a key ocular transparent tissue for vision that can be bio-printed, due its relatively simple structural disposition, into five independent layers. In normal conditions, the different hydrophilic and hydrophobic permeability of such layers, along with the interconnected tight junctions in epithelial cells, can severely limit the access of external agents into inner ocular structures, acting as a potent biological barrier [21]. However, severe alterations in the corneal thickness along with keratitis of multiple causes can lead to advanced stages of corneal tissue damage, where corneal transplant is the last medical choice. In this scenario, 3D bio-printed corneal tissue could emerge as an interesting medical option, bearing in mind that severe corneal disorders are the main cause of blindness worldwide [20]. In addition, it is worth mentioning that nowadays there is a lack of full-structure corneal in vitro models for both drug screening and toxicological testing, and that the deficit of donated corneas has increased the urgency of transplantable corneal substitutes. On the other hand, there are other relevant ocular tissues such as the retina, where the application of 3D bioprinting technology is more challenging from a scientific point of view, due to its complexity, neurological origin and connections with other areas of the central nervous system [22]. Some retinal dystrophies that dramatically hamper human life and for which there are no currently effective treatments include retinitis pigmentosa, Stargardt disease and age-related macular degeneration, to name just the most representative. Therefore, the possibility of bio-printing functional retinal tissue for both drug testing and graft implantation purposes has recently caught the attention of the scientific community in order to offer an alternative medical approach against such devastating retinal pathologies.

In any case, the field of 3D bioprinting for regenerative medicine is in its early stages and there are still several technological challenges to overcome, as well as some relevant ethical and regulatory concerns to be addressed, before fabricating large scale organs of all levels of complexity [23]. For instance, to become a realistic medical option, several parameters still need to be deeply considered such as the biocompatibility and mechanical properties of engrafts along with the biological behavior and attachment properties of cells, to name just the most relevant [22]. Nevertheless, if improvement and evolution in 3D bioprinting technology continues to progress exponentially, the creation of artificial biosynthetic and customizable full eyeballs in the near future is likely, along with other applications that have not yet been fathomed [24,25].

This review further discusses the current status and implementation of 3D bioprinting technology in the ophthalmology field in order to manufacture relevant tissue-engineering items such as the cornea, retina and conjunctiva. Special attention will be paid to the description of the most commonly employed bioprinting methods, and the most relevant eye tissue engineering studies performed by 3D bioprinting technology at preclinical level. In addition, regulatory, ethical and future directions related to the use of this "game-changer" technology in ophthalmology will be addressed.

2. 3D Bioprinting for Eye Tissue Engineering

The eye is a very complex organ formed by different structures within which are the orbit, the sclera, the conjunctiva, the cornea, the iris, the pupil, the lens, the vitreous humor, the retina and the optic nerve [26]. Generally, each of the diseases that occur in the eyes affect only one of the aforementioned structures [27]. In this sense, the approximations carried out to date using 3D bioprinting have as their main objective the production of structures that resemble the characteristics and properties of the affected tissue. Such 3D-structures would allow the replacement of the entire damaged tissue or a part of it, in order to restore the patient's vision. So far, the three main target tissues have been the cornea, the retina and the conjunctiva.

2.1. Cornea

The cornea is an innervated and avascular tissue located in front of the pupil and iris [28]. Its main characteristic is its transparency, which allows the transmittance and refraction of the light entering the eye [20]. It acts as a mechanical and chemical barrier protecting the inner eye from external agents such as mechanical damage, microorganisms or ultraviolet radiation [29]. As a complex tissue, it is divided into five differentiated layers (Figure 3): epithelium, Bowman's membrane, stroma, Descement's membrane and endothelium [28,30].

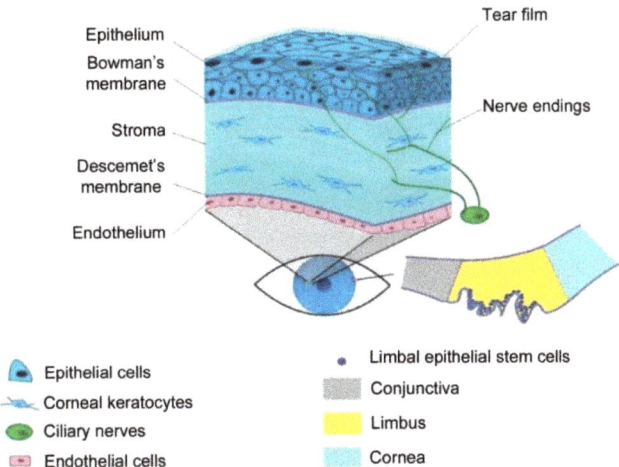

Figure 3. Anatomy of the cornea. Reproduced with permission from [20], Elsevier, 2019.

The corneal epithelium is composed of a few layers of epithelial cells that form the outermost area of the cornea. The epithelial cells are constantly renewed from the basal layer, which is formed by limbal stem cells (LSCs) [31,32]. However, any damage in the basal area would lead to a dysfunction of the LSCs that would result in overgrowth of the conjunctiva and blood vessels, photophobia and pain [32]. The Bowman's membrane is a thin acellular layer that separates the epithelium from the stroma [31]. The stroma is the widest part of the cornea. It is composed of laminin and collagen I fibrils that align perfectly to form a complex structure. This structural complexity is the key to its transparency and mechanical resistance [33,34]. In addition, it is composed of keratinocyte cells, which are responsible for maintaining the ECM [31]. These cells have little mitotic activity and present dendritic morphology. Nevertheless, in case of trauma, they are activated as a fibroblast that can differentiate into myofibroblasts [34,35]. Myofibroblasts express proteins that can alter the ECM causing opacity of the cornea, contraction and a corneal scar formation [31,35]. Descement's membrane is an acellular layer that separates the stroma from the endothelium [31]. The endothelium is the deepest layer and is composed of endothelial cells that are responsible for maintaining the fluid balance of the cornea [31]. They have very little capacity of regeneration in vivo, therefore any damage in this area would cause irreversible blindness [36].

Taking into account the structural complexity of the cornea, degeneration of any of its parts could lead to serious diseases. In fact, bilateral blindness due to corneal damage has a high prevalence worldwide [29] and it is estimated that more than four million people suffer from a corneal disease [35]. With this demand, keratoplasty or corneal transplantation is the treatment of choice. However, the possibility of rejection, the poor survival of the explanted tissue, the absence of corneal banks, the high cost and scarce accessibility to transplantation necessitate the consideration alternative treatments [29,37].

Cell therapy [38] and the manufacturing of structures such as acellular membranes [39] have been proposed in order to supply high transplantation demand. However, it has been impossible to obtain a fully functional corneal substitute. In this context, 3D bioprinting has emerged as a promising technology since complex multilayer tissues, such as the cornea, can be easily reproduced. Furthermore, this technique can be advantageous over other techniques, since scaffolds with characteristics similar to those of the native cornea can be obtained. These characteristics are listed below.

Transparency. Transparency is its greatest characteristic. Previously proposed manufactured therapies, such as decellularized membranes, have had difficulties in achieving a transparency similar to that of the native cornea. As the key to transparency resides in a perfectly arranged structure, the use of 3D bioprinting that deposits layers exactly, as a pre-designed form, could be the solution.

Biomechanics. The biomechanical properties of the cornea affect corneal curvature, strength, and conformability [40]. Previously proposed treatments, such as cell therapy, have paid little attention to these parameters. The mechanical strength can be adjusted by combining different biomaterials. Conventional treatments, such as membranes, use a single material, thereby limiting the control of the biomechanical properties. On the contrary, 3D bioprinting is a technology that allows the use of a great diversity of materials with very diverse properties. In this way, the mechanical properties can be adjusted to the needs of the corneal tissue.

Curvature. Optical parameters of the cornea, such as light refraction, are due to its curvature [41]. Based on corneal geometrical information and using computer designed programs, a corneal prototype can be perfectly fabricated. This could be easily carried into the bioprinter achieving what would be hard to obtain with conventional techniques.

Multilayer structure. The cornea is a complex multilayer tissue. It is composed of different layers in which different materials, cells and internal structure are found. Conventional cell therapies have been shown ineffective due to the poor survival rate and functionality of the implanted cells [36]. Furthermore, single material membranes have not achieved the multilayer complexity of the cornea. Thus, 3D bioprinting overcomes this problem as it is based on the deposition of materials layer by layer. In addition, different cell types (epithelial, keratocytes and endothelial cells) can be embedded into biocompatible biomaterials increasing cell viability and functionality. As a result, a corneal native-mimicking structure with the five differentiated layers could be performed.

In this context, many studies have been carried out using 3D bioprinting technology for corneal tissue fabrication. Overall, these research studies have focused on the main part of the cornea, the stroma. Isaacson et al. [42] used extrusion based bioprinting for the development of a structure mimicking the stroma by embedding human keratocyte cells into an alginate/methacrylate type I collagen ink. They proposed the application of a rotational Scheimpflug camera in order to design patient-specific corneal model. Likewise, they developed a supportive structure to maintain the scaffold curvature during the bioprinting procedure. Consequently, they were able to reproduce the curved corneal geometry (Figure 4A-a) and cell viability was high for 7 days after bioprinting (Figure 4A-b). However, properties of great importance such as transparency and mechanical properties were not mentioned. These parameters were taken into a mixture of cells and ink placed onto slabs as a control. The study demonstrated that transparency and mechanical properties of bio-printed scaffolds were higher than those in the slabs, and data were similar to the native human cornea. Nevertheless, when analysing cellular studies, results were not as promising. Although cell viability was high in both systems, in both bio-printed scaffold and in slabs, cells were elongated and showed a dendritic morphology associated with keratocytes (Figure 4B-b). Therefore, cells' metabolic activity and protein expression was low. It is believed that the high crosslinking density of 3D bio-printed scaffolds together with the absence of a curve geometry could negatively affect cell behaviour.

Kim et al. [43] studied this abnormal cell behaviour exhaustively after extrusion bioprinting. They wanted to analyze how the shear stress, applied when extruding through the printing nozzle, affects cell behaviour. To do so, they proposed to bio-print, by using different nozzle diameters, human keratocytes into a bio-ink based on decellularized corneal ECM in order to reproduce corneal stroma. Results demonstrated that not only shear stress affected cell behaviour, but also the deposition of collagen fibrils. In fact, by bioprinting with wide nozzle diameters, no aligned collagen fibrils were observed in scaffolds, which decreased transparency. Furthermore, cell dendritic morphology and keratocyte specific gene expression were not found. In contrast, after bioprinting using narrower nozzles, the shear stress increased and, as a result, highly structured collagen fibrils were shown. Nevertheless, cells were damaged and showed fibroblastic behaviour. The authors concluded that with the application of proper force, they could achieve scaffolds with both characteristics: structured collagen fibrils and cells with keratocyte behaviour. Thus, they bio-printed scaffolds with the proper extrusion nozzle (25G) and, after demonstrating that they met the adequate characteristics, scaffolds were implanted into rabbits. In vivo studies showed that implanted scaffolds were optically more transparent than the control (the not printed implant). In addition, keratocytes' cellular behaviour was activated, which enhanced collagen production simulating a lattice pattern similar to the structure of native human cornea stroma [43].

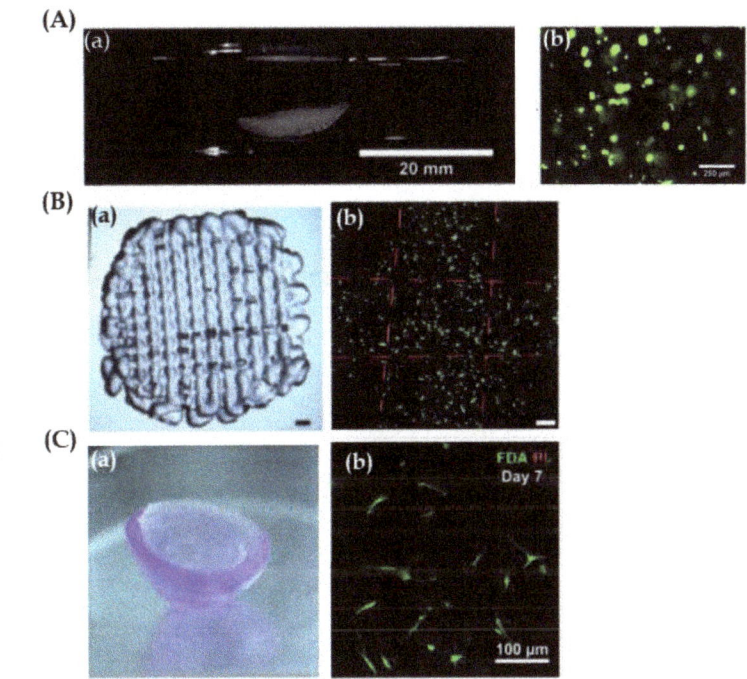

Figure 4. Corneal stroma structures and keratocytes. (**A**) Reproduced with permission form [42], Elsevier, 2018. (**a**) Images of extrusion bio-printed corneal stroma. Scale bar 20 mm. (**b**) Representative live/dead stain images using fluorescence microscopy after 3D bioprinting, showing live (green) and dead (red) cells. Scale bar 250 μm. (**B**) Reproduced with permission from [44], IOP Science, 2019. (**a**) Stereomicrographs of the methacrylate gelatin scaffold. Scale bar 1 mm. (**b**) Live/dead cell viability assay of 3D printed GelMA scaffolds on day 21, showing live (green) and dead (red) cells. Scale bar 100 μm. (**C**) Reproduced with permission from [37], Wiley, 2019. (**a**) Macrograph of ink-jet bio-printed 3D type I collagen/agarose scaffold. (**b**) Human corneal stroma keratocytes (CSK) stained with live/dead staining 7 days after bioprinting, showing live (green) and dead (red) cells. It is noticeable that the CSK is spreading and shows typical dendritic shapes in the scaffold. Scale bar 100 μm.

In order to avoid keratocyte stress through the nozzle when extrusion bioprinting is used, Duarte et al. [37] proposed another approach; the use of the inkjet bioprinting technique. This study focused on bioprinting a stroma-mimicking structure by using type I collagen/agarose and human keratocytes bio-ink. After bioprinting, biomechanical properties, transparency, and cell viability and behaviour were analyzed. Results showed good printability using inkjet bioprinting, achieving curved and transparent scaffolds (Figure 4C-a). Moreover, cell viability was high. Rounded morphology was observed at day 1 after bioprinting. Nevertheless, cells became dendritic and showed keratocyte phenotype after 7 days (Figure 4C-b). In contrast, mechanical strength was lower than that of the human native cornea, so, improving mechanical properties would be their next main objective.

When the objective is to bio-print the corneal epithelium, fewer studies have been published so far. Wu et al. [45] proposed to bio-print human corneal epithelial cells embedded into alginate/gelatin ink, in which different concentrations of collagen I were added. Extrusion bioprinting was the technique that they selected in order to bio-print square grid-like scaffolds (Figure 5A-a). Results showed that the collagen concentration of 0.82 mg/mL was optimal for achieving scaffolds with high transparency and good resolution. In addition, cell viability was high after bioprinting, but cells showed rounded morphology (Figure 5A-b). The authors argued that cells embedded into alginate bio-inks were not able to degrade it and, therefore, they could not proliferate, elongate and differentiate. Thus, they proposed to add sodium citrate as a degradation system, so achieving controllable degradable scaffolds in which cell proliferation rate and epithelial specific protein expression were increased.

Another study was performed by Zhang et al. [30]. They focused on simulating a corneal structure by combining two manufacturing techniques, digital light processing (DLP) and extrusion bioprinting. They applied the first technique to create an acellular supportive corneal structure using methacrylate gelatin on which different concentrations of sodium alginate/gelatin ink mixed with human epithelial cells were deposited with the extrusion bioprinter. Parameters such as geometry, thickness, mechanical properties and transparency were analyzed. Besides, cell viability was assayed. Results showed that the DLP technique significantly improved the manufacturing accuracy. The geometry, curvature and thickness of the obtained scaffold were more similar to those of the native human cornea than those obtained in the other studies carried out so far. In contrast, extrusion bio-printed layers showed high diversity among alginate/gelatin bio-ink mixtures developed in this study, in terms of printability and mechanical properties, even though, the overall transparency was good. Cell viability was high but, as the authors focused mainly on improving the manufacturing precision and geometrical control, more in vitro studies should be carried out prior to taking these scaffolds into in vivo studies.

The previous studies made an approach towards manufacturing different parts of the cornea with different materials and techniques. However, to date, the only study in which the bioprinting of two different cellular parts of the cornea has been tried is that by Sorkio et al. [32]. They proposed the development of a corneal epithelium and a stroma using laser-assisted bioprinting (LaBP), and the use of stem cells, which show high differentiation capacity into epithelial stem cells and keratocytes. The authors argued that the LaBP technique may protect cells from the damage caused by nozzle stress. In addition, more viscous bio-inks can be used with this technique. In this study, two different bio-inks were developed, one based on human recombinant laminin, hyaluronic acid and human embryonic stem cells for corneal epithelium tissue, and another one composed of human collagen type I, blood plasma, thrombin and human adipose tissue derived stem cells for corneal stroma tissue. First, the scaffolds were bio-printed separately. Results showed that the bio-ink for bioprinting epithelium was printable using LaBP and that the cells embedded into the scaffolds showed high viability (Figure 5B-b). Moreover, epithelial cell morphology and expression of corneal epithelial markers were observed after 12 days. On the other hand, although the stroma-mimicking scaffold could be fabricated through LaBP without any difficulty, scaffolds lost their shape after a few days of culture, which indicated lost mechanical strength and the necessity of a supportive structure. Cells in the stromal scaffold showed high viability and expression of proliferative markers. In addition, cell organization resembled the native human corneal stroma. On the other hand, stroma scaffolds were implanted into explanted porcine eyes, which were maintained in culture, and a proper interaction and attachment to the host tissue was observed. Finally, a scaffold containing both layers, stroma and epithelium, was bio-printed in order to simulate native human cornea. The resulting structure was opaque due to the supportive membrane that was needed to avoid the stroma layer's shape loss (Figure 5B-a). This opacity made its application difficult as cornea substitute as it did not meet with the main corneal characteristic of being functional. Thus, other supportive structures for the bio-printed corneal scaffold were needed in order to improve both transparency and stability.

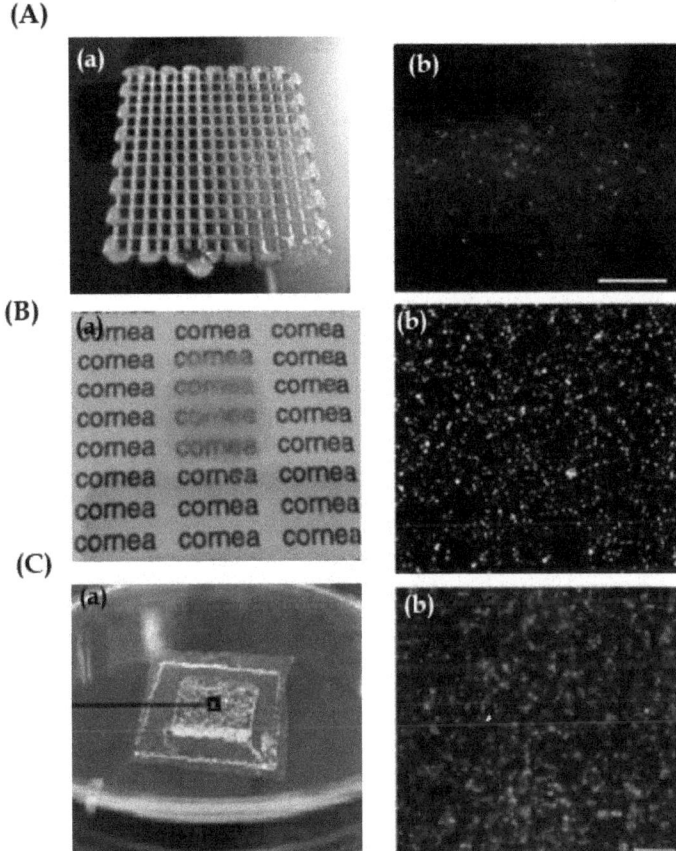

Figure 5. (**A**) Reproduced with permission from [45], Nature, 2016. Cornea epithelial structures: (**a**) Top view of a 3D human corneal epithelial cells/gelatin/alginate construct. (**b**) Epithelial cell viability after extrusion bioprinting by live/dead staining, showing live (green) and dead (red) cells. Scale bar 500 µm. (**B**) Reproduced with permission from [32], Elsevier, 2018. Cornea stroma and epithelium structure. (**a**) 3D bio-printed cornea from human embryonic stem cells and human adipose tissue derived stem cells fabricated onto supportive membrane using laser-assisted bioprinting. This shows moderate transparency. (**b**) Cell viability of human embryonic stem cells seven days after printing shown with live-dead-staining. Live cells are visualized with green and dead cells with red. Scale bar 1 mm. (**C**) Reproduced with permission from [46], Wiley, 2019. Cornea endothelium structures. (**a**) Image of the bio-printed genetically modified human corneal endothelial cells (HCECs)/gelatin scaffold on an amniotic membrane. (**b**) The seeded live HCECs were densely and evenly distributed just after bioprinting. Scale bar: 500 µm.

Diseases affecting the corneal endothelium are the main cause of corneal transplantation [36]. Nevertheless, to date, only the study proposed by Kim et al. [46] has been focused on bioprinting. An interesting gene therapy approach was performed in which human corneal endothelial cells were genetically modified to express ribonuclease 5 (R5). R5 increases angiogenesis and facilitates endothelial cells' mitotic capacity. Therefore, cell survival rate and wound healing ability are promoted. Cells were embedded into a gelatin ink and were bio-printed by extrusion onto a bovine decellularized amniotic membrane (AM) simulating the Descement's membrane. After bioprinting, transparency, cell morphology and functional phenotype were assayed. Results showed that the scaffolds maintained their transparency for 10 days after bioprinting. Moreover, endothelial cells showed their usual shape and the R5 expression was high (Figure 5C). Then, scaffolds were implanted into rabbit's cornea. Cell injection and an acellular membrane were used as controls. After surgery, there was an improvement in transparency in rabbits where a bio-printed scaffold had been implanted. Furthermore, four weeks later, levels of transparency near to normal cornea were achieved. In contrast, inflammation and persistent corneal oedema were observed in rabbits treated with cells and the acellular membrane. In addition, the endothelial corneal cells of the scaffold maintained their activity and shape, and rabbit native cell attachment to the scaffold was observed. Results were promising since they presented 3D bioprinting as a good alternative to the conventional treatments of corneal diseases.

As we have seen, to date advances have been made in the field of 3D bioprinting to create corneal tissue, and in most of them, extrusion bioprinting is the most commonly used technique (Table 1). However, it has been demonstrated that alternative techniques, such as inkjet or laser assisted bioprinting, could also be advantageous since they can in some cases be more cell friendly. The studies are recent and are focused on the most extensive layer of the cornea, the stroma. Even so, the development of corneal epithelial and endothelial tissues also seems quite promising. Until now, due to the complex characteristics of the cornea, it has not been possible to obtain a complete multilayer corneal tissue through 3D bioprinting. Nevertheless, this technique is in its beginnings and studies have shown interesting advances over common therapies. Therefore, more research should be carried out in order to achieve a functional corneal tissue.

Table 1. Current studies of 3D bioprinting for cornea tissue engineering.

3D Bioprinting Technique	Materials of the Bio-Inks and Inks	Cells	Scaffold Function/Study Objective	In Vivo	Most Relevant Results	Ref.
Extrusion 3D bioprinting	Sodium alginate and methacrylated type I collagen	Human corneal keratocytes	Tissue replication. Corneal stroma structure	No	• Reproduce corneal curvature • Good printability • High cell viability after 7 days of bioprinting	[42]
Extrusion 3D bioprinting	Methacrylated gelatin (GelMA)	Human corneal keratocytes	Tissue replication. Corneal stroma structure	No	• Excellent transparency • Adequate mechanical strength • High cell viability but rounded morphology and low metabolic activity	[44]
Extrusion 3D bioprinting	Decellularized corneal extracellular matrix based bio-ink	Human corneal keratocytes differentiated from human turbinate derived mesenchymal stem cells	Tissue replication. Corneal stroma structure	New Zealand white rabbits	• Establishment of the best nozzle diameter in order to bio-print aligned collagen fibrils similar to cornea • Establishment of the best nozzle diameter in order to maintain keratocyte morphology and phenotypic characteristics • Transplanted scaffold showed good transparency in rabbit eyes • Keratocytes' cellular behaviour was activated after transplantation	[43]
Drop-on-demand inkjet bioprinting	Type I collagen and agarose	Human corneal keratocytes	Tissue replication. Corneal stroma structure	No	• Good transparency and optical density but low mechanical properties • Good cell viability. Cells became dendritic and achieved typical keratocyte shape. • Cells maintained their phenotype after bioprinting.	[37]
Extrusion 3D bioprinting	Sodium alginate, gelatin and type I collagen	Human corneal epithelial cells	Tissue replication. Corneal epithelium structure	No	• Good printability and high transparency • High cell viability after bioprinting but round morpholog • Fabrication of degradation-controllable systems using sodium citrate • Improvement of cell proliferation, growth and epithelial specific marker protein expression with the degradation system	[45]

Table 1. Cont.

3D Bioprinting Technique	Materials of the Bio-Inks and Inks	Cells	Scaffold Function/Study Objective	In Vivo	Most Relevant Results	Ref.
Combination of digital light processing (DLP) and extrusion 3D bioprinting	Methacrylated gelatin (GelMA) for DLP Sodium alginate and gelatin for extrusion 3D-bioprinting	Human corneal epithelial cells	Tissue replication. Development of supportive structure with DLP technique in order to bio-print corneal epithelium structure on it	No	• Good development of cornea structure with digital light processing (DLP) in terms of geometry, thickness and curvature. • Overall, good transparency of epithelium scaffolds but high diversity in mechanical properties • High cell viability and distribution	[30]
Laser-assisted 3D bioprinting	2 Types: Human recombinant laminin and Hyaluronic acid sodium Human collagen type I and Human blood plasma + Thrombin	Human embryonic stem cells (hESC) Human adipose derived stem cells (hASC)	Tissue replication. Cornea epithelium structure Corneal stroma structure	No Explanted porcine corneas	• Good printability with laser-assisted bioprinting • High hESC viability and epithelial specific marker protein expression • High proliferative protein expression in hASC • Strong adhesion, cell migration and good attachment to the host tissue in explanted porcine corneas • Opacity when both layers were combined	[32]
Extrusion 3D bioprinting	Gelatin based bio-ink	Human corneal endothelial cells genetically modified to express ribonuclease (R5)	Tissue replication. Corneal endothelium structure.	New Zealand white rabbits. Descemet's membrane-denuded corneal disorder model.	• High transparency • High cell viability, usual endothelial shape and high R5 expression. • Improvement of rabbit corneal transparency in vivo. • High functional phenotype expression and native cell attachment in vivo.	[46]

2.2. Retina

The retina is a multilayered vascularized complex tissue situated at the back of the eye, opposite to the pupil [47] (Figure 6). Its main function is to convert the light signals that reach the eye into electrical signals that are conducted to the brain [48]. This function is possible thanks to the photoreceptor cells that make up this tissue. The retina is formed by more than 130 million cells of at least 60 different types [24,49]. They are generated from the fetal retinal progenitor cells [48]. Some of these cells are rod and cone photoreceptor cells, bipolar cells, horizontal cells, retinal ganglion cells and the glial cells, among others [50]. All these cell types work together to convert the light signals into electrical signals. Under the retina there is a monolayer known as the retinal pigment epithelium (RPE) formed by pigment epithelial cells. This specialized monolayer is a physical support for the retina. In addition, it provides nutrients and growth factors that create a suitable biological microenvironment for the cells of the retina [51,52].

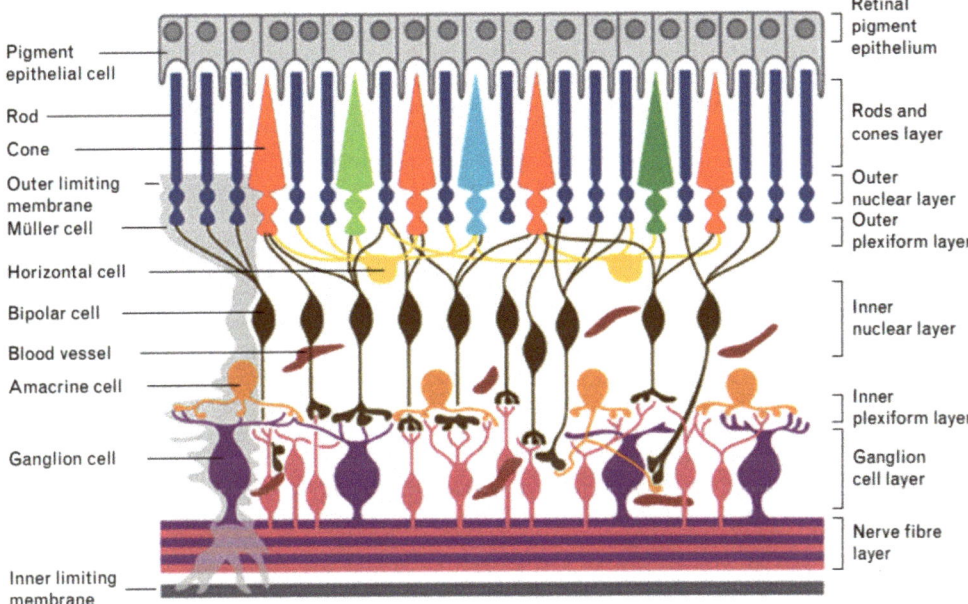

Figure 6. Diagram of the structure of the retina. The different cell types are located in different layers. The light reaches the nerve fiber layer. Ganglion cells transmit signals to bipolar and horizontal cells. Finally, they reach the rods and cones that transform it into electrical signals. The retinal pigment epithelium, formed by the epithelial pigment cells, served as physical, nutritional and signal support to the rest of the retina. Reproduced with permission from [53], Lippincott Williams and Wilkins Ltd., 2016.

The degeneration of the cells of the retina can lead to the appearance of different eye diseases. Some of these diseases are associated with a single cell type while others are associated with larger areas of the retina that involve different cell types. Some examples of the first type of disease are glaucoma [54], associated with retinal ganglion cells, and retinitis pigmentosa [55], associated with photoreceptor cells. An example of the latter is age-related macular degeneration (AMD) that arises because of mild and chronic inflammation of the central area of the retina [56]. The degenerations produced in the cells of the retina can lead to a progressive loss of vision until a total and irreversible loss is produced [27].

It is considered that many retinal diseases could be reversed if new cells from the retina were transplanted into the damaged area [57]. That is why many of the proposed therapies advocate the implantation of cells in the retina [58,59]. The administration of photoreceptor cells, progenitor cells, retinal sheets and RPE cells, among others, has been studied, although with not very clear results [60]. In fact, there is a considerable cell loss and a lack of control over cell behavior once implanted [61–63]. Therefore, appearance of abnormal behaviors and structures have been observed. As a solution to the problems involved in the implantation of cells in the retina, different scaffolds have been developed [64–66]. These scaffolds allow the transplantation of cells in a more controlled way. Solvent casting, electrospinning and molecular templating, among other techniques, have been used to produce these scaffolds [57]. Until now, none of the traditional microfabrication techniques have allowed the obtaining of 3D scaffolds with good structural properties and with the ability to incorporate the number of required cells in the correct position and orientation [24].

In this context, 3D bioprinting has been postulated as an excellent alternative for the design and production of scaffolds with characteristics that meet the needs of a tissue such as the retina. Some of the advantages that this technique offers are mentioned below.

Cell culture. It is very difficult to seed retinal cells in vitro [67]. Many of them undergo apoptosis and those that do not undergo dedifferentiation or stop producing the signals that they produce naturally in the eye [68]. Cells used for retinal regeneration have to be properly integrated and differentiated in the case of progenitor cells, or have to remain differentiated in the case of mature retinal cells. 3D bio-printed scaffolds allow the solving of these problems since they improve the viability and the maintenance of the phenotype of the implanted cells. Moreover, these 3D scaffolds provide mechanical and physical support for the adhesion, proliferation and differentiation of the retinal cells.

Complexity of scaffolds. The retina is a tissue with great structural complexity. It has several layers of diverse thicknesses and with different properties. 3D bioprinting allows the obtaining of precise scaffolds with highly complex designs (unlike previously used techniques that did not allow such control) [57]. The number of layers, their thickness and their spatial arrangement can be easily controlled by making a proper design and adjusting the printing parameters. It is necessary to replicate this spatial arrangement and thickness of the tissue so that the functions of the retina are not altered.

Cell types. The retina is a tissue with a high cell diversity. In particular, it has more than 60 different cell types [24,49]. 3D bioprinting allows the incorporation of different cell types to the scaffold [69]. These cells can be incorporated into different layers, thus resembling the original tissue. In this way, a possible approach could be the incorporation of ganglion cells in a first layer, bipolar cells in a second, cones and rods in a third, and RPE cells in a fourth layer. This arrangement would be very difficult to achieve by other current manufacturing techniques.

Cell orientation. The cells of the retina need a very specific orientation to be able to carry out their function properly [70,71]. The correct orientation of the cells is one of the most difficult aspects to achieve when making a scaffold. Although the new approaches that will emerge over time might allow more precise control of cell deposition, 3D bioprinting already allows a relative control over cell orientation. This can be achieved by adjusting the printing parameters, such as the printing orientation and layer thickness.

Stiffness. The average stiffness of the retina is 10–20 kPa [72]. Although this parameter is not as limiting as the previous limitations, it is important when trying to create a tissue to replace the one that is damaged [73]. 3D bioprinting works with a myriad of materials and their mixtures. This allows the achieving of a stiffness as similar as possible to that of the natural retina.

Taking into account all these advantages, different research groups have carried out approaches for retinal regeneration using 3D bioprinting and printing technology. Lorber et al. [74] used piezoelectric inkjet bioprinting to print retinal ganglion cell (RGC) neurons and retinal glial cells. The viability and effect of cell bioprinting on outgrowth in culture were studied. An abundant settlement of cells was detected in the nozzle. This fact significantly reduced the number of cells incorporated into the scaffolds. Nevertheless, the viabilities obtained were adequate compared to the control (69% and 78% for glial cells and 69% and 74% for retinal cells, respectively). Bioprinting did not appear to have a negative effect on the survival/regeneration properties of the cells in culture. Likewise, when used as a substrate, the glia cells that had been printed using 3D piezoelectric inkjet bioprinting retained their growth promoting properties. Kador et al. [60] used another 3D bioprinting technique to obtain their scaffold: the thermal inkjet bio-printing. In this study, they proposed a very novel approach since they evaluated the possibility of bioprinting RGC cells on an electro-spun matrix of polylactic acid. Different parameters were modified during bioprinting, such as the ejection energies and the cell densities. The results were promising. As in the previous study, good cell viabilities were obtained indicating that thermal inkjet bioprinting can effectively be used for obtaining scaffolds for retina regeneration. Furthermore, the bio-printed RGCs maintained adequate electrophysiological properties. One of the main goals of this study was to achieve a proper orientation of the cells. The microscopy images showed how the design of the matrix and the 3D bioprinting allowed the achievement of a radial arrangement of the axons of the printed cells. In this way, the orientation of the RGC was significantly improved compared to the control. Specifically, 72% of the axons were aligned with the scaffold while, in the case of the dendrites, 49% were aligned. Only 11% of the cells of the control group were aligned.

Another study in which great importance was given to the orientation of the cells was that carried out by Worthington et al. [57]. In this study, different scaffolds using two photon polymerization were obtained. The studied variables were the pore size, the hatching distance, the hatching type and the slicing distance. The time necessary for printing and the fidelity of the obtained scaffolds with respect to the original designs were analyzed and optimized. In addition, induced pluripotent stem cells (iPSCs) were differentiated into retinal progenitor cells and incorporated into the printed scaffolds (Figure 7). The obtained results made it possible to clarify that those scaffolds with larger diameter pores were better for use in retinal regeneration. In these scaffolds, retinal progenitor cells could be incorporated. Besides, cells formed neural structures aligned in parallel to the vertical pores of the scaffolds. In contrast, in the scaffolds with smaller diameter pores, cells remained on top of the surface and did not align in parallel to the pores.

Other studies have focused their attention on reproducing the structure of the retina. They have proposed different approaches to obtain different layers seeded with different cell types. Two examples of this type of approach are the ones proposed by Shi et al. [24,75]. Using microvalve-based bioprinting, a structure equivalent to that of the retina was created. A first monolayer was printed, made up of alginate and pluronic-containing RPE cells (ARPE-19) on a preformed membrane (Figure 8A). This structure simulated the RPE monolayer. Over it, a second layer was bio-printed. This was also made up of the same materials and contained photoreceptor cells (Y79) (Figure 8B,C). Two types of pattern were created for the top layer, one with a higher density of cells in the center and another with a higher density at the perimeter. The bio-ink printed with Y79 cells preserved its structure during the culture process. Viability was not compromised and cell density increased over time. This proof of concept demonstrated that a structure with characteristics similar to those of the retina can be obtained, achieving good cell viability and cytocompatibility. Wang et al. [76] made a similar approach. In this case, the 3D bioprinting technique used was laser assisted 3D. They obtained a two-layer scaffold similar to the retina. The bio-ink used in both layers was the same HA-GM (hyaluronic acid with methacrylation by glycidyl-hydroxyl reaction) and polyethylene-glycol-Arg-Gly-Asp-Ser peptide (PEG-RGDS). The difference between the two layers lay in the thickness and in the incorporated cells. For the RPE layer, RPE cells and a thickness of 125 um were used, while for the upper layer fetal retinal progenitor cells (fRPCs) were used that were differentiated to retina photoreceptors (PR), along with a layer thickness of 250 um. The porosity of the scaffold was analyzed as a function of the degree of methacrylation of the hyaluronic acid (low, medium or high), the swelling ratio, the rigidity of the scaffold, the viability of the cells, the formation of the two layers in the scaffold and the differentiation of fRPCs cells into PR cells within the scaffold. Results were encouraging since the stiffness of the scaffold was similar to that of the native retina, the viability remained above 70%, the microscopy images showed that two well-differentiated layers had been obtained (Figure 8D), and the fRPCs did differentiate into PR. Therefore, it was concluded that tis co-cultivation system allowed the development of an environment similar to that of the native retina, which promoted the maturation of PRs.

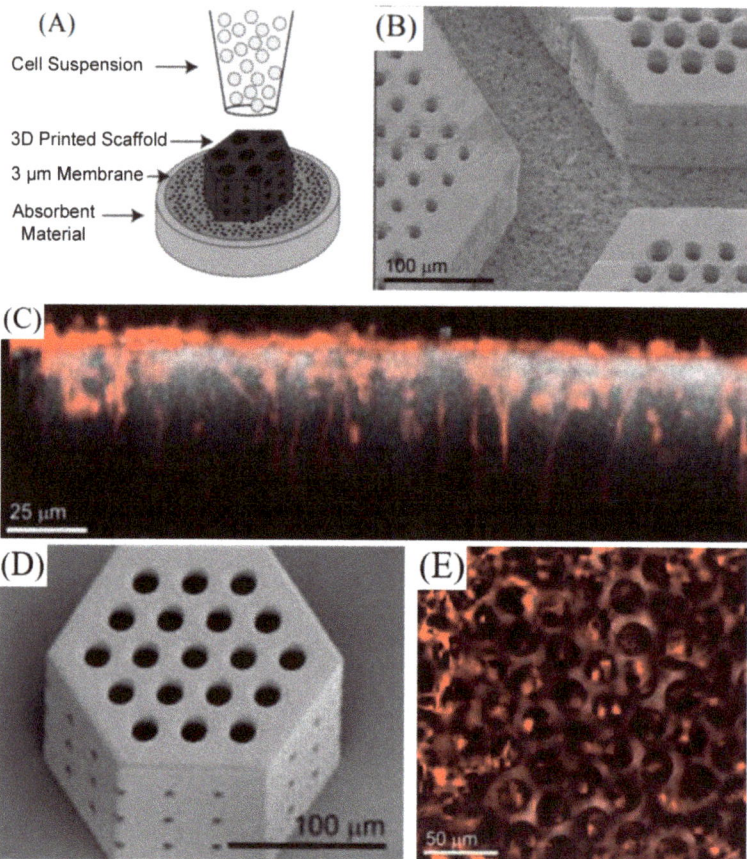

Figure 7. (**A**) Schematic of the retinal progenitor cell loading strategy. (**B**) Large photoreceptor cell porous membrane adhered to the membrane after processing. (**C**) Side view of retinal neurons (marked in red) settled in and aligned with 25 μm vertical pores. (**D**) Representative scanning electron microscopy (SEM) image of a small retinal progenitor cell scaffold used to determine design-to-structure fidelity. (**E**) Sequential top-down images of retinal neurons (marked in red) on the surface of photoreceptor scaffolds and nestled in 25 μm pores. Reproduced with permission from [57], Elsevier, 2017.

To date, these studies have made it possible to determine: (i) the cell viability after printing; (ii) the structure of the scaffolds; (iii) the orientation of the cells within the scaffolds; and (iv) their arrangement in different layers (different levels or heights) (Table 2). Still, much more research is needed. Among the steps to be taken in the near future are the bioprinting of more layers, the use of more cell types and the study of the ability of the bio-printed cells to transmit signals within the scaffold itself. In addition, it is expected that in the future the scaffolds obtained using 3D bioprinting will be more complex and similar to the native retina. Finally, these bio-printed tissues will serve as autologous retinal cell grafts to treat those patients suffering from retinal degeneration.

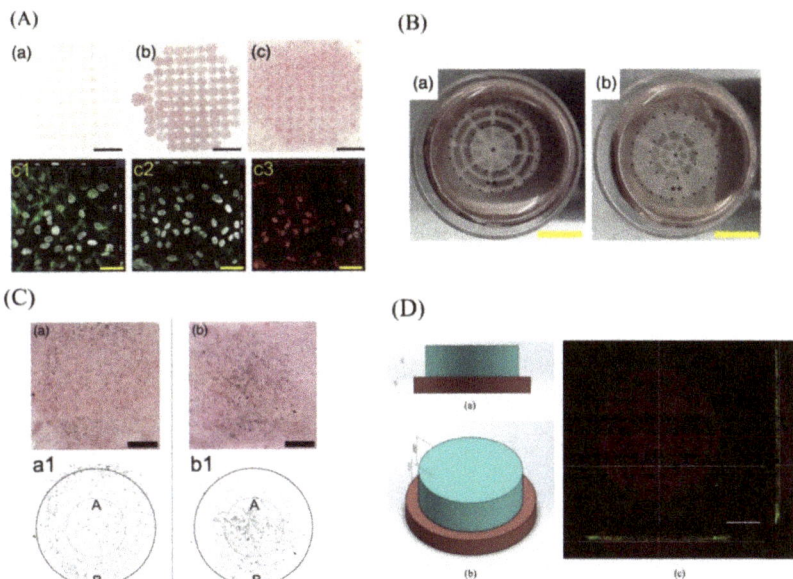

Figure 8. (**A**) Bio-printed ARPE-19 cells (**a–c**): hematoxylin and eosin staining at days 1, 7, and 14, respectively, scale bar: 5 mm. Confocal images of ARPE-19 cell layers at Day 14: F-actin cytoskeleton immunofluorescence staining (**c1**), Zonula occludens-1 (**c2**) in green, Claudin-1 (**c3**) in red, and nuclei in grey, scale bar: 50 µm. Reproduced with permission form [75], Wiley, 2018. (**B**) The bio-printed retinal equivalents with two distinctive Y79 cell-seeding density: high average cell density at the center (**a**) and high average cell density at the periphery (**b**); *: central area, **: periphery; scale bar: 10 mm. Reproduced with permission from [24], Whioce Publishing Pte. Ltd., 2017. (**C**) Hematoxylin and eosin staining of the bio-printed Y79 cells with two distinctive patterns on ARPE-19 cell monolayer at Day 14: high density at periphery (**a**) and high density at the central area (**b**). Data analysis (integrated intensity) of bio-printed Y79 proliferation after 14 days, high density at periphery (**a1**), and high density at the central area (**b1**); A = area of the inner circle; B = area of the annulus; diameters: small circle (10 mm) and large circle (20 mm); scale bar: 5 mm. Reproduced with permission from [75], Wiley, 2018. (**D**) Bilayer printing of fluorescent labelled hydrogels: (**a**) Top view and (**b**) side view of structural design from SolidWorks® (**c**) Confocal fluorescent images showing bilayer construct. The printed structure recapitulated the structural design, indicating ability to construct multi-layered structure. Scale bar = 500 µm. Reproduced with permission from [76], Elsevier, 2018.

Table 2. Current studies of 3D bioprinting for retina tissue engineering.

3D Bioprinting Technique	Materials of the Bio-Inks and Inks	Cells	Scaffold Function/Study Objective	In Vivo	Most Relevant Results	Ref.
Laser assisted 3D bioprinting	HA-GM (hyaluronic acid with methacrylation by glycidyl-hydroxyl reaction) and PEG-RGDS (Arg-Gly-Asp-Ser peptide)	Retinal pigment epithelial cells (RPE) Human fetal retinal progenitor cells (fRPCs)	Tissue equivalent replication. Retina made up of two layers	No	• Development of a structure of two layers: one assembling the retina (using fetal retinal progenitor cells (fRPCs)) and the other assembling the pigment epithelium (using RPE) • Good cell viability • Differentiation of fRPCs to PRs (photoreceptor cells) within the scaffold	[76]
Piezoelectric inkjet bioprinting	DMEM (Dulbecco's Modified Eagle's Medium) (not structural function)	Retinal ganglion cell (RGCs) neurons Retinal glial cells.	Study the effect of piezoelectric inkjet bioprinting in the viability of the printed cells.	No	• Piezoelectric inkjet allows printing of retinal cells with similar survival/regeneration properties to controls • Printed glial cells retain their growth promoting capability when used as substrate • Cell sedimentation occurred in the nozzle area	[74]
Microvalve-based inkjet bioprinting	DMEM:F12 (not structural function) Alginate and Pluronic	Human retinal pigmented epithelial cell line (ARPE-19) Human retinoblastoma cell line (Y79)	Tissue replication. Retina made up of two layers.	No	• Development of a structure formed by a monolayer with ARPE-19 cells (representing the Brunch's membrane and the RPE monolayer) and a second with a human retinoblastoma cell line (Y79) • The obtained structure is stable • Viability is not compromised and cell density increases with time	[24]

Table 2. Cont.

3D Bioprinting Technique	Materials of the Bio-Inks and Inks	Cells	Scaffold Function/Study Objective	In Vivo	Most Relevant Results	Ref.
Two-photon lithography	Indium tin oxide (ITO)-coated glass	Human induced pluripotent stem cell (iPSC)	Development of scaffolds to deliver correctly oriented retinal progenitor cells	No	• Establishment of the best parameters to print scaffolds using two-photon lithography with adequate and reproducible characteristics • Differentiation of iPSCs to retinal progenitor cells and incorporation of these last into the scaffold • The retinal progenitor cells formed neural structures parallel to the vertical pores of the scaffolds	[57]
Thermal inkjet 3D bioprinting combined with electrospinning	Alginate and culture Medium for 3D bioprinting Polylactic acid (PLA) dissolved in 1,1,1,3,3,3 hexafluoro-isopropanol (HFIP) and matrigel for electrospinning	Retinal ganglion Cells (rgcS)	Development of scaffolds to deliver correctly oriented retinal progenitor cells	No	• Determination of printing parameters, materials and cell density in order to print a pattern with an organization similar to that of the human retina • Good cell viability, adequate orientation of the cells in the pattern and correct guidance of the axons within the scaffold • The cells maintained their functional electrophysiological properties after being printed	[60]

2.3. Conjunctiva

The conjunctiva is a mucosal tissue that covers the sclera and provides lubrication and protection to the eye by producing tears and mucus [77]. It consists of a goblet cell rich in highly vascularized stratified epithelium [78]. This tissue suffers from different injuries caused by ocular thermal or chemical abrasions, conjunctival lacerations, autoimmune diseases, inflammation, foreign bodies or surgery, etc. [79]. To treat the damaged conjunctiva the usually employed strategies are surgery and autologous grafts or allograft tissues such as AM and pericardium [80]. These approaches have some limitations: (i) unavailability of healthy conjunctiva (in the case of autologous grafts); (ii) immune responses; (iii) keratinization; (iv) goblet cell loss; (v) microbial infections; (vi) low level of stratifications, and (vii) opacification of the site, etc. [78]. These limitations make necessary the development of new strategies among which 3D printing has been postulated as an excellent alternative. 3D printing can act as an improvement for the development of structures similar to the conjunctiva as it allows the achievement of the following characteristics.

Thickness. It is crucial to develop a 3D structure with an adequate thickness; that is, as close as possible to the original (average thickness of 33 µm). By determining the number of layers and their thickness, the size of the 3D printed structure can be controlled very precisely.

Cell density. 3D bioprinting allows control of the density of goblet cells included in the 3D developed membrane.

Transparency, elasticity and slight rigidity. The large number of materials that can be used in 3D bioprinting allows the controlling and adjusting of the color and transparency of the construct. These materials also make possible the obtaining of elastic properties similar to that of the healthy tissue. In addition, the rigidity of the scaffold can also be adjusted. One of the problems related with the grafts used so far is the difficulty of handling in operations because of their fineness. 3D bioprinting makes it possible to achieve scaffolds with sufficient rigidity to facilitate manipulation, without this, in turn, having a negative biological effect.

Biological activity. The use of materials of biological origin allows the adjustment of the re-epithelization capacity, decreasing scar formation and fornix foreshortening, adjusting biodegradability and achieving good biocompatibility.

So far, the only approach that has used 3D printing to obtain a structure that allows regeneration of the damaged conjunctiva is the one carried out by Dehghani et al. [81]. They developed a membrane by extrusion 3D printing using gelatin, elastin and hyaluronic acid as materials. They carried out multiple rheological and texturometry tests to guarantee that the ink and the membrane obtained had the necessary properties to be implanted in the conjunctiva. Biological properties were also analyzed in terms of cytocompatibility, adhesiveness and cell proliferation in vitro, and epithelialization, inflammation, scar tissue formation and presence of granulation tissue in vivo. All these results were compared with an AM (frequently used in injuries of conjunctiva). The results obtained were promising. The ink could be properly printed and the obtained membrane had adequate color and transparency, and its handling was simpler than that of the AM. Furthermore, in vitro good cytocompatibility, adhesion and cell proliferation were obtained. In vivo, the results were also positive. The epithelization time was similar in the printed membrane and in the AM. However, the data regarding inflammation, cell density, degradation and granulomatous reaction were better in the 3D printed membrane group.

These results show that this technique is suitable for the development of membranes for the regeneration of damaged conjunctiva. In this sense, it is reasonable to think that in the near future more research into the application of 3D printing to conjunctiva regeneration will be carried out.

3. 3D Printing for Ocular Drug Delivery

The main objective in the field of pharmacology is to achieve the maximum therapeutic effect with the minimum toxicity [82]. In this regard, the development of personalized patient specific drugs or doses is booming. 3D printing has recently been postulated as the appropriate technology to accomplish this goal due to its ease of use, fast speed, and accessibility [83]. In this way, the possibility of developing pharmaceutical forms containing various drugs, adjusting the doses to each patient and modifying drugs' pharmacokinetic profiles has become a reality in preclinical studies thanks to 3D printing technology [83]. This personalized medicine would bring a huge advantage to patients suffering from chronic eye pathologies, since current treatments require the constant application of eye drops and, in the worst cases, repetitive intravitreal injections that can cause devastating intraocular inflammation [84].

In this context, although there have been several studies in which 3D printing devices have been developed as drug delivery systems, only the one proposed by Won et al. [84] focuses on the eye. In this study, a flexible coaxial printing was used in order to develop a system that contained two drugs for the treatment of retinal vascular disease (RVD), which is based on an abnormal vascularization of the retina. The drug delivery system consisted of an external shell composed of polycaprolactone and bevacizumab (PCL-BEV), a drug that prevents excessive angiogenesis. The interior part was composed of sodium alginate and dexamethasone (ALG-DEX), an anti-inflammatory drug. In vitro assays showed a continuous release of BEV and DEX. Moreover, good biocompatibility and a reduction in the growth rate of human umbilical vein endothelial cells was observed. Then, the printed drug delivery system was intravitreally injected into two animal models: rabbits, in order to study the release kinetics, and choroid neovascularization (CVC) rat models, to determine its therapeutic effects. Intravitreal drug injections were used as control. Results corroborated that the printed drug delivery system prolonged the release of BEV and DEX compared to control. Interestingly, higher angiogenic inhibition over time was observed in CVC rats compared to controls and a reduction of inflammation was achieved.

As reflected in this study, the implementation of 3D printing technology for the development of specific drug delivery systems in ophthalmology can be valuable. In addition, the manufacture of artificial tissues similar to native tissues with this technology can be useful when it comes to screening new drugs for eye diseases. However, before this technology can be extensively applied in clinics, multiple regulatory questions should be addressed.

4. Ethical Issues and Commercialization Regulatory Aspects

Although the previously mentioned technical requirements can be fulfilled by increased research knowledge, there are still some relevant concerns related to both ethical and regulatory aspects that jeopardize the road to clinic of this "game changer" technology [1,2].

From an ethical point of view, a clear benefit of this technology includes the use of 3D bio-printed ocular organs or tissues for academic or research applications, as intermediate drug testing models between in vitro conditions and in vivo probing of concepts. Such models could work as a promising alternative to minimize the use of animals in the laboratory. In addition, patients' own cells reprogrammed into induced pluripotent stem cells (iPSCs) and bio-printed into 3D ocular structures could represent a more efficient and reliable model for drug testing than the use of experimental animals. However, there are also risks and ethical issues that should be considered, especially when 3D bioprinting technology is aimed at tissue engineering purposes. In this case, the composition of biological inks raises some concerns, not only associated with the security of the grafts implanted, but also related to the biological origin of such cells [3]. In the clearest scenario, where patient's autologous cells are included in the bio-ink composition, a random migration of cells from implanted ocular grafts could arise in different parts of the body, leading to potential undesired effects [5,8]. It is also likely that the biological behavior of such cells can be altered due to the mechanical stress that cells suffer by the transient forces applied during the bioprinting process. Therefore, although 3D bioprinting technology holds huge potential in tissue engineering clinical practice, the benefit-risk balance should be considered, in the same way as in other advanced therapies such as cell and gene therapy. In case non-autologous cells are implanted, apart from previously mentioned concerns, the possibility of inflammatory response against implanted ocular graft also needs to be analyzed. In this scenario, it should not be forgotten that the donor of cells for the implementation of 3D bio-printed grafts needs to sign an informed consent to allow the use of such cells. The situation is more delicate if non-autologous stem cells at the embryonic status are manipulated and bio-printed to become part of a grafted ocular tissue or organ, due to the ethical dilemma that arises with the use of embryonic cells. Another more challenging possibility is the use of cells derived from animal models to print ocular tissues implanted in humans. In this case, in addition to the previously mentioned biological concerns, the risk of developing zoonosis diseases should also be considered [20].

However, not only the origin and status of bio-printed cells rise ethical issues. We should also consider if any biological "item" can be printed [21]. For instance, and leaving apart any technological consideration, strictly from an ethical point of view, when implanting bio-printed tissues, a retina can be more problematic than a cornea, due to the neuronal structure of the retina and its direct connection to specific areas of the brain. This issue also generates the discussion as to whether specific areas of the brain, or even the brain or the eye as a whole, could be bio-printed and implanted into human beings.

Another ethical concern for the application of 3D bioprinting technology into regular clinical practice arises from the design and implementation of clinical trials for personalized medicines. Traditionally, clinical trials are designed and classified into different phases to evaluate the safety of the treatment in the early stages, and later the efficacy in a large population, before the introduction of a drug into the market. However, this approach is not feasible in the case of patient-tailored medical products for ophthalmic purposes, due to interindividual variability among human beings, which hampers any extrapolation of the results obtained in a specific patient, although experience accumulated in clinical cases could serve to gain progressive knowledge in order to apply the technology in medical practice [22]. Furthermore, the irreversible nature of grafts implanted by bioprinting technology impedes the patient's withdrawal from the trial after implantation, in the case of complications. In this sense, the development of 4D bio-printable organs, that can be biodegraded under physiological conditions after having performed the desired effect, merits special attention [24,25]. However, it should be also borne in mind that enrolling in this kind of clinical trial involves the acceptance of high risks associated with the implementation of the technology. Therefore, only advanced stages of diseases that have been unsuccessfully treated with conventional approaches should be amenable for this kind of treatment.

When dealing with health and financial resources, it is logical to expect ethical conflicts. In this sense, the technological possibility to bio-print and implant specific organs or tissues as an alternative solution to face advanced stages of diseases could stratify society. In this sense, even though the manufacturing of bio-inks and 3D bio-printing are not expensive items, the multidisciplinary nature of the global process, as well as the surveillance of this approach, makes it a high-cost procedure [85]. Hence, its implementation would be not affordable for all strata of society, only being obtainable for a particular subgroup of the total population with access to financial resources. Therefore, only those who can afford to pay for the bio-impression of their own organs would presumably enjoy a longer and better quality of life, minimizing for instance the use of immune-suppressant drugs indicated to avoid rejections of conventionally transplanted organs. In addition, relevant organs or tissues specifically designed with better biological properties could be implanted not only to deal with advanced stages of diseases, but also to enhance their physiological performance, which at the end could result in the elaboration of "super" bio-items for eugenic goals [86], such as "super" eyes or retinas.

Considering all the risks and benefits that 3D bioprinting technology can offer in the coming years, not only to the research and medical community but also to patients affected by ocular diseases, legal and regulatory aspects related to the implementation of the technology need also to be also deeply analyzed to avoid illicit and fraudulent use if the technology finally ends up in the "wrong hands". However, actually, the scale-up of 3D bioprinting technology and its clinical application for medical purposes does not fit into any of the current regulatory categories, despite that, from a global point of view, it could be considered as a specific tissue engineering approach [87]. In addition, the patient-tailored application of the technology hampers the compliance with global regulatory requirements for commercialization purposes that at moment are limited to recommendations, notifications and reports provided by European and American agencies, the EMA and FDA, respectively. Although nowadays both agencies aim to legislate the application of this innovate technology into clinical practice, they lack a specific regulatory framework [88]. From a more world-wide point of view, only a few regulatory agencies in countries such as Japan and South Korea have developed broad regulatory measures that can be applied to 3D bioprinting technology. This initiative could work as a starting point and reference for other countries. In any case, such regulatory measures are mainly focused on the application of these technologies for academic and research purposes or for the development of acellular devices in ophthalmology such us spectacles, lenses or smartphone-based fundus cameras, etc. [88]. Therefore, in order to implement this technology regularly in medical practice, it is necessary to start working on the design of a multidisciplinary and world-wide panel to provide a global regulatory framework. It also should be borne in mind that, in order to find a solution and resolve legal problems associated with the technology, all related tenets need to be addressed. In this sense, due to the complexity of the technology, a "whole" legal approach would be preferred, rather than a "piecemeal" approach.

5. Current Challenges and Future Perspectives of Ocular 3D Bioprinting

Recent advances in ocular 3D bioprinting have brought new opportunities for eye tissue engineering with potential biomedical applications, and nowadays it seems unquestionable that this field will continue to grow and evolve in future years. However, there are still relevant challenges to overcome before ocular and, in general, 3D bioprinting becomes a real clinical option.

First, the materials for bio-ink preparation should be biologically functional while maintaining robust and controllable post-printing mechanical properties and should enable adequate physiological, bio-chemical and mechanical interactions with the cellular component [89]. One strategy to find a desirable balance between biological activity and mechanical characteristics is the use of hybrid constructs that contain, on the one hand, synthetic materials that provide structural integrity and, on the other hand, natural materials that provide a cell-friendly environment for cellular growth. Other approaches are based on the chemical modification of the scaffold or on the use of synthetic peptides such as Arg-Gly-Asp (RGD) in order to prompt the crosslinking of the material and control its mechanical properties or its degradation time. For instance, a similar strategy was used for retinal bioprinting using a bio-ink based on HA with methacrylation by glycidyl-hydroxyl reaction and PEG-RGDS, with encouraging results, since the mechanical properties achieved allowed the bioprinting of two retinal layers with suitable rigidity and high cell viability [76]. In addition, cell differentiation occurred within the scaffold, which indicated that the hydrogel was biologically active and enabled biochemical interactions with the cell component. In this regard, appropriate cell orientation within the scaffold has also been achieved in retinal bioprinting using retinal ganglion cells that maintained their functional electrophysiological properties after being printed, demonstrating that the scaffold provided suitable physiological, biochemical and mechanical interactions for that purpose [60].

Cell sourcing constitutes another important challenge for 3D bioprinting of tissues and organs. In fact, a high number of regeneration-competent cells are needed and, due to tissue heterogeneity, different types of cells are also required. In fact, most organs are more complex than current 3D bioprinters can reproduce and achieving their intricate composition and functionality is still far from clinical translation [4,90]. In eye 3D bioprinting, most ocular structures bio-printed so far are limited to one or two cell types and, in the case of cornea and retina, only one or two layers have been bio-printed in the same construct, which is far from the authentic complex configuration of these ocular structures. In any case, regarding the challenges related to limited cell availability in forming the scaffolds, some of the solutions carried out to date are based on the use of stem cells or progenitor cells such as mesenchymal cells or induced pluripotent stem cells (iPSC), which, ideally, should be autologous or non-immunogenic [89]. In this sense, human fetal retinal progenitor cells have been used for retinal bioprinting and successful differentiation into photoreceptor cells was achieved [76]. In addition, human iPSC have also been used for retinal bioprinting and differentiated into retinal progenitor cells [57]. Considering all this, important advances have been made in order to overcome specific challenges related to cell sourcing, but more fundamental research is still needed in order to be able to bio-print a whole functional ocular structure such as the cornea or the retina with all the required different cell types and layers and the necessary biomechanical cues. These advances would contribute in the future to mimicking the complexity of the desired organ structures in a more precise manner.

In addition to the difficulties in obtaining a highly complex and similar to native bio-printed construct, another key aspect to consider before clinical translation could occur would be the vascularization and innervation of such tissue-engineered constructs after transplantation. So far, most tissue constructs obtained by 3D bioprinting lack a functional vascularization network, which would hinder the oxygen and nutrient supply after implantation in vivo [89]. Different strategies have been postulated in order to solve this issue in different types of tissue, including the use of angiogenic growth factors, the embedding of microchannels that would enhance the diffusion of oxygen and nutrients, or the direct fabrication of vasculature [89]. However, the reproduction of the complex and complete vascular network necessary for clinical translation remains very challenging. Regarding the eye, bioprinting a full ocular structure has still not been accomplished, so that would be the first step before moving to vascularization and innervation of the tissue construct. However, this aspect would acquire special relevance in the case of the retina, where the light signals captured by the photoreceptors must be processed into electrical impulses and transmitted through the optic nerve to the brain. In this regard, the functional electrophysiological properties of bio-printed retinal ganglion cells achieved so far [60] hold promise for future functional retinal constructs with appropriate connections among cells of the different retinal layers, capable of completing the complex visual phototransduction process.

In summary, recent advances in the field of 3D bioprinting and, particularly, for ocular tissue-engineering show promise for future biomedical applications, although there are still many challenges that need to be overcome before clinical translation can occur. Mimicking the complexity and heterogeneity of organs and providing them with the diversity of functional and supporting cell types, as well as with the essential functional elements such as vasculature and innervation, represent the major difficulties that 3D bioprinting is currently facing. In addition, for future commercialization, further aspects such as standardization of protocols, regulation of the process, the cost-effectiveness for scaling and the logistics of 3D bio-printed products would need to be taken into consideration. The key benefits of 3D bioprinting include the possibility of more targeted and personalized medicine, automated tissue fabrication and the flexibility of incorporating a wide variety of cells and materials in a precise anatomical 3D geometry. Further research for in vitro optimization and in vivo implementation of bio-printed tissue constructs and the combined efforts of different multidisciplinary fields would enhance the progress of 3D bioprinting towards clinically relevant bio-printed organs.

6. Conclusions

In recent years, great advances have been made while using 3D bioprinting for eye tissue engineering. Different ocular tissues with various layers and various cell types have been replicated. Nevertheless, we are still far from achieving complete tissues similar to healthy ones. It is expected that, in the future, the different ocular components will be completely replicated using 3D bioprinting. This progress could allow the combination of the structures obtained and to integrate them into a single construct, as a complete ocular model [27], which would require the consideration of corresponding ethical and biological aspects. Furthermore, as previously mentioned, the generated models would allow planning of operations before performing them, understanding the interaction between cells and the progression of different diseases affecting the tissue, or analyzing the effects of diverse drugs.

Funding: This research was fundedby the Basque Country Government (Department of Education, University and Research, Consolidated Groups IT907-16 and grant number PRE_2020_2_0143), and forms part of the Nanogrow project RTC-2017-6696-1. Additional funding was provided by the CIBER of Bioengineering, Biomaterials and Nanomedicine (CIBER-BBN), and initiative of the Carlos III Health Institute (ISCIII) and by the University of the Basque Country (UPV/EHU), postdoctoral grant number ESPDOC19/47). The APC was funded by the Basque Country Government (Department of Education, University and Research, Consolidated Groups IT907-16).

Acknowledgments: The authors wish to thank the intellectual and technical assistance from the ICTS "NANBIOSIS," more specifically by the Drug Formulation Unit (U10) of the CIBER in Bioengineering, Biomaterials and Nanomedicine (CIBER-BBN) at the University of Basque Country (UPV/EHU). I.V.B. thanks the University of the Basque Country (UPV/EHU) for the granted postdoctoral fellowship (ESPDOC19/47) from the call for the Specialization of Doctor Researcher Personnel. S.R.A thanks the Basque Government for the granted predoctoral fellowship (PRE_2020_2_0143).

Conflicts of Interest: The authors declare no conflict of interest.

References

1. Corsi, A.; de Souza, F.F.; Pagani, R.N.; Kovaleski, J.L. Big Data Analytics as a Tool for Fighting Pandemics: A Systematic Review of Literature. *J. Ambient. Intell. Hum. Comput.* **2020**, 1–18. [CrossRef] [PubMed]
2. Smith, V.; Warty, R.R.; Sursas, J.A.; Payne, O.; Nair, A.; Krishnan, S.; da Silva Costa, F.; Wallace, E.M.; Vollenhoven, B. The Effectiveness of Virtual Reality in Managing Acute Pain and Anxiety for Medical Inpatients: Systematic Review. *J. Med. Internet Res.* **2020**, *22*, e17980. [CrossRef] [PubMed]
3. Bova, L.; Billi, F.; Cimetta, E. Mini-Review: Advances in 3D Bioprinting of Vascularized Constructs. *Biol. Direct* **2020**, *15*, 1–5. [CrossRef]
4. Loai, S.; Kingston, B.; Wang, Z.; Philpott, D.; Tao, M.; Cheng, H. Clinical Perspectives on 3D Bioprinting Paradigms for Regenerative Medicine. *Regen. Med. Front.* **2019**, *1*, e190004.
5. Tan, C.T.; Liang, K.; Ngo, Z.H.; Dube, C.T.; Lim, C.Y. Application of 3D Bioprinting Technologies to the Management and Treatment of Diabetic Foot Ulcers. *Biomedicines* **2020**, *8*, 441. [CrossRef] [PubMed]
6. Di Marzio, N.; Eglin, D.; Serra, T.; Moroni, L. Bio-Fabrication: Convergence of 3D Bioprinting and Nano-Biomaterials in Tissue Engineering and Regenerative Medicine. *Front. Bioeng. Biotechnol.* **2020**, *8*, 326. [CrossRef]
7. Poomathi, N.; Singh, S.; Prakash, C.; Patil, R.V.; Perumal, P.T.; Barathi, V.A.; Balasubramanian, K.K.; Ramakrishna, S.; Maheshwari, N.U. Bioprinting in Ophthalmology: Current Advances and Future Pathways. *Rapid Prototyp. J.* **2019**, *25*, 496–514. [CrossRef]
8. Fonseca, A.C.; Melchels, F.P.W.; Ferreira, M.J.S.; Moxon, S.R.; Potjewyd, G.; Dargaville, T.R.; Kimber, S.J.; Domingos, M. Emulating Human Tissues and Organs: A Bioprinting Perspective Toward Personalized Medicine. *Chem. Rev.* **2020**, *120*, 11128–11174. [CrossRef] [PubMed]
9. Murphy, S.V.; Atala, A. 3D Bioprinting of Tissues and Organs. *Nat. Biotechnol.* **2014**, *32*, 773–785. [CrossRef] [PubMed]
10. Hölzl, K.; Lin, S.; Tytgat, L.; Van Vlierberghe, S.; Gu, L.; Ovsianikov, A. Bioink Properties before, during and After 3D Bioprinting. *Biofabrication* **2016**, *8*, 032002. [CrossRef]
11. Gopinathan, J.; Noh, I. Recent Trends in Bioinks for 3D Printing. *Biomater. Res.* **2018**, *22*, 11. [CrossRef]
12. Yang, Y.; Song, X.; Li, X.; Chen, Z.; Zhou, C.; Zhou, Q.; Chen, Y. Recent Progress in Biomimetic Additive Manufacturing Technology: From Materials to Functional Structures. *Adv. Mater.* **2018**, *30*, 1706539. [CrossRef] [PubMed]
13. Kyle, S.; Jessop, Z.M.; Al-Sabah, A.; Whitaker, I.S. 'Printability' of Candidate Biomaterials for Extrusion Based 3D Printing: State-of-the-Art. *Adv. Healthc. Mater.* **2017**, *6*. Epub 30 May 2017. [CrossRef] [PubMed]
14. Li, J.; Chen, M.; Fan, X.; Zhou, H. Recent Advances in Bioprinting Techniques: Approaches, Applications and Future Prospects. *J. Transl. Med.* **2016**, *14*, 271. [CrossRef] [PubMed]
15. Yue, Z.; Liu, X.; Coates, P.T.; Wallace, G.G. Advances in Printing Biomaterials and Living Cells: Implications for Islet Cell Transplantation. *Curr. Opin. Organ. Transplant.* **2016**, *21*, 467–475. [CrossRef] [PubMed]

16. Malda, J.; Visser, J.; Melchels, F.P.; Jüngst, T.; Hennink, W.E.; Dhert, W.J.A.; Groll, J.; Hutmacher, D.W. 25th Anniversary Article: Engineering Hydrogels for Biofabrication. *Adv. Mater.* **2013**, *25*, 5011–5028. [CrossRef] [PubMed]
17. Bhattacharjee, N.; Urrios, A.; Kang, S.; Folch, A. The Upcoming 3D-Printing Revolution in Microfluidics. *Lab Chip* **2016**, *16*, 1720–1742. [CrossRef] [PubMed]
18. Visser, J.; Melchels, F.P.W.; Weinans, H.; Kruyt, M.C.; Malda, J. Applications of 3D Printing in Medicine; 5 Years Later. *Ned. Tijdschr. Geneeskd.* **2019**, *163*, D3683. [PubMed]
19. Sommer, A.C.; Blumenthal, E.Z. Implementations of 3D Printing in Ophthalmology. *Graefes Arch. Clin. Exp. Ophthalmol.* **2019**, *257*, 1815–1822. [CrossRef] [PubMed]
20. Zhang, B.; Xue, Q.; Li, J.; Ma, L.; Yao, Y.; Ye, H.; Cui, Z.; Yang, H. 3D Bioprinting for Artificial Cornea: Challenges and Perspectives. *Med. Eng. Phys.* **2019**, *71*, 68–78. [CrossRef] [PubMed]
21. Sorbara, L.; Maram, J.; Fonn, D.; Woods, C.; Simpson, T. Metrics of the Normal Cornea: Anterior Segment Imaging with the Visante OCT. *Clin. Exp. Optom.* **2010**, *93*, 150–156. [CrossRef] [PubMed]
22. Cunha-Vaz, J. The Blood-Ocular Barriers. *Surv. Ophthalmol.* **1979**, *23*, 279–296. [CrossRef]
23. Mandrycky, C.; Wang, Z.; Kim, K.; Kim, D.H. 3D Bioprinting for Engineering Complex Tissues. *Biotechnol. Adv.* **2016**, *34*, 422–434. [CrossRef] [PubMed]
24. Shi, P.; Edgar, T.Y.S.; Yeong, W.Y.; Laude, A. Hybrid Three-Dimensional (3D) Bioprinting of Retina Equivalent for Ocular Research. *Int. J. Bioprint* **2017**, *3*, 008. [CrossRef]
25. Cubo-Mateo, N.; Podhajsky, S.; Knickmann, D.; Slenzka, K.; Ghidini, T.; Gelinsky, M. Can 3D Bioprinting be a Key for Exploratory Missions and Human Settlements on the Moon and Mars? *Biofabrication* **2020**, *12*, 043001. [CrossRef]
26. Nayak, K.; Misra, M. A Review on Recent Drug Delivery Systems for Posterior Segment of Eye. *Biomed. Pharmacother.* **2018**, *107*, 1564–1582. [CrossRef] [PubMed]
27. Fenton, O.S.; Paolini, M.; Andresen, J.L.; Müller, F.J.; Langer, R. Outlooks on Three-Dimensional Printing for Ocular Biomaterials Research. *J. Ocul. Pharmacol. Ther.* **2020**, *36*, 7–17. [CrossRef] [PubMed]
28. Willoughby, C.E.; Ponzin, D.; Ferrari, S.; Lobo, A.; Landau, K.; Omidi, Y. Anatomy and Physiology of the Human Eye: Effects of Mucopolysaccharidoses Disease on Structure and Function—A Review. *Clin. Experiment. Ophthalmol.* **2010**, *38*, 2–11. [CrossRef]
29. Ludwig, P.E.; Huff, T.J.; Zuniga, J.M. The Potential Role of Bioengineering and Three-Dimensional Printing in Curing Global Corneal Blindness. *J. Tissue Eng.* **2018**, *9*, 2041731418769863. [CrossRef] [PubMed]
30. Zhang, B.; Xue, Q.; Hu, H.; Yu, M.; Gao, L.; Luo, Y.; Li, Y.; Li, J.; Ma, L.; Yao, Y.; et al. Integrated 3D Bioprinting-Based Geometry-Control Strategy for Fabricating Corneal Substitutes. *J. Zhejiang Univ. B Sci.* **2019**, *20*, 945–959. [CrossRef] [PubMed]
31. Shiju, T.M.; Carlos de Oliveira, R.; Wilson, S.E. 3D in Vitro Corneal Models: A Review of Current Technologies. *Exp. Eye Res.* **2020**, *200*, 108213. [CrossRef]
32. Sorkio, A.; Koch, L.; Koivusalo, L.; Deiwick, A.; Miettinen, S.; Chichkov, B.; Skottman, H. Human Stem Cell Based Corneal Tissue Mimicking Structures using Laser-Assisted 3D Bioprinting and Functional Bioinks. *Biomaterials* **2018**, *171*, 57–71. [CrossRef]
33. McKay, T.B.; Hutcheon, A.E.K.; Guo, X.; Zieske, J.D.; Karamichos, D. Modeling the Cornea in 3-Dimensions: Current and Future Perspectives. *Exp. Eye Res.* **2020**, *197*, 108127. [CrossRef] [PubMed]
34. Gibney, R.; Matthyssen, S.; Patterson, J.; Ferraris, E.; Zakaria, N. The Human Cornea as a Model Tissue for Additive Biomanufacturing: A Review. *Procedia Cirp.* **2017**, *65*, 56–63. [CrossRef]
35. Prina, E.; Mistry, P.; Sidney, L.E.; Yang, J.; Wildman, R.D.; Bertolin, M.; Breda, C.; Ferrari, B.; Barbaro, V.; Hopkinson, A.; et al. 3D Microfabricated Scaffolds and Microfluidic Devices for Ocular Surface Replacement: A Review. *Stem Cell Rev. Rep.* **2017**, *13*, 430–441. [CrossRef] [PubMed]
36. Fuest, M.; Yam, G.H.; Mehta, J.S.; Duarte Campos, D.F. Prospects and Challenges of Translational Corneal Bioprinting. *Bioengineering* **2020**, *7*, 71. [CrossRef] [PubMed]
37. Duarte Campos, D.F.; Rohde, M.; Ross, M.; Anvari, P.; Blaeser, A.; Vogt, M.; Panfil, C.; Yam, G.H.; Mehta, J.S.; Fischer, H.; et al. Corneal Bioprinting Utilizing Collagen-based Bioinks and Primary Human Keratocytes. *J. Biomed. Mater. Res. Part A* **2019**, *107*, 1945–1953. [CrossRef] [PubMed]
38. Kao, W.; Coulson-Thomas, V. Cell Therapy of Corneal Diseases. *Cornea* **2016**, *35* (Suppl. 1), S9–S19. [CrossRef]
39. Meller, D.; Pauklin, M.; Thomasen, H.; Westekemper, H.; Steuhl, K. Amniotic Membrane Transplantation in the Human Eye. *Dtsch. Ärzteblatt Int.* **2011**, *108*, 243–248. [CrossRef] [PubMed]
40. Wallace, H.B.; McKelvie, J.; Green, C.R.; Misra, S.L. Corneal Curvature: The Influence of Corneal Accommodation and Biomechanics on Corneal Shape. *Transl. Vis. Sci. Technol.* **2019**, *8*, 5. [CrossRef] [PubMed]
41. Iyamu, E.; Iyamu, J.; Obiakor, C.I. The Role of Axial Length-Corneal Radius of Curvature Ratio in Refractive State Categorization in a Nigerian Population. *ISRN Ophthalmol.* **2011**, *2011*, 138941–138946. [CrossRef] [PubMed]
42. Isaacson, A.; Swioklo, S.; Connon, C.J. 3D Bioprinting of a Corneal Stroma Equivalent. *Exp. Eye Res.* **2018**, *173*, 188–193. [CrossRef]
43. Kim, H.; Jang, J.; Park, J.; Lee, K.; Lee, S.; Lee, D.; Kim, K.H.; Kim, H.K.; Cho, D. Shear-Induced Alignment of Collagen Fibrils using 3D Cell Printing for Corneal Stroma Tissue Engineering. *Biofabrication* **2019**, *11*, 035017. [CrossRef] [PubMed]
44. Kilic Bektas, C.; Hasirci, V. Cell Loaded 3D Bioprinted GelMA Hydrogels for Corneal Stroma Engineering. *Biomater. Sci.* **2020**, *8*, 438–449. [CrossRef] [PubMed]
45. Wu, Z.; Su, X.; Xu, Y.; Kong, B.; Sun, W.; Mi, S. Bioprinting Three-Dimensional Cell-Laden Tissue Constructs with Controllable Degradation. *Sci. Rep.* **2016**, *6*, 24474. [CrossRef] [PubMed]

46. Kim, K.W.; Lee, S.J.; Park, S.H.; Kim, J.C. Ex Vivo Functionality of 3D Bioprinted Corneal Endothelium Engineered with Ribonuclease 5-Overexpressing Human Corneal Endothelial Cells. *Adv. Healthc. Mater.* **2018**, *7*, 1800398. [CrossRef]
47. Eiraku, M.; Takata, N.; Ishibashi, H.; Kawada, M.; Sakakura, E.; Okuda, S.; Sekiguchi, K.; Adachi, T.; Sasai, Y. Self-Organizing Optic-Cup Morphogenesis in Three-Dimensional Culture. *Nature* **2011**, *472*, 51–56. [CrossRef] [PubMed]
48. Grossniklaus, H.E.; Geisert, E.E.; Nickerson, J.M. Chapter Twenty-Two—Introduction to the Retina. In *Progress in Molecular Biology and Translational Science*; Hejtmancik, J.F., Nickerson, J.M., Eds.; Academic Press: Cambridge, MA, USA, 2015; Volume 134, pp. 383–396.
49. Thoreson, W.B.; Dacey, D.M. Diverse Cell Types, Circuits, and Mechanisms for Color Vision in the Vertebrate Retina. *Physiol. Rev.* **2019**, *99*, 1527–1573. [CrossRef]
50. Holmes, D. Reconstructing the Retina. *Nature* **2018**, *561*, S2–S3. [CrossRef]
51. Ao, J.; Wood, J.P.; Chidlow, G.; Gillies, M.C.; Casson, R.J. Retinal Pigment Epithelium in the Pathogenesis of Age-Related Macular Degeneration and Photobiomodulation as a Potential Therapy? *Clin. Exp. Ophthalmol.* **2018**, *46*, 670–686. [CrossRef]
52. Yvon, C.; Ramsden, C.M.; Lane, A.; Powner, M.B.; da Cruz, L.; Coffey, P.J.; Carr, A.F. Using Stem Cells to Model Diseases of the Outer Retina. *Comput. Struct. Biotechnol. J.* **2015**, *13*, 382–389. [CrossRef] [PubMed]
53. Lorber, B.; Hsiao, W.; Martin, K.R. Three-Dimensional Printing of the Retina. *Curr. Opin. Ophthalmol.* **2016**, *27*, 262–267. [CrossRef] [PubMed]
54. Gupta, D.; Chen, P.P. Glaucoma. *Am. Fam. Physician* **2016**, *93*, 668–674. [PubMed]
55. Tsang, S.H.; Sharma, T. Retinitis Pigmentosa (Non-Syndromic). *Adv. Exp. Med. Biol.* **2018**, *1085*, 125–130.
56. Mitchell, P.; Liew, G.; Gopinath, B.; Wong, T.Y. Age-Related Macular Degeneration. *Lancet* **2018**, *392*, 1147–1159. [CrossRef]
57. Worthington, K.S.; Wiley, L.A.; Kaalberg, E.E.; Collins, M.M.; Mullins, R.F.; Stone, E.M.; Tucker, B.A. Two-Photon Polymerization for Production of Human iPSC-Derived Retinal Cell Grafts. *Acta Biomater.* **2017**, *55*, 385–395. [CrossRef] [PubMed]
58. Hertz, J.; Qu, B.; Hu, Y.; Patel, R.D.; Valenzuela, D.A.; Goldberg, J.L. Survival and Integration of Developing and Progenitor-Derived Retinal Ganglion Cells Following Transplantation. *Cell Transplant.* **2014**, *23*, 855–872. [CrossRef]
59. Singhal, S.; Bhatia, B.; Jayaram, H.; Becker, S.; Jones, M.F.; Cottrill, P.B.; Khaw, P.T.; Salt, T.E.; Limb, G.A. Human Müller Glia with Stem Cell Characteristics Differentiate into Retinal Ganglion Cell (RGC) Precursors in Vitro and Partially Restore RGC Function in Vivo Following Transplantation. *Stem Cells Transl. Med.* **2012**, *1*, 188–199. [CrossRef] [PubMed]
60. Kador, K.E.; Grogan, S.P.; Dorthé, E.W.; Venugopalan, P.; Malek, M.F.; Goldberg, J.L.; D'lima, D.D. Control of Retinal Ganglion Cell Positioning and Neurite Growth: Combining 3D Printing with Radial Electrospun Scaffolds. *Tissue Eng. Part A* **2016**, *22*, 286–294. [CrossRef] [PubMed]
61. Barber, A.C.; Hippert, C.; Duran, Y.; West, E.L.; Bainbridge, J.W.B.; Warre-Cornish, K.; Luhmann, U.F.O.; Lakowski, J.; Sowden, J.C.; Ali, R.R.; et al. Repair of the Degenerate Retina by Photoreceptor Transplantation. *Proc. Natl. Acad. Sci. USA* **2013**, *110*, 354–359. [CrossRef]
62. Ballios, B.G.; Cooke, M.J.; Donaldson, L.; Coles, B.L.K.; Morshead, C.M.; van der Kooy, D.; Shoichet, M.S. A Hyaluronan-Based Injectable Hydrogel Improves the Survival and Integration of Stem Cell Progeny Following Transplantation. *Stem Cell Rep.* **2015**, *4*, 1031–1045. [CrossRef] [PubMed]
63. MacLaren, R.E.; Pearson, R.A.; MacNeil, A.; Douglas, R.H.; Salt, T.E.; Akimoto, M.; Swaroop, A.; Sowden, J.C.; Ali, R.R. Retinal Repair by Transplantation of Photoreceptor Precursors. *Nature* **2006**, *444*, 203–207. [CrossRef]
64. Hynes, S.R.; Lavik, E.B. A Tissue-Engineered Approach towards Retinal Repair: Scaffolds for Cell Transplantation to the Subretinal Space. *Graefes Arch. Clin. Exp. Ophthalmol.* **2010**, *248*, 763–778. [CrossRef] [PubMed]
65. Yao, J.; Tao, S.; Young, M. Synthetic Polymer Scaffolds for Stem Cell Transplantation in Retinal Tissue Engineering. *Polymers* **2011**, *3*, 899–914. [CrossRef]
66. Treharne, A.J.; Grossel, M.C.; Lotery, A.J.; Thomson, H.A. The Chemistry of Retinal Transplantation: The Influence of Polymer Scaffold Properties on Retinal Cell Adhesion and Control. *Br. J. Ophthalmol.* **2011**, *95*, 768–773. [CrossRef] [PubMed]
67. Sorkio, A.E.; Vuorimaa-Laukkanen, E.; Hakola, H.M.; Liang, H.; Ujula, T.A.; Valle-Delgado, J.; Österberg, M.; Yliperttula, M.L.; Skottman, H. Biomimetic Collagen I and IV Double Layer Langmuir-Schaefer Films as Microenvironment for Human Pluripotent Stem Cell Derived Retinal Pigment Epithelial Cells. *Biomaterials* **2015**, *51*, 257–269. [CrossRef]
68. Baranov, P.; Michaelson, A.; Kundu, J.; Carrier, R.L.; Young, M. Interphotoreceptor Matrix-Poly(E-Caprolactone) Composite Scaffolds for Human Photoreceptor Differentiation. *J. Tissue Eng.* **2014**, *5*, 2041731414554179. [CrossRef] [PubMed]
69. Munaz, A.; Vadivelu, R.K.; St. John, J.; Barton, M.; Kamble, H.; Nguyen, N. Three-Dimensional Printing of Biological Matters. *J. Sci. Adv. Mater. Devices* **2016**, *1*, 1–17. [CrossRef]
70. Chui, T.Y.P.; Song, H.; Clark, C.A.; Papay, J.A.; Burns, S.A.; Elsner, A.E. Cone Photoreceptor Packing Density and the Outer Nuclear Layer Thickness in Healthy Subjects. *Investig. Ophthalmol. Vis. Sci.* **2012**, *53*, 3545–3553. [CrossRef]
71. Song, H.; Chui, T.Y.P.; Zhong, Z.; Elsner, A.E.; Burns, S.A. Variation of Cone Photoreceptor Packing Density with Retinal Eccentricity and Age. *Investig. Ophthalmol. Vis. Sci.* **2011**, *52*, 7376–7384. [CrossRef] [PubMed]
72. Worthington, K.S.; Wiley, L.A.; Bartlett, A.M.; Stone, E.M.; Mullins, R.F.; Salem, A.K.; Guymon, C.A.; Tucker, B.A. Mechanical Properties of Murine and Porcine Ocular Tissues in Compression. *Exp. Eye Res.* **2014**, *121*, 194–199. [CrossRef]
73. Hertz, J.; Robinson, R.; Valenzuela, D.A.; Lavik, E.B.; Goldberg, J.L. A Tunable Synthetic Hydrogel System for Culture of Retinal Ganglion Cells and Amacrine Cells. *Acta Biomater.* **2013**, *9*, 7622–7629. [CrossRef]

74. Lorber, B.; Hsiao, W.; Hutchings, I.M.; Martin, K.R. Adult Rat Retinal Ganglion Cells and Glia can be Printed by Piezoelectric Inkjet Printing. *Biofabrication* **2014**, *6*, 015001. [CrossRef] [PubMed]
75. Shi, P.; Tan, Y.S.E.; Yeong, W.Y.; Li, H.Y.; Laude, A. A Bilayer Photoreceptor-Retinal Tissue Model with Gradient Cell Density Design: A Study of Microvalve-Based Bioprinting. *J. Tissue Eng. Regen. Med.* **2018**, *12*, 1297–1306. [CrossRef] [PubMed]
76. Wang, P.; Li, X.; Zhu, W.; Zhong, Z.; Moran, A.; Wang, W.; Zhang, K.; Chen, S. 3D Bioprinting of Hydrogels for Retina Cell Culturing. *Bioprinting* **2018**, *12*, e00029. [CrossRef]
77. Taurone, S.; Spoletini, M.; Ralli, M.; Gobbi, P.; Artico, M.; Imre, L.; Czakò, C.; Kovàcs, I.; Greco, A.; Micera, A. Ocular Mucous Membrane Pemphigoid: A Review. *Immunol. Res.* **2019**, *67*, 280–289. [CrossRef] [PubMed]
78. Witt, J.; Mertsch, S.; Borrelli, M.; Dietrich, J.; Geerling, G.; Schrader, S.; Spaniol, K. Decellularised Conjunctiva for Ocular Surface Reconstruction. *Acta Biomater.* **2018**, *67*, 259–269. [CrossRef]
79. Yamaguchi, T. Inflammatory Response in Dry Eye. *Investig. Ophthalmol. Vis. Sci.* **2018**, *59*, DES192–DES199. [CrossRef] [PubMed]
80. Alam, J.; de Paiva, C.S.; Pflugfelder, S.C. Immune—Goblet Cell Interaction in the Conjunctiva. *Ocul. Surf.* **2020**, *18*, 326–334. [CrossRef]
81. Dehghani, S.; Rasoulianboroujeni, M.; Ghasemi, H.; Keshel, S.H.; Nozarian, Z.; Hashemian, M.N.; Zarei-Ghanavati, M.; Latifi, G.; Ghaffari, R.; Cui, Z.; et al. 3D-Printed Membrane as an Alternative to Amniotic Membrane for Ocular Surface/Conjunctival Defect Reconstruction: An in Vitro & in Vivo Study. *Biomaterials* **2018**, *174*, 95–112. [PubMed]
82. Mathew, E.; Pitzanti, G.; Larrañeta, E.; Lamprou, D.A. 3D Printing of Pharmaceuticals and Drug Delivery Devices. *Pharmaceutics* **2020**, *12*, 266. [CrossRef] [PubMed]
83. Peng, W.; Datta, P.; Ayan, B.; Ozbolat, V.; Sosnoski, D.; Ozbolat, I.T. 3D Bioprinting for Drug Discovery and Development in Pharmaceutics. *Acta Biomater.* **2017**, *57*, 26–46. [CrossRef]
84. Won, J.Y.; Kim, J.; Gao, G.; Kim, J.; Jang, J.; Park, Y.; Cho, D. 3D Printing of Drug-Loaded Multi-Shell Rods for Local Delivery of Bevacizumab and Dexamethasone: A Synergetic Therapy for Retinal Vascular Diseases. *Acta Biomater.* **2020**, *116*, 174–185. [CrossRef] [PubMed]
85. Reid, J.A.; Mollica, P.A.; Johnson, G.D.; Ogle, R.C.; Bruno, R.D.; Sachs, P.C. Accessible Bioprinting: Adaptation of a Low-Cost 3D-Printer for Precise Cell Placement and Stem Cell Differentiation. *Biofabrication* **2016**, *8*, 025017. [CrossRef] [PubMed]
86. Velasco Fernandez, R. The Philosophical Basis of Eugenesia. *Medicina* **1960**, *40*, 2.
87. Pashkov, V.; Harkusha, A. 3-D Bioprinting Law Regulation Perspectives. *Wiad. Lek.* **2017**, *70*, 480–482. [PubMed]
88. Gilbert, F.; O'Connell, C.D.; Mladenovska, T.; Dodds, S. Print Me an Organ? Ethical and Regulatory Issues Emerging from 3D Bioprinting in Medicine. *Sci. Eng. Ethics* **2018**, *24*, 73–91. [CrossRef]
89. Murphy, S.V.; De Coppi, P.; Atala, A. Opportunities and challenges of translational 3D bioprinting. *Nat. Biomed. Eng.* **2020**, *4*, 370–380. [CrossRef] [PubMed]
90. Heinrich, M.A.; Liu, W.; Jimenez, A.; Yang, J.; Akpek, A.; Liu, X.; Pi, Q.; Mu, X.; Hu, N.; Schiffelers, R.M.; et al. 3D Bioprinting: From Benches to Translational Applications. *Small* **2019**, *15*, e1805510. [CrossRef] [PubMed]

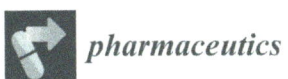

Article

Material Characterisation and Stratification of Conjunctival Epithelial Cells on Electrospun Poly(ε-Caprolactone) Fibres Loaded with Decellularised Tissue Matrices

Lucy A. Bosworth [1,*], Kyle G. Doherty [1], James D. Hsuan [1,2], Samuel P. Cray [1], Raechelle A. D'Sa [3], Catalina Pineda Molina [4,5], Stephen F. Badylak [4,5,6] and Rachel L. Williams [1]

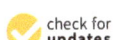

Citation: Bosworth, L.A.; Doherty, K.G.; Hsuan, J.D.; Cray, S.P.; D'Sa, R.A.; Pineda Molina, C.; Badylak, S.F.; Williams, R.L. Material Characterisation and Stratification of Conjunctival Epithelial Cells on Electrospun Poly(ε-Caprolactone) Fibres Loaded with Decellularised Tissue Matrices. *Pharmaceutics* **2021**, *13*, 318. https://doi.org/10.3390/pharmaceutics13030318

Academic Editor: Yolanda Diebold

Received: 27 January 2021
Accepted: 24 February 2021
Published: 28 February 2021

Publisher's Note: MDPI stays neutral with regard to jurisdictional claims in published maps and institutional affiliations.

Copyright: © 2021 by the authors. Licensee MDPI, Basel, Switzerland. This article is an open access article distributed under the terms and conditions of the Creative Commons Attribution (CC BY) license (https://creativecommons.org/licenses/by/4.0/).

[1] Department of Eye and Vision Science, Institute of Life Course and Medical Sciences, Faculty of Health and Life Sciences, University of Liverpool, Liverpool L7 8TX, UK; K.Doherty@liverpool.ac.uk (K.G.D.); JAMES.HSUAN@liverpoolft.nhs.uk (J.D.H.); hlscray@liverpool.ac.uk (S.P.C.); rlw@liverpool.ac.uk (R.L.W.)
[2] Liverpool University Hospitals NHS Foundation Trust, Liverpool L9 7AL, UK
[3] Department of Mechanical, Materials and Aerospace Engineering, Faculty of Science and Engineering, University of Liverpool, Liverpool L69 3GH, UK; rdsa@liverpool.ac.uk
[4] McGowan Institute for Regenerative Medicine, University of Pittsburgh, Pittsburgh, PA 15219, USA; CAP131@pitt.edu (C.P.M.); badylaks@upmc.edu (S.F.B.)
[5] Department of Surgery, School of Medicine, University of Pittsburgh, Pittsburgh, PA 15213, USA
[6] Department of Bioengineering, University of Pittsburgh, Pittsburgh, PA 15261, USA
* Correspondence: lucy.bosworth@liverpool.ac.uk

Abstract: The conjunctiva, an under-researched yet incredibly important tissue, plays key roles in providing protection to the eye and maintaining homeostasis of its ocular surface. Multiple diseases can impair conjunctival function leading to severe consequences that require surgical intervention. Small conjunctival defects can be repaired relatively easily, but larger defects rely on tissue grafts which generally do not provide adequate healing. A tissue engineering approach involving a biomaterial substrate capable of supporting a stratified epithelium with embedded, mucin-secreting goblet cells offers a potential solution. As a first step, this study aimed to induce stratification of human conjunctival epithelial cells cultured on electrospun scaffolds composed from poly(ε-caprolactone) (PCL) and decellularised tissue matrix (small intestinal submucosa (SIS) or urinary bladder matrix (UBM)) and held at the air/liquid interface. Stratification, up to 5 cell layers, occurred more frequently on scaffolds containing PCL + UBM. Incorporation of these decellularised tissue matrices also impacted material properties, with significant changes occurring to their fibre diameter, tensile properties, and chemical composition throughout the scaffold structure compared to PCL alone. These matrix containing scaffolds warrant further long-term investigation as a potential advanced therapy medicinal product for conjunctiva repair and regeneration.

Keywords: electrospinning; conjunctiva; decellularized tissue matrix; small intestinal submucosa; urinary bladder matrix; polycaprolactone; fiber; tissue engineering; stratification; conjunctival epithelial cells

1. Introduction

The conjunctiva is a mucous membrane that has an important role in maintaining a normal ocular surface and motility of the eye and eyelids. The palpebral conjunctiva lines the posterior surfaces of the eyelids and is reflected in the fornices to become the bulbar conjunctiva overlying the anterior sclera until it merges with the cornea. The total surface area is approximately 15 cm^2 [1]. It has a stratified epithelium up to six layers thick with numerous goblet cells, and an underlying basement membrane. Beneath is the stroma, which comprises loose, vascular connective, and lymphoid tissue as well as the accessory lacrimal glands of Krause and Wolfring.

The conjunctiva serves to protect the eye and contributes to a healthy ocular surface and tear film through mucin production by the goblet cells. These not only stabilise the epithelium—tear film interface which helps to lubricate the ocular surface, but also have some antimicrobial activity [2]. A healthy conjunctiva is necessary for normal ocular motility, and has innate and adaptive immune responses to defend against pathogens [3].

Conjunctival diseases are numerous, but of greatest interest to tissue engineering are those that result in significant loss of healthy conjunctiva, which may in turn cause corneal problems with loss of vision, or double vision. These include mucous membrane pemphigoid, Stevens-Johnson syndrome, trauma including burns, malignancy, and complicated glaucoma or socket surgery. Of these, malignancy potentially offers the greatest scope for engineered conjunctival substitutes as following complete resection of a tumour there may be an extensive defect but the remaining tissue is healthy and provides a good host environment for a transplant. Other conditions may affect the whole conjunctiva or recur in the transplant [4].

Small conjunctival defects can be closed directly or repaired with an autologous graft, but larger defects have traditionally required either amniotic or mucous membrane grafting. In this instance, amniotic membrane acts as an inlay graft or basement membrane substitute to promote overgrowth of host conjunctival epithelial cells. However, where defects are very large or involve opposing conjunctival surfaces, there is a risk of scarring and symblepharon developing before epithelialisation has occurred, which can lead to diplopia from limited motility and lid malposition (Figure 1) [5]. Oral mucous membrane largely overcomes this problem, but is quite different to conjunctiva being much thicker and lacking goblet cells. It does not support the tear film, is cosmetically poor and can impair detection of recurrent disease. At present, local resection of very extensive conjunctival tumours is limited by the current reconstructive techniques. Tissue engineered conjunctival substitutes offer the potential to overcome this barrier, and reduce the risk of post-operative diplopia and ocular surface problems due to conjunctival deficiency.

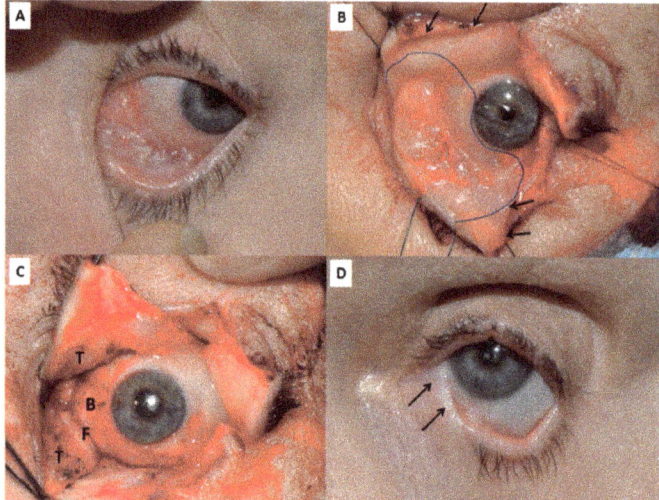

Figure 1. (**A**) Conjunctival squamous cell carcinoma affecting the infero-medial quadrant of the left eye. (**B**) Same patient during surgery. The upper and lower eyelids have undergone a full-thickness vertical lid-split procedure (arrows mark the cut edges) to improve visualisation and access to the tumour. The intended resection margin is shown by the curved line. (**C**) Following resection of the tumour there is an extensive conjunctival defect involving the tarsal plates and conjunctiva (T), the inferior fornix (F) and the bulbar conjunctiva (B). (**D**) Late post-operative image of the same patient showing symblepharon between the lower lid and globe (arrows), despite reconstruction with amniotic membrane, a free tarsal graft to the lower lid and temporary Gore-tex sheets as spacers.

To be clinically-usable and with demonstrable long-term positive outcome, an advanced therapy medicinal product (ATMP) for the conjunctiva needs to possess a number of essential properties, including:

- robust enough to handle with surgical instruments without becoming disrupted or compromised
- able to retain a suture for fixation
- manufactured within a limited time frame
- non-allergenic and provoking minimal inflammatory/scarring response
- have an intact epithelium sufficient to prevent symblepharon/adhesions, and which allows eventual transition to a normal conjunctival epithelium including goblet cells
- a sufficiently mobile stroma to allow full extraocular movements

These criteria build on those previously outlined by Schrader et al. [6], who also commented on a conjunctival ATMP needing to mimic the natural tissue architecture and possess sufficient elasticity to prevent or reduce contraction. As discussed in several detailed reviews, a number of biological and synthetic materials have been researched and developed with the aim of creating the optimal ATMP for *ex vivo* culture of conjunctival epithelial and goblet cells, which, following transplantation, should lead to repair and regeneration of the conjunctiva [6–8]. However, whilst biological or synthetic materials are frequently selected due to their known key benefits, they often possess other less favourable properties that can limit their success as an ATMP.

In recent years, research in tissue decellularisation has significantly increased and there are multiple decellularised tissue products that are commercially available [9]. Decellularisation of mammalian tissues and organs involves the complete removal of cells to leave the tissue's 3D structural architecture that may then be re-populated with a different source of cells (e.g., allogeneic) to create new, engineered tissues. With application of complex, multi-step decellularisation protocols to efficiently eliminate all cellular antigens, the remaining extracellular matrix (ECM) structure should provide a near-perfect blueprint of appropriate dimensional scale and ideal combination of biomolecules (i.e., proteins and polysaccharides) to support cell adhesion, proliferation and, importantly, phenotype and differentiation [10]. Yet, as described in the detailed review by Gilbert et al. [11], the need to completely remove all cellular components requires both physical (e.g., sonication, snap-freezing, mechanical force) and chemical (e.g., enzymatic digestion, ionic solutions, detergents) processing, which can adversely affect the tissue's natural structure and hence impact its resulting biological and mechanical properties. Changes to the tissue's microstructure may impede its mechanical and functional properties, resulting in a fragility that makes it difficult to handle without incurring further damage [12–14]. To overcome this, it is possible to mill lyophilised decellularised tissue (dECM) into a powder, retaining its unique cocktail of biological properties, and subsequently form a hydrogel via its solubilisation and neutralisation, as described by Saldin et al. [15]. 3D dECM-hydrogels support the encapsulation of viable cells and overcome the difficulties associated with successfully recellularising bulk decellularised tissues [16]. The development of dECM powders used to create these biological hydrogels is an active area of research and have been sourced from a wide variety of tissues and whole organ systems, including (but not limited to) musculoskeletal, cardiac, liver, kidney, and skin. Porcine-derived small intestinal submucosa (SIS) and urinary bladder matrix (UBM) are two other tissues commonly used to create dECM hydrogels. Not surprisingly, the different anatomical locations of these two tissues renders differences in their structural, functional and biochemical properties. For example, SIS-matrices comprise approximately 90% collagen, being predominantly type I with minor quantities of types III, IV, V, and VI, whereas UBM-matrices contain almost identical collagen types, but with a greater quantity of type III and the addition of type VII, which are essential components of epithelial basement membranes [17].

Whilst exploration of these dECM hydrogels continues in research groups worldwide, they remain mechanically weak which can restrict their clinical usability [18]. These mechanical changes may be overcome by incorporating the dECM powder with other, more durable biomaterial substrates, such as electrospun fibres. Electrospinning is a popular technique for fabricating fibre scaffolds that mimic the structural properties of tissues [19]. This approach therefore offers several advantages: the fibrous substrate confers structural support and topographical cues, and the powdered dECM provides the cells with a specific mix of biomolecules known to support and maintain that particular cell phenotype [20,21].

In this study, decellularised tissue powders (SIS or UBM) with poly(ε-caprolactone) (PCL; a biodegradable, synthetic polymer) were electrospun to create bioactive, fibre scaffolds with the aim of developing a novel conjunctival ATMP. Research findings demonstrated dECM-containing PCL scaffolds exhibited notable differences both in terms of material properties (fibre morphology, mechanical) and in vitro cell response (cell morphology, stratification) compared to PCL alone.

2. Materials and Methods

2.1. Tissue Decellularisation

UBM and SIS scaffolds were prepared at the University of Pittsburgh, from porcine tissue sources at Animal Biotech Industries (Doylestown, PA, USA), as outlined in Keane et al. [22]. Briefly, for UBM preparation, the urethra and ureter were removed from the bladders. Bladders were opened along their length and mechanically scraped to remove the tunica serosa, tunica muscularis externa, tunica submucosa, and tunica muscularis mucosa. Further, rinsing with deionised water was used to remove the urothelial cells on the surface of the tunica mucosa. For SIS preparation, intestines were flushed with distilled water, opened along their length and mechanically scraped to remove the tunica mucosa, tunica serosa, and tunica muscularis externa. Decellularisation of the remaining tissues was performed using a solution of 0.1% v/v peracetic acid (Rochester Midland Corporation, Rochester, NY, USA) and 4% v/v ethanol (200 proof; Decon Laboratories Inc., King of Prussia, PA, USA) in type I water (Thermo Scientific, Waltham, MA, USA), with agitation at 300 rpm in a shaker, for 2 h. The resulting UBM and SIS were then washed three times, alternating between phosphate buffered saline (PBS; Fisher BioReagents, Pittsburgh, PA, USA) and sterile water, for 15 min on an orbital shaker at 300 rpm each time. The UBM and SIS scaffolds were lyophilised and milled into powder using a #60 mesh screen on a Wiley Mill (GE Motors & Industrial Systems, Houston, TX, USA) [23].

2.2. Solution Preparation

Powdered decellularised porcine tissues (small intestinal submucosa (SIS) and urinary bladder matrix (UBM)) were received at the University of Liverpool. Solutions of poly(ε-caprolactone) (PCL; Purasorb PC12, Corbion, Amsterdam, The Netherlands) dissolved in 1,1,1,3,3,3-hexafluoroisopropanol (HFIP; Merck, Gillingham, UK) were prepared at concentrations of 12%w/v plus 1% or 10% SIS or UBM and stirred continuously for 48 h at room temperature.

2.3. Scaffold Fabrication

Solutions were loaded into separate capillary-ended syringes with an applied flow rate of 1 mL/h and subsequently electrospun (50 min per run) using an IME Technologies EC-CLI unit with controlled ambient environment (temperature 21 °C, relative humidity 50%) and applied spinning parameters: needle voltage +15 kV, collector voltage −4 kV, and distance 17 cm. Emitted fibres were collected on a mandrel lined with wax paper (PME, Enfield, UK) and rotating at 100 rpm.

2.4. Material Characterisation

2.4.1. Fibre Morphology and Diameter

Scanning electron microscopy (SEM) was used to obtain high magnification images of the fibre scaffolds. Scaffolds were mounted on carbon-tabbed SEM stubs (Agar Scientific

Ltd., Stansted, UK) and AuPd sputter-coated for an even coverage. Scaffolds were imaged using a FEI Quanta 250 FEG SEM operating at high vacuum with 5 kV electron beam.

Fibre diameters were measured by analysing the SEM images using ImageJ software (v.1.53c, National Institutes of Health, Bethesda, MD, USA). This was achieved by using the line draw tool and the scale bar of each image to initially set the scale. Measured diameters were statistically analysed using GraphPad Prism v9 (San Diego, CA, USA). Fibre diameters for each group ($N = 3$; $n = 900$) were not normally distributed and were subsequently analysed using a Kruskal–Wallis test with Dunn's multiple comparisons test. Data are presented as the median and interquartile range.

2.4.2. Tensile Testing

For tensile testing, fibre scaffolds were cut into 3×1 cm rectangles and placed and secured (using sticky tape) over a paper window to give final test dimensions of 2×1 cm. Scaffold thickness was measured using an electronic micrometer. Paper windows allowed easy handling and positioning of the scaffold within tensile grips. Window sides were cut prior to commencement of the tensile test to ensure only the fibre scaffold was loaded. A UniVert (CellScale; Waterloo, ON Canada) in tensile mode was used with 1 N load cell and 10% strain ($n = 6$). Data were processed in MS Excel and Graphpad Prism (v.9, GraphPad Software, Inc., San Diego, CA, USA), where a one-way ANOVA with Tukey's multiple comparisons test was applied.

2.4.3. Chemical Spectroscopy (FTIR, Imaging-Mass Spectrometry)

Chemical composition of the scaffolds was initially determined using a Fourier transform infra-red spectrometer (Bruker Vertex 70v; Bruker, Durham, UK) with diamond attenuated total reflection. A background scan was taken prior to scaffold analysis and subsequently subtracted from that scaffold's spectrum. The scaffold was pressed into close contact with the diamond and the spectrum measured. Data were obtained in the range of 450–4000 cm^{-1}, with 4 cm^{-1} resolution and scan number 32. Data were analysed with OPUS software (v8.2.28; Bruker, Durham, UK).

For imaging-mass spectrometry, data were collected on a Waters Synapt G2-Si in MALDI using HD Imaging 1.4 (Waters UK, Elstree, UK) to set acquisition parameters and MassLynx 4.1 SCN9509 (Agilent, Stockport, UK) to process the data for PCL, PCL + SIS10% and PCL + UBM10%. Acquisition parameters were set to collect masses over the 100–2000 mass/charge (m/z) range in positive resolution mode. Scan time per pixel was 0.5 s at 250 Laser Energy and a repetition rate of 500 Hz. An area of 14 mm^2 was collected with a pixel size of 50×50 µm.

2.5. In Vitro Set-Up and Cell Culture

A human conjunctival epithelial cell (HCjE) line [24] was cultured at 37 °C and 5% CO_2 in 75 cm^2 sterile flasks (Greiner Bio-one, Stonehouse, UK) with keratinocyte serum-free medium (KSFM; Thermo Fisher, Loughborough, UK) supplemented with 25 µg/mL bovine pituitary extract (Thermo Fisher), 0.4 mM calcium chloride (Merck, Gillingham, UK), 0.2 ng/mL recombinant human epidermal growth factor (rEGF, Thermo Fisher, Loughborough, UK), 100 U penicillin and 0.1 mg/mL streptomycin (Merck, Gillingham, UK) and 2.5 µg/mL amphotericin B (Merck, Gillingham, UK).

Within a sterile, laminar flow cabinet the membranes of 24-well transwells (Millicell; Merck, Gillingham, UK) were removed and replaced with the fibre scaffolds. Scaffolds were secured by using silicone glue (Dowsil 732 (clear); Dow Corning, Penarth, UK), which was limited to the side of the transwell and not present within the new fibrous base of the transwell. Transwells were irradiated with ultraviolet light for 30 min on both sides and then disinfected by submerging in 70% v/v Ethanol (VWR, Lutterworth, UK) overnight. Ethanol was removed and transwells washed twice in sterile phosphate buffered saline solution (PBS; Thermo Fisher, Loughborough, UK) before being transferred to new, sterile 24-well plates (Greiner Bio-One, Stonehouse, UK).

A density of 1×10^5 cells per cm^2 were seeded directly onto each scaffold and after 30 min topped-up with KSFM. After 14 days of growth, samples were switched to stratification media as outlined in Gipson et al. [24]. Stratification media was composed of: Dulbeccos modified Eagles media/Ham's nutrient buffer F-12 (DMEM/F12 1:1; Merck, Gillingham, UK), 10% foetal calf serum (Biosera, Nuaille, France), 10 ng/mL rEGF, 100 U penicillin and 0.1 mg/mL streptomycin, and 2.5 μg/mL amphotericin B. Following 7 days in stratification media cultures were switched to air/liquid interface, where media was removed from the apical chamber and received on the basal-side only to further promote stratification over an extra 7 days. Figure 2 provides a schematic of the in vitro experimental set-up.

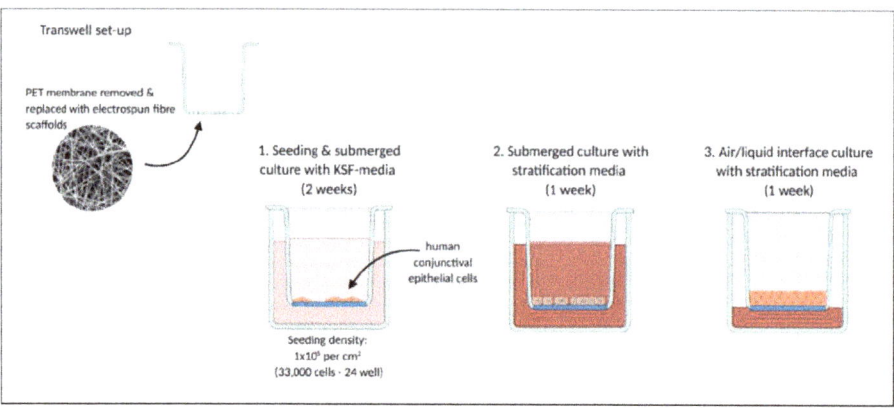

Figure 2. Experimental set-up for in vitro culture of human conjunctival epithelial cells demonstrating preparation of transwells with removal of polyester (PET) membrane and replacement with electrospun scaffolds. Cells were seeded and cultured fully submerged for two weeks with keratinocyte serum free media (KSF-media), followed by one week with stratification media and a further week at the air/liquid interface with media received on the cells' basal side. Created with BioRender.com.

2.6. In Vitro Characterisation

2.6.1. Assessing Cell Morphology by SEM

Cell-seeded scaffolds were washed in sterile PBS and fixed in 1.5% v/v glutaraldehyde (TAAB Laboratories, Aldermaston, UK) in PBS for 30 min at 4 °C. Scaffolds (n = 2) were subsequently dehydrated in increasing concentrations of Ethanol; 50, 70 and 90% v/v for 2 × 3 min and 100% v/v for 2 × 5 min. Finally, scaffolds were chemically dried in hexamethyldisilazane (Sigma, UK) for 2 × 5 min. Scaffolds were mounted on carbon-tabbed SEM stubs, AuPd sputter-coated, and imaged on a Hitachi TM4000 Plus (Hitachi, Warrington, UK) at 15 kV in BSE mode and high vacuum.

2.6.2. Assessing Cell Stratification by Confocal Microscopy

Cell-seeded scaffolds were washed in sterile PBS and fixed in 10% neutral buffered formalin (Merck, Gillingham, UK) for 10 min at room temperature. Samples were washed several times in PBS, permeabilised with 0.5% Triton-X for 5 min and washed three times in PBS. DAPI (1:1000; Thermo Fisher, Loughborough, UK) was applied for 20 min at room temperature (in the dark) to stain the cells' nuclei. Scaffolds were washed in PBS and subsequently mounted on glass microscope slides. Substrates were imaged by confocal microscopy (Zeiss LSM800; Cambridge, UK) at ×40 magnification and images processed using Fiji ImageJ (v.1.53c, National Institutes of Health, Bethesda, MD, USA). Three set coordinates within the XY image were randomly selected and applied to images for all scaffold groups. This generated 6 regions of interest (area = 298.46 × 40.80 μm) per sample

(n = 3) that were viewed in the orthogonal slice: 3 in the XZ plane (co-ordinates: 190, 256, 500) and 3 in the YZ plane (co-ordinates: 180, 256, 400). Distinctly separated nuclei were counted and instances of cell nuclei in close proximity and stacking on top of each other noted, for example, 3 nuclei stacked on top of each other would be 3 cells counted and 1 instance of a triple cell layer. The number of instances, where cells were present either as a monolayer or 2-, 3-, 4-, 5-layers, were totalled and the proportion for each type of layer presented as a percentage of this total. The labelling of images was removed prior to processing to blind the operator and remove the potential for bias. Data were processed in Graphpad Prism v.9 (San Diego, CA, USA) and a one-way ANOVA with Tukey's multiple comparisons test applied for the total cell number within each group (n = 3).

3. Results
3.1. Material Characterisation
3.1.1. Fibre Morphology and Diameter

There were no observable issues during the electrospinning process. The rotating mandrel, which was used to target and collect the emitted polymeric jet following its propulsion across the air-gap, was evenly covered following a 50-min spin time for each of the five solutions that were electrospun. Gross inspection of the collected fibres revealed differences between the groups (Figure 3A). Electrospun PCL presented uniform coverage across the sheet of wax paper (used to easily remove collected fibres for analysis), with an even white colour and smooth texture. The inclusion of decellularised tissue powders (dECM) to the PCL, however, demonstrated numerous droplets throughout the collected area, which increased in number with greater dECM content. Inspection by SEM revealed these droplets to have dried on top and within the surrounding fibres to create areas of flattened topography (Figure 3B). Removal of fibres did, on occasion, result in tearing of the scaffold where droplets had contacted and dried to the wax-backing paper. This only occurred in scaffolds containing larger quantities of dECM.

Separate to these droplets, the bulk of polymer deposition on the collector sheet revealed fibres with rounded and smooth morphologies (Figure 4). High magnification SEM images revealed a shift in fibre morphology, where PCL alone demonstrated two distinct fibre sizes, but the inclusion of dECM resulted in the fabrication of finer and more uniform fibres. This was particularly noticeable for PCL + UBM10%. Measurement of fibre diameter for all groups supported these visual findings, with fibres in all groups containing dECM being significantly finer than pure PCL fibres. PCL fibres possessed a median fibre diameter of 0.65 μm (IQR 0.28–1.46 μm). Addition of 1% dECM powder, resulted in a notable reduction, with median fibre diameters measuring 0.36 μm (IQR 0.22–0.82 μm) upon addition of SIS and 0.21 μm (IQR 0.15–0.29 μm) for UBM. Increasing the quantity of dECM to 10% demonstrated a further decrease in fibre diameter for SIS (median 0.22 μm (IQR 0.15–0.38 μm)), but a similar distribution of fibre diameters for UBM (median 0.22 μm (IQR 0.16–0.31 μm)). UBM10% was the only group to produce a fibre range below 1 μm.

3.1.2. Chemical Spectroscopy (FTIR and Imaging-Mass Spectrometry)

In order to detect the presence of decellularised tissue within the PCL fibres, FTIR and Imaging-Mass Spectrometry were performed. Comparison of the scaffolds' complete spectra revealed no obvious differences (Figure 5A). Characteristic chemical bonds for esters were identified C=O (1750–1735 cm^{-1}) and C–O (1260–1000 cm^{-1}), in addition to C–H bonds (2960–2850 cm^{-1}). Closer examination demonstrated a distinct peak within 1650–1590 cm^{-1} which was most apparent for PCL + SIS10% and PCL + UBM10%.

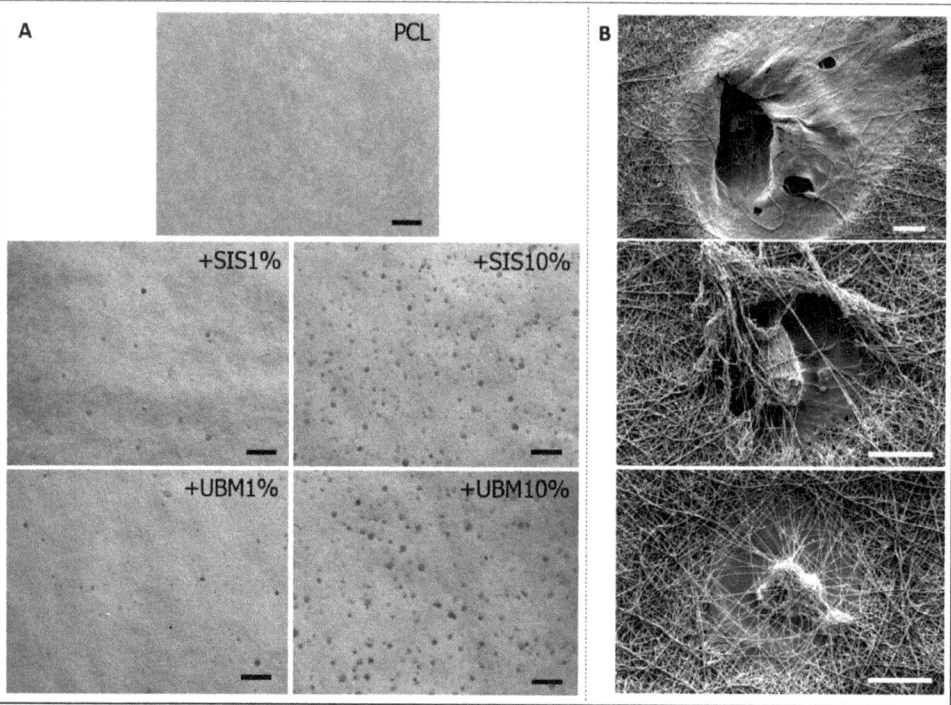

Figure 3. (**A**) Gross images of as-spun electrospun fibres for poly(ε-caprolactone) (PCL) and with the addition of 1% or 10% decellularised tissue powder (dECM—small intestinal submucosa (SIS) and urinary bladder matrix (UBM)) (scale = 5 mm). Images converted to greyscale for observation of 'wet' droplets on dECM containing fibre scaffolds. (**B**) Scanning electron microscopy images highlighting the 'wet' droplets present within the PCL + SIS10% fibres and the holes these create. Scale bar = 40 μm, magnification ×1000 (top image) and ×2000 (middle and bottom images).

Imaging-mass spectrometry (Imaging-MS) allowed the spatial distribution of molecular species to be visualised between PCL and those containing the greatest quantity of dECM powder (Figure 5B). Normalisation of the data to 10,000 counts demonstrated clear differences in the heat map for each group. Minimal ionisation was detected across the surface for PCL fibres, but this increased with inclusion of 10%SIS, where low to mid counts (~5000) were detected, and increasing further from low to high counts (~10,000) for 10%UBM. Presence of UBM and SIS increased the ionisation of the fibres at several mass-to-charge (m/z) values, including a m/z peak at 523.25. The imaging element of this technique revealed these increased intensities to be distributed throughout the fibre scaffolds.

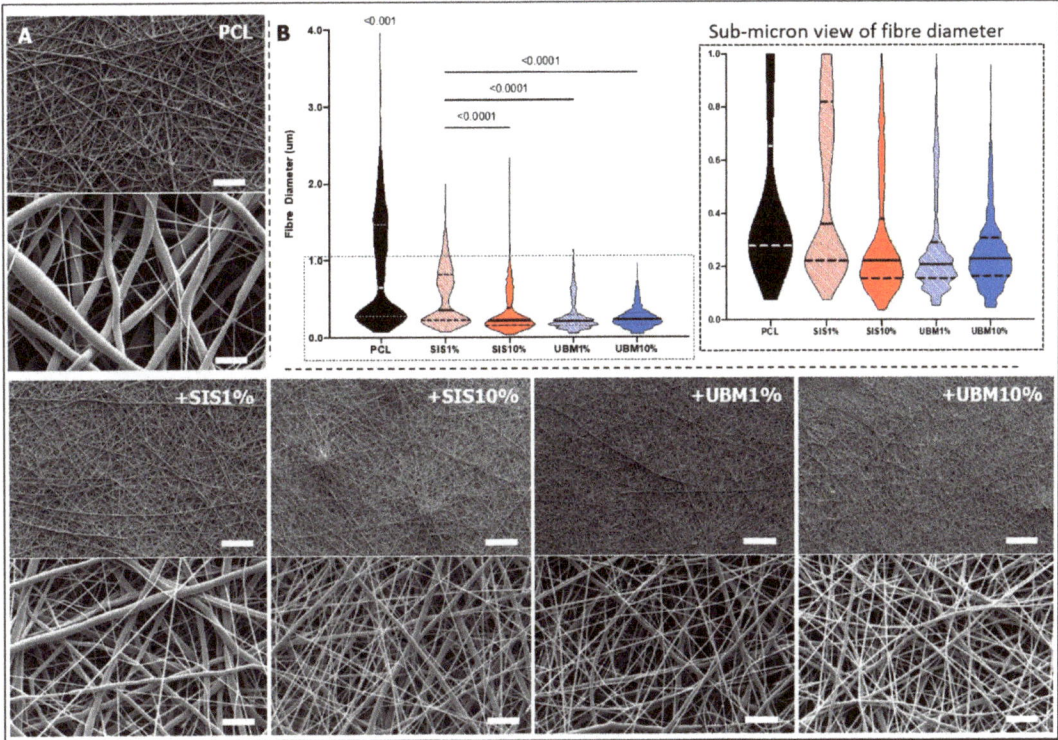

Figure 4. (**A**) Scanning electron microscopy images of electrospun poly(ε-caprolactone) (PCL) scaffolds and following the addition of 1% or 10% decellularised tissue powder (small intestinal submucosa (SIS) and urinary bladder matrix (UBM)). Low magnification images ×1000, scale = 50 µm; high magnification images ×10,000, scale = 5 µm. (**B**) Measured fibre diameter presented as a violin plot for each group with magnified view of data spread within the sub-micron range ($n = 900$). Kruskal–Wallis statistical test with Dunn's multiple comparisons ($p < 0.05$). PCL was significantly different in all groups.

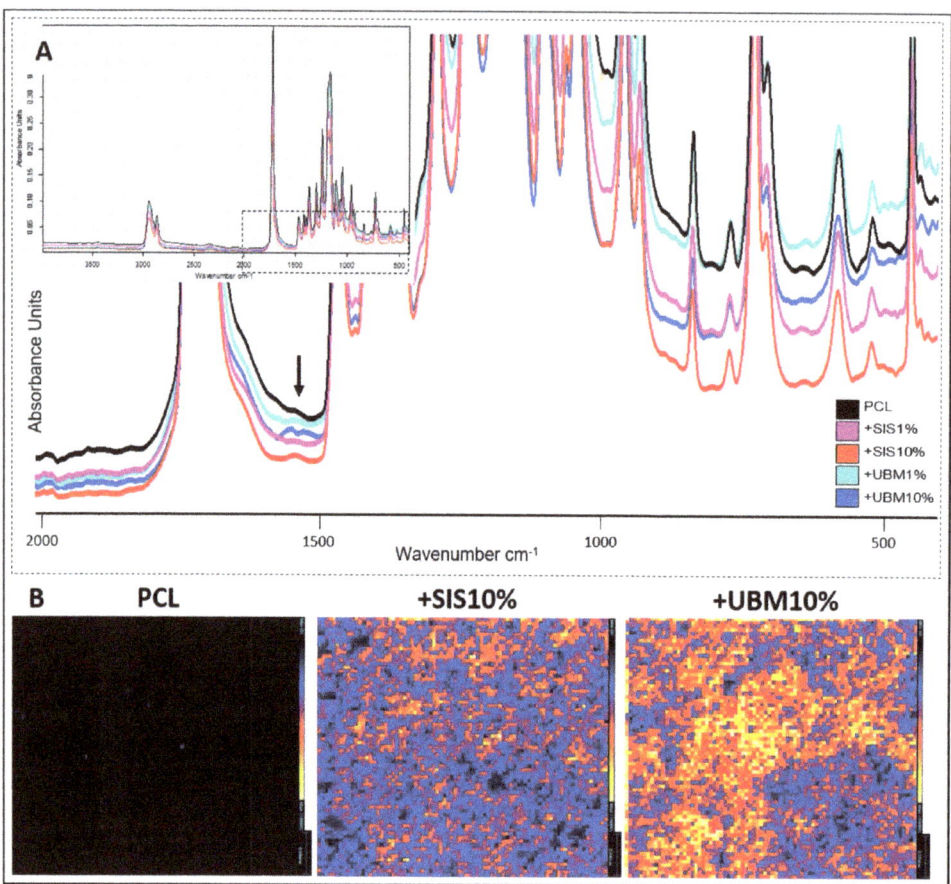

Figure 5. Spectroscopic analysis of electrospun poly(ε-caprolactone) (PCL) scaffolds and following the addition of decellularised tissue powder (small intestinal submucosa (SIS) and urinary bladder matrix (UBM)). (**A**) Fourier transform infra-red spectroscopy with inset demonstrating complete spectra for each group, and magnified view of chemical change at 1590 cm^{-1} representative of a primary amine (N-H bend), which was most noticeable for SIS10% and UBM10% groups. (**B**) Imaging-mass spectrometry demonstrating greater ionisation (and even distribution) in SIS10% and UBM10% groups compared to PCL at *m/z* 523. Maximum number of counts = 10,000. Scale for PCL = 0.58 mm, SIS10% = 0.54 mm, UBM10% = 0.55 mm.

3.1.3. Tensile Properties

Scaffolds were subjected to mechanical testing to determine any change in their tensile properties following addition of dECM (Figure 6). In terms of Young's modulus, electrospun PCL scaffolds yielded a stiffness of 8.29 ± 0.94 MPa (Figure 6A). The inclusion of 1% dECM resulted in a significant increase in scaffold stiffness compared to PCL alone, where SIS1% and UBM1% were 10.16 ± 0.89 MPa (p = 0.0280) and 11.25 ± 0.64 MPa (p = 0.0003), respectively. However, a similar trend was not observed for either 10% dECM groups, with Young's modulus calculated as 8.17 ± 0.84 MPa (SIS10%) and 8.58 ± 1.53 MPa (UBM10%). The yield stress (i.e., the maximum tensile load before plastic deformation) of PCL was 0.37 ± 0.07 MPa (Figure 6B). The addition of dECM powders revealed a general increase in the maximum load that the scaffolds were able to withstand. This was particularly evident for UBM-containing scaffolds with UBM1% yielding at 0.57 ± 0.06 MPa (p = 0.0006) and UBM10% at 0.54 ± 0.07 MPa (p = 0.0049). Blends of PCL and SIS resulted in yield stresses of 0.49 ± 0.08 MPa (not significant) and 0.50 ± 0.09 MPa (p = 0.036) for 1% and 10% dECM, respectively. The ultimate tensile strength (UTS) of PCL scaffolds was 1.12 ± 0.14 MPa (Figure 6C). All scaffolds containing dECM had a significantly greater UTS compared to PCL ($p < 0.0001$). Inclusion of SIS increased the UTS to 1.70 ± 0.15 MPa and 1.82 ± 0.18 MPa for 1% and 10%, respectively. UBM1% had the highest UTS overall (2.31 ± 0.18 MPa) and was significantly different to all other scaffolds ($p < 0.0001$ vs. SIS1%, $p = 0.0002$ vs. SIS10%, and $p = 0.0031$ vs. UBM10%). UBM10% scaffolds had a UTS of 1.92 ± 0.17 MPa. The maximum strain reached at the UTS also presented significant decreases following dECM blending (Figure 6D). Maximum strain for PCL scaffolds was 1.21 ± 0.36 mm/mm. For SIS1% and SIS10%, scaffold extension reduced to 0.80 ± 0.03 mm/mm ($p = 0.0092$) and 0.54 ± 0.08 mm/mm ($p < 0.0001$), respectively. Similarly, UBM1% and UBM10% yielded strains of 0.57 ± 0.07 mm/mm ($p < 0.0001$) and 0.61 ± 0.15 mm/mm ($p < 0.0001$).

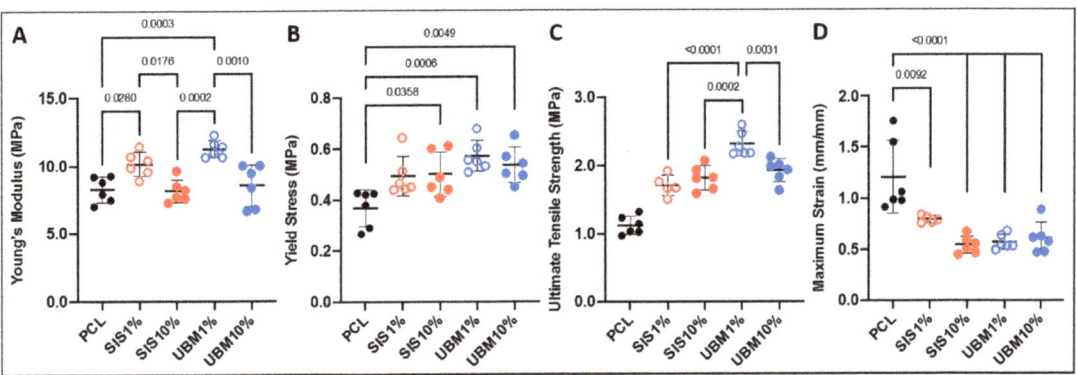

Figure 6. Tensile testing data for scaffolds of electrospun poly(ε-caprolactone) (PCL) and with the addition of 1% or 10% decellularised tissue powder (small intestinal submucosa (SIS) and urinary bladder matrix (UBM)): (**A**) Young's modulus, (**B**) yield stress, (**C**) ultimate tensile strength and (**D**) maximum strain at break. One-way ANOVA with Tukey's multiple comparisons ($n = 6$), significance for $p < 0.05$. Statistical differences shown by p values.

3.2. Air/Liquid Interface Culture and Stratification

The response of human conjunctival epithelial cells (HCjE), in terms of their ability to stratify on the different scaffolds was investigated. HCjE cells were cultured on the scaffolds for a total of four weeks, where the final week was at the air/liquid interface. SEM imaging revealed a difference in cell response to the fibre scaffolds (Figure 7). Low magnification (×1000) images for the PCL scaffold revealed patches of electrospun fibres with limited presence of cells. In contrast, dECM-containing scaffolds demonstrated complete cell coverage over the fibre surface at the same magnification. HCjE cells on PCL-only scaffolds appeared well spread with flattened morphologies. In some regions, it was possible to view the shape of fibres situated beneath the cells. Cellular processes enabling cell-to-cell contact were evident. Indication of HCjE stratification on PCL fibres appeared limited. Observation through the z-plane of PCL scaffolds and DAPI-stained cell nuclei by confocal microscopy revealed occasions of two (40.47 ± 6.45%) and three (13.26 ± 6.03%) cell nuclei loosely-stacked on top of each other (Figure 8A,B). Single nuclei accounted for 46.37 ± 5.88% and the total number of nuclei (180 ± 28) counted from the six regions of interest ($n = 3$) was lowest on PCL scaffolds overall (Figure 8B,C). SEM images for dECM-containing scaffolds identified two main morphologies: small, rounded cells with multiple cellular processes, and larger, elongated cells with flattened appearances (Figure 7). These flattened cells appeared in greater numbers within the SIS1% cohort. A breakdown of cell layers for SIS1% from the total number of counted nuclei (202 ± 39) revealed single cells accounting for 63.86 ± 15.60%, two-layers 31.35 ± 13.13% and three stacked-nuclei occurring 4.79 ± 2.16%. A greater number of cell nuclei (321 ± 85) were counted in the SIS10% group, with observed instances of one, two, three and even four-layers from the regions of interest being 33.46 ± 17.95%, 46.91 ± 5.88%, 18.50 ± 11.33% and 1.13 ± 0.99%, respectively. UBM-containing groups supported superior stratification with greater instances of four and occasionally five layers of cell nuclei evident in the regions of interest. For UBM1% 329 ± 50 cell nuclei were counted, with 22.31 ± 5.08% being single nuclei, 51.44 ± 3.43% two nuclei, 22.82 ± 4.09% three nuclei and 3.43 ± 2.45% four-stacked nuclei. For UBM10%, from 392 ± 81 counted nuclei, 13.80 ± 10.52% were single, 37.02 ± 7.85% two-layers, 33.13 ± 9.07% three-layers, 13.48 ± 8.87% four-layers, and 2.57 ± 1.10% five-layers.

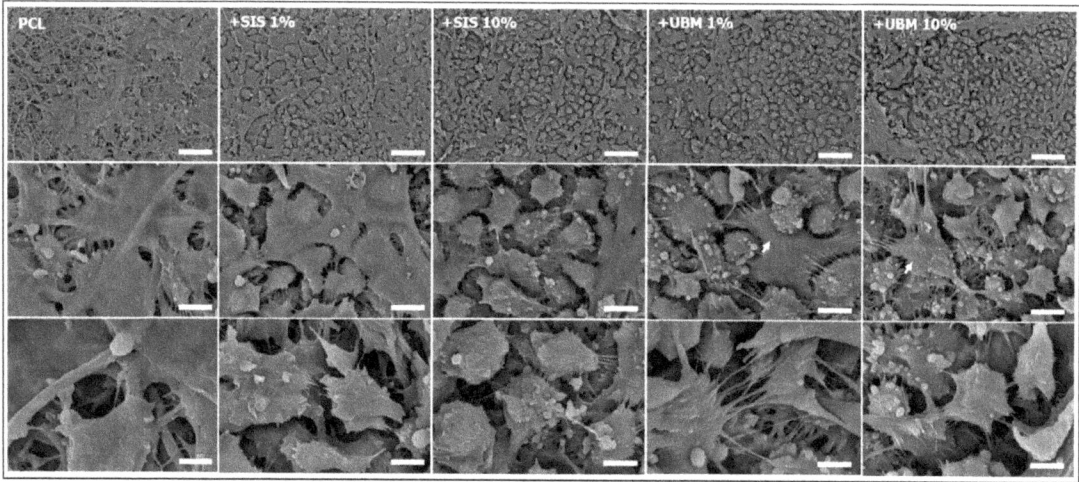

Figure 7. Representative scanning electron microscopy images of human conjunctival epithelial cells cultured on electrospun scaffolds fabricated from poly(ε-caprolactone) (PCL) and PCL with addition of 1% or 10% decellularised tissue powder (small intestinal submucosa (SIS) and urinary bladder matrix (UBM)). Images: top row = ×1000 (scale = 50 µm), middle row = ×5000 (scale = 10 µm), bottom row = ×10,000 (scale = 5 µm); arrows indicate presence of microvilli.

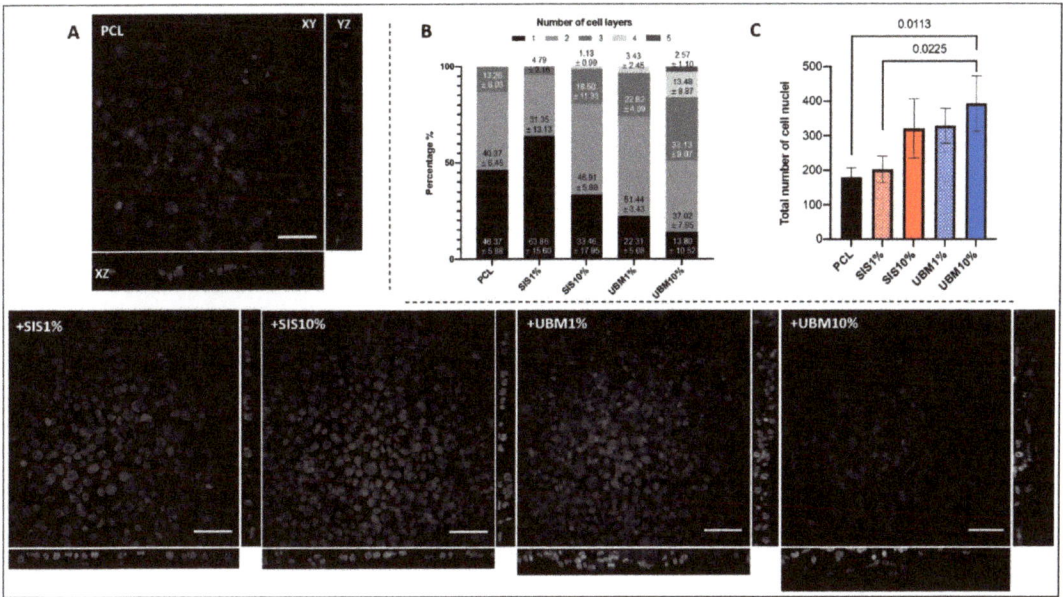

Figure 8. (**A**) Representative confocal images of DAPI-stained human conjunctival epithelial cell nuclei cultured on electrospun scaffolds fabricated from poly(ε-caprolactone) (PCL) and PCL with addition of 1% or 10% decellularised tissue powder (small intestinal submucosa (SIS) and urinary bladder matrix (UBM)). Images shown; XY z-stack (scale = 50 μm), XZ side view and YZ side view. (**B**) Cell layers observed from 6 set regions of interest presented as percentages within each group (n = 3). (**C**) Total number of cell nuclei counted within 6 regions of interest for each group (n = 3). One-way ANOVA with Tukey's multiple comparisons, significance for $p < 0.05$. Statistical differences shown by p values.

4. Discussion

This study investigated the incorporation of dECM powders with PCL to fabricate bioactive fibre scaffolds. The prepared solutions all yielded fibres when electrospun using the same parameters. Examination of the collected fibre sheets demonstrated macroscopic differences upon the addition of dECM to the PCL solution (Figure 3A). Instead of a uniform coverage of fibres, droplets spread randomly throughout the deposited area were visible, and these increased in number with greater dECM quantity. SEM imaging revealed these droplets to present flat/wet-looking regions located within a network of otherwise smooth, bead-free fibres (Figure 3B). Instability of the polymer jet during electrospinning can result in the formation of "beads-on-a-string", though this was not evident from these SEM images. Yet, this phenomenon does suggest periods of jet instability giving rise to occasional electrospraying as opposed to continuous electrospinning. Another theory could be non-solubilised dECM components accelerating along the emitted polymer jet before contacting with the collector system. Inspection of the polymer/dECM solutions did reveal a granular sediment, suggesting the dECM had not fully dissolved in the solvent. To our knowledge, this presentation of droplets has not been previously reported in the literature and our findings are in contrast with studies that suggest the direct dissolution of dECM in solvent is sufficient [25–28]. Other studies initially solubilise the dECM powder in solutions of acetic acid and/or pepsin prior to dissolution with the synthetic polymer and solvent [29–31]. Although a study by Stankus et al. [20] does suggest that dECM agglomerates may contain proteins that remain insoluble in the selected electrospinning solvent. It is worth noting that we were later able to achieve droplet-free, uniform fibre sheets following the initial dissolution of dECM in 0.5M acetic acid and pepsin at a 1:10 with dECM (Figure S1).

Continuing with direct addition of dECM powders with PCL in solution, a significant decrease ($p < 0.0001$) in fibre diameter was determined following its incorporation (Figure 4). This was achieved irrespective of tissue source and quantity included. However, further statistically different reductions in diameter were achieved when comparing SIS1% to SIS10% and to both UBM groups. For SIS1%, the fibres presented a more bimodal distribution compared to all other dECM-containing groups with an IQR of 0.22–0.82 μm and range of 1.92 μm. As indicated in the violin plot, the majority of dECM-containing fibres measured below 1 μm, though only UBM10% yielded a fibrous network that was completely submicron and with tightest range (0.91 μm). This is considerably different to PCL which had a range of 3.88 μm. Comparison of these findings to the literature is mixed. A couple of articles (using the same method of fabrication) state no quantified change in fibre diameter following dECM inclusion [26,27], whereas Kim et al. [32] reported a significant reduction in fibre diameter (45%) following the inclusion of 1% SIS with poly(lactic-*co*-glycolic) acid (PLGA). Hong et al. [25] attributed these decreases to the elevated conductivity of solutions following addition of dECM. Solution conductivity is a known parameter that influences fibre formation during electrospinning. Solutions of higher conductivity possess greater charge and upon application of a high voltage, the emitted polymeric jet undergoes considerable stretching and thinning due to the charge repulsion, resulting in the formation of finer diameter fibres [33].

Spectroscopic analysis is a routine way to locate the presence of molecular species and FTIR and Imaging-MS were undertaken in this study. Comparison of molecular spectra by FTIR revealed no change to the chemical groups of PCL but also the identity of a new peak in dECM-containing scaffolds (Figure 5A). For SIS10% and UBM10%, a new peak was observed in the region 1650–1590 cm^{-1}, which is associated with a primary amine (specifically NH bend) [34]. Imaging-MS demonstrated clear changes in scaffold composition following inclusion of dECM, which were distributed throughout the fibrous network (Figure 5B). Intensities were 100x greater than PCL alone and more notable for UBM over SIS, suggesting the slight differences in the make-up of these tissues had a direct impact on the ionisation of the scaffold. In order to ascertain what these changes may be ascribed to, Raman spectroscopy, which allows whole molecule vibrations to be analysed, is required.

When designing an ATMP for tissue repair and regeneration, the mechanical properties also need to be considered. Whilst not a load-bearing tissue per se, ATMPs for conjunctival replacement still need to possess physical characteristics sufficient enough to enable its handling and transplantation during surgery, and resist tearing when secured in place by sutures. Furthermore, a transplanted ATMP will need to be sufficiently elastic in order to support eye movements and blinking [35]. The addition of dECM powders to electrospun PCL scaffolds resulted in significant increases in Young's modulus, yield stress and UTS, but significant decreases in maximum strain. Our findings are in general agreement with the literature, where increases in modulus [25,31,32,36], yield strength [26,37] and UTS [32], and decrease in strain [31] have also been reported. However, several other studies demonstrate different findings: Stankus et al. [20] described a linear decrease in modulus and UTS with increasing mass of UBM to poly(ester-urethane) urea; Fernandez-Perez et al. [28] found addition of decellularised cornea with PCL had no impact on scaffold stiffness; Hong et al. [29] determined increasing quantities of dECM yielded a general decrease in UTS but scaffolds were stiffer. Separate to the addition of dECM, fibre diameter is known to have a direct impact on tensile properties. A study by Wong et al. [38] demonstrated an abrupt shift in the stiffness and strength of electrospun PCL fibres at ~0.7 μm, with these properties increasing with decreasing fibre diameter. PCL fibres in this study presented a median diameter of 0.65 μm (IQR 0.28–1.46 μm), which were significantly larger than dECM-containing PCL fibres and hence likely contributed to the shift observed in the obtained tensile properties. Of further note, the Young's modulus for both SIS10% and UBM10% did not yield significant increases as per their 1% counterparts. This can most likely be attributed to the deposition of droplets during the electrospinning process.

Unfortunately, the removal of these scaffolds from the wax paper was very difficult as some of these droplets fused to the paper during drying and were unable to be removed without creating small holes in the scaffold (Figure 3B). Consequently, these defects will have contributed to the lower tensile performance of these 10% dECM scaffolds. Comparison of tensile properties for these groups to conjunctiva tissue reveals a general mismatch as the tensile strength and stiffness of human conjunctiva was reported as 0.7 MPa and 3.9 MPa, respectively [14]. Whilst these electrospun scaffolds may be considerably stronger and stiffer, further comparison to human amniotic membrane (a graft for conjunctiva) demonstrates their similarity—amnion UTS and modulus being 1.7 MPa and 11.5 MPa, respectively [14], which would suggest their general suitability.

An immortalised cell line of human conjunctival epithelial cells was cultured on these different scaffold groups [24]. This involved submerged culture for the first three weeks, with the initial two-week period using keratinocyte serum-free media and the third week switching to stratification media. At the start of the fourth week, scaffolds were cultured at the air/liquid interface, where stratification media was received by the cells on their basal side only (Figure 2). Culture at the air/liquid interface provides a better mimic of the natural in vivo environment and has been proven to promote cell proliferation, stratification and differentiation of epithelial cells [39]. Despite being cultured for the same period of time different cell morphologies were apparent between PCL and dECM-containing scaffolds (Figure 7). Low magnification SEM images revealed PCL-only scaffolds to be sparsely populated by HCjE cells despite a four-week period in culture. This is in contrast to dECM-containing scaffolds where cells had fully covered the available fibre surface. Inclusion of SIS and UBM in polyester electrospun scaffolds has previously been shown to increase cell attachment [20,32]. Furthermore, cells on PCL scaffolds appeared thinly spread and with flattened morphologies. Whilst a two-dimensional technique, it is possible to gauge a sense of depth from SEM images and for PCL scaffolds these images presented limited evidence of cell layering suggestive of stratification. Comparison to side profiles of nuclei-stained confocal images presented a slightly different view (Figure 8A). Whilst the majority of nuclei counted from the six regions of interest were located as single cells ($46.37 \pm 5.88\%$), there were many instances of two ($40.37 \pm 6.45\%$) and even three ($13.26 \pm 6.03\%$) layers of cell nuclei located within close proximity to each other (Figure 8B). However, the number of cell nuclei totalled from these regions was lowest out of the five scaffold groups and was significantly different to UBM10% (cohort with greatest number of nuclei) with a difference of 74.12% (Figure 8C). Without surface treatment, PCL alone is not an ideal substrate for cellular expansion due to its inherent hydrophobicity [40]. Ang et al. [41] similarly reported lower cell density and less stratification of primary rabbit conjunctival cells on untreated-PCL compared to PCL treated with Sodium Hydroxide, which made the material more hydrophilic. For dECM-containing scaffolds, two dissimilar morphologies were apparent. Cells either presented as small and rounded with numerous filopodia that contacted with neighbouring cells, or they appeared larger, flatter, and more elongated. This latter morphology was particularly noticeable within the SIS1% group, though stacking of cells was also visible from SEM images. Corroboration with z-plane views did support instances of two ($31.35 \pm 13.13\%$) and three ($4.79 \pm 2.16\%$) layers, though the majority of nuclei were held as a monolayer ($63.86 \pm 15.60\%$). It should be noted that the total number of cell nuclei counted within the regions of interest was markedly lower (63.53% difference) than for UBM10%. The number of cell nuclei counted for SIS10% was also low compared to UBM10% with a difference of 20.22%. Yet a larger proportion of these cell nuclei were stacked in two ($46.91 \pm 5.88\%$), three ($18.50 \pm 11.33\%$) or even four ($1.13 \pm 0.99\%$) layers, which suggests a greater quantity of SIS triggered an increase in cell proliferation and a tendency to stratify, though further investigation is needed to confirm this. However, incorporation of UBM did lead to a change in cell response, where a greater number of microvilli were observed on these scaffolds (Figure 7). Microvilli are an indication of epithelial cell polarity [42]. Microvilli at the ocular surface help stabilise the tear film and either their complete absence or limited presence has been noted in patients affected by tear film abnormalities and ocular surface diseases [43–45]. Both 1% and 10% UBM scaffolds yielded respective total cell nuclei counts of 329 ± 50 and 392 ± 81, and a shift from monolayers to more than three quarters of all nuclei being held in two, three, four, and even five layers. UBM10% demonstrated the greatest presence of cell stratification with 37.02 ± 7.85% representing two nuclei layers, 33.13 ± 9.07% for three layers, 13.48 ± 8.87% for four layers, and 2.57 ± 1.10% for five layers, where 2, 6, and 4 separate instances of 5 nuclei stacked on top of each other were evident in each sample (n = 3, 6 regions of interest).

The number of epithelial cell layers varies across the distinct regions of the conjunctiva: typically, 6 in the bulbar, 3 in the fornix, 2–3 in the upper tarsus, and 4–5 in the lower tarsus of the palpebral [3]. With this in mind, these scaffolds appear to provide suitable mimicry of the conjunctiva by supporting a similar degree of stratification. Replication of three or more cell layers was most evident in scaffolds containing UBM. It should be noted, however, that the z-plane view was for cell nuclei only and thus does not take account of the whole cell body. It is therefore likely that stratification may have occurred to a greater extent, with cell cytoplasm (free from the nucleus) covering a larger area and this potentially being positioned directly on top of other cells. For healthy conjunctival epithelial cells in the bulbar region, the relative size ratio of the cell nucleus compared to the cytoplasm has been reported as 1:4 [46]. Furthermore, the culture time at the air/liquid interface was likely insufficient to support development of an established and more mature epithelium. Several research groups have achieved various layers of stratification for HCjE cells grown on biological substrates, including Gipson et al. [24] where 2–3 layers of HCjE cells were achieved following their culture on transwells coated with collagen type I, and Zorn-Kruppa et al. [47] who similarly demonstrated stratification up to 3 layers for HCjE cells when seeded at high density (750,000) on collagen stromal layers and cultured at the air/liquid interface for 6 days. Other groups have demonstrated the benefit of co-culture systems of HCjE cells and fibroblasts to stimulate stratification, for example, García-Posadas et al. [48] observed 3–5 layers of primary conjunctival epithelial cells following air/liquid interface culture on fibrin-hydrogels containing conjunctival fibroblasts. It is therefore promising that our dECM-PCL electrospun scaffolds have demonstrated the ability to support several cell layers without the need of co-cultures, which may be a consequence of these dECM powders providing a more complete biological cocktail of biomolecules (proteins, glycoproteins, proteoglycans, growth factors, chemokines and cytokines [15]), which would not all be present in these singular biomolecular structures. Whether the extent of this stratification could be enhanced, both in terms of coverage and number of layers, with culture of HCjE cells and fibroblasts would be an interesting study, however.

The subtle differences in UBM composition to SIS do appear to have a played role, but overall, the incorporation of dECM to PCL has provided a level of bioactivity that HCjE cells have responded to. Coupled with notable differences to material composition, particularly fibre diameter and tensile properties, these dECM-containing scaffolds warrant further exploration as potential ATMP substrates for conjunctiva replacement and regeneration. In particular, the ability to support mucin-secreting goblet cells is an essential feature that these, or any, potential ATMPs would need to demonstrate.

The subtle differences in UBM composition to SIS do appear to have played a role. A proteomic study on decellularised UBM tissue suggests that the collective grouping of different collagen types (I, II, III, VI, and XIV) coupled with high quantities of proteoglycans, such as perlecan (essential component for epithelial cell basement membrane formation [49] and therefore predominant in conjunctival basement membrane-ECM [50,51]), make them useful biomaterials for promoting cell growth and tissue remodelling and regeneration, and would be advantageous as constructs to support skin remodelling [52]. To the authors' knowledge, there is no similar proteomics study for SIS, which would allow a better comparison of the composition of these two tissues; however, a study by Lindberg and Badylak [53] reported lyophilised SIS did not support growth and attachment of epidermal cells as well as non-lyophilised SIS and suggested detrimental structural and/or compositional changes had occurred. As a lyophilised powder, this may have been a contributing factor in this study. Whilst further elucidation of UBM and SIS composition is necessary to truly ascertain the biological effects, this study has demonstrated the incorporation of dECM to PCL has provided a level of bioactivity that HCjE cells have responded to. Coupled with notable differences to material composition, particularly fibre diameter and tensile properties, these dECM-containing scaffolds warrant further exploration as potential ATMP substrates for conjunctiva replacement and regeneration. In particular, the ability to support mucin-secreting goblet cells is an essential feature that these, or any, potential ATMPs would need to demonstrate.

5. Conclusions

This study aimed to determine the impact of including powders of decellularised tissue matrices with a synthetic polymer to create electrospun fibre scaffolds. Several differences occurred with fibre fabrication (reduced diameter) and their chemical composition (amine presence, uniform distribution) and tensile properties (increased stiffness, yield stress, strength at break, and decreased extension). These scaffolds also influenced the response of HCjE cells, with greater presence of rounded and clustered cells and their stratification up to five layers high. With development and longer-term culture, these dECM-containing PCL scaffolds may lead to the creation of an innovative ATMP for repair and regeneration of damaged conjunctiva.

Supplementary Materials: The following is available online at https://www.mdpi.com/1999-4923/13/3/318/s1, Figure S1: Scanning electron microscopy images of electrospun poly(ε-caprolactone) scaffolds with the addition of pepsin-solubilised decellularised tissue powder (dECM): (A) 1% small intestinal submucosa (SIS), (B) 10% SIS, (C) 1% urinary bladder matrix (UBM), and (D) 10% UBM. Magnification ×10,000, scale = 5 µm. (E) Measured fibre diameter presented as a violin plot for each group (n = 50).

Author Contributions: Conceptualization, L.A.B., K.G.D., and R.L.W.; Methodology, L.A.B., K.G.D., S.P.C., and C.P.M.; Formal analysis, L.A.B.; Resources, S.F.B., R.A.D., and R.L.W.; Data curation, L.A.B., K.G.D., and S.P.C.; Writing—original draft preparation, L.A.B., K.G.D., and J.D.H.; Writing—review and editing, L.A.B., K.G.D., J.D.H., R.L.W., R.A.D., C.P.M., and S.F.B.; Funding acquisition, L.A.B., R.L.W., and R.A.D. All authors have read and agreed to the published version of the manuscript.

Funding: This research was funded by The Ulverscroft Foundation, The Geoffrey and Pauline Martin Trust and EPSRC (EP/M002209/1 and EP/P023223/1).

Institutional Review Board Statement: Not applicable

Informed Consent Statement: Not applicable

Data Availability Statement: The data presented in this study are available on request from the corresponding author.

Acknowledgments: The authors' wish to thank Lisa White (University of Nottingham, UK) for helpfully couriering the decellularised tissue powders from Badylak's research laboratories. HCjE cells were kindly provided by Professor Ilene Gipson from the Schepens Eye Research Institute at Harvard Medical School in Boston, Massachusetts, USA.

Conflicts of Interest: The authors declare no conflict of interest.

References

1. Nelson, J.; Cameron, J. The conjunctiva: Anatomy and physiology. In *Cornea Fundam. Diagnosis Management*, 3rd ed.; Krachmer, J., Mannis, M., Holland, E., Eds.; Elsevier-Mosby: Philadelphia, PA, USA, 2011; pp. 25–31.
2. Mantelli, F.; Argüeso, P. Functions of ocular surface mucins in health and disease. *Curr. Opin. Allergy Clin. Immunol.* **2008**, *8*, 477–483. [CrossRef]
3. Harvey, T.; Alzaga Fernandez, A.G.; Patel, R.; Goldman, D.; Ciralsky, J. Conjunctival anatomy and physiology. In *Ocular Surface Disease Cornea, Conjunctiva Tear Film*; Holland, E., Mannis, M., Lee, W., Eds.; W.B. Saunders: London, UK, 2013; pp. 23–27.

4. Foster, C.S.; De La Maza, M.S. Ocular cicatricial pemphigoid review. *Curr. Opin. Allergy Clin. Immunol.* **2004**, *4*, 435–439. [CrossRef]
5. Lee, K.H.; Rhiu, S.; Yoon, S.C.; Seo, K.Y. Conjunctival Mini-flap Operation for Restrictive Strabismus After Periocular Surgery. *Am. J. Ophthalmol.* **2013**, *156*, 1244–1251.e2. [CrossRef]
6. Schrader, S.; Notara, M.; Beaconsfield, M.; Tuft, S.J.; Daniels, J.T.; Geerling, G. Tissue Engineering for Conjunctival Reconstruction: Established Methods and Future Outlooks. *Curr. Eye Res.* **2009**, *34*, 913–924. [CrossRef] [PubMed]
7. Lu, Q.; Al-Sheikh, O.; Elisseeff, J.H.; Grant, M.P. Biomaterials and tissue engineering strategies for conjunctival reconstruction and dry eye treatment. *Middle East Afr. J. Ophthalmol.* **2015**, 428–434. [CrossRef]
8. Eidet, J.R.; Dartt, D.A.; Utheim, T.P. Concise Review: Comparison of Culture Membranes Used for Tissue Engineered Conjunctival Epithelial Equivalents. *J. Funct. Biomater.* **2015**, *6*, 1064–1084. [CrossRef]
9. Scarritt, M.; Murdock, M.; Badylak, S.F. Biologic Scaffolds Composed of Extracellular Matrix for Regenerative Medicine. In *Principles of Regenerative Medicine*; Elsevier: Amsterdam, The Netherlands, 2019; pp. 613–626. [CrossRef]
10. Agmon, G.; Christman, K.L. Controlling stem cell behavior with decellularized extracellular matrix scaffolds. *Curr. Opin. Solid State Mater. Sci.* **2016**, *20*, 193–201. [CrossRef]
11. Gilbert, T.W.; Sellaro, T.L.; Badylak, S.F. Decellularization of tissues and organs. *Biomaterials* **2006**, *27*, 3675–3683. [CrossRef] [PubMed]
12. Liao, J.; Joyce, E.M.; Sacks, M.S. Effects of decellularization on the mechanical and structural properties of the porcine aortic valve leaflet. *Biomaterials* **2008**, *29*, 1065–1074. [CrossRef]
13. Bautista, C.A.; Park, H.J.; Mazur, C.M.; Aaron, R.K.; Bilgen, B. Effects of Chondroitinase ABC-Mediated Proteoglycan Digestion on Decellularization and Recellularization of Articular Cartilage. *PLoS ONE* **2016**, *11*, e0158976. [CrossRef] [PubMed]
14. Kasbekar, S.; Kaye, S.B.; Williams, R.L.; Stewart, R.M.; Leow-Dyke, S.; Rooney, P. Development of decellularized conjunctiva as a substrate for the ex vivo expansion of conjunctival epithelium. *J. Tissue Eng. Regen. Med.* **2018**, *12*, e973–e982. [CrossRef]
15. Saldin, L.T.; Cramer, M.C.; Velankar, S.S.; White, L.J.; Badylak, S.F. Extracellular matrix hydrogels from decellularized tissues: Structure and function. *Acta Biomater.* **2017**, *49*, 1–15. [CrossRef]
16. Fernández-Pérez, J.; Ahearne, M. The impact of decellularization methods on extracellular matrix derived hydrogels. *Sci. Rep.* **2019**, *9*, 1–12. [CrossRef]
17. Cramer, M.C.; Badylak, S.F. Extracellular Matrix-Based Biomaterials and Their Influence Upon Cell Behavior. *Ann. Biomed. Eng.* **2020**, *48*, 2132–2153. [CrossRef]
18. Spang, M.T.; Christman, K.L. Extracellular matrix hydrogel therapies: In vivo applications and development. *Acta Biomater.* **2018**, *68*, 1–14. [CrossRef]
19. Bosworth, L.A.; Downes, S. *Electrospinning for Tissue Regeneration*; Elsevier: Amsterdam, The Netherlands, 2011.
20. Stankus, J.J.; Freytes, D.O.; Badylak, S.F.; Wagner, W.R. Hybrid nanofibrous scaffolds from electrospinning of a synthetic biodegradable elastomer and urinary bladder matrix. *J. Biomater. Sci. Polym. Ed.* **2008**, *19*, 635–652. [CrossRef] [PubMed]
21. Gibson, M.; Beachley, V.; Coburn, J.; Bandinelli, P.A.; Mao, H.-Q.; Elisseeff, J. Tissue Extracellular Matrix Nanoparticle Presentation in Electrospun Nanofibers. *BioMed Res. Int.* **2014**, *2014*, [CrossRef]
22. Keane, T.J.; Swinehart, I.T.; Badylak, S.F. Methods of tissue decellularization used for preparation of biologic scaffolds and in vivo relevance. *Methods* **2015**, *84*, 25–34. [CrossRef]
23. Mehrban, N.; Molina, C.P.; Quijano, L.M.; Bowen, J.; Johnson, S.A.; Bartolacci, J.; Chang, J.T.; Scott, D.A.; Woolfson, D.N.; Birchall, M.A.; et al. Host macrophage response to injectable hydrogels derived from ECM and α-helical peptides. *Acta Biomater.* **2020**, *111*, 141–152. [CrossRef] [PubMed]
24. Gipson, I.K.; Spurr-Michaud, S.; Argüeso, P.; Tisdale, A.; Ng, T.F.; Russo, C.L. Mucin Gene Expression in Immortalized Human Corneal-Limbal and Conjunctival Epithelial Cell Lines. *Investig. Ophthalmol. Vis. Sci.* **2003**, *44*, 2496–2506. [CrossRef]
25. Hong, S.; Kim, G. Electrospun micro/nanofibrous conduits composed of poly(ε-caprolactone) and small intestine submucosa powder for nerve tissue regeneration. *J. Biomed. Mater. Res. Part B Appl. Biomater.* **2010**, [CrossRef]
26. Reid, J.A.; Callanan, A. Influence of aorta extracellular matrix in electrospun polycaprolactone scaffolds. *J. Appl. Polym. Sci.* **2019**, *136*, 48181. [CrossRef]
27. Reid, J.A.; Callanan, A. Hybrid cardiovascular sourced extracellular matrix scaffolds as possible platforms for vascular tissue engineering. *J. Biomed. Mater. Res. Part B Appl. Biomater.* **2020**, *108*, 910–924. [CrossRef]
28. Fernández-Pérez, J.; Kador, K.E.; Lynch, A.P.; Ahearne, M. Characterization of extracellular matrix modified poly(ε-caprolactone) electrospun scaffolds with differing fiber orientations for corneal stroma regeneration. *Mater. Sci. Eng. C* **2020**, *108*, 110415. [CrossRef] [PubMed]
29. Hong, Y.; Takanari, K.; Amoroso, N.J.; Hashizume, R.; Brennan-Pierce, E.P.; Freund, J.M.; Badylak, S.F.; Wagner, W.R. An Elastomeric Patch Electrospun from a Blended Solution of Dermal Extracellular Matrix and Biodegradable Polyurethane for Rat Abdominal Wall Repair. *Tissue Eng. Part C Methods* **2012**, *18*, 122–132. [CrossRef]
30. Feng, B.; Ji, T.; Wang, X.; Fu, W.; Ye, L.; Zhang, H.; Li, F. Engineering cartilage tissue based on cartilage-derived extracellular matrix cECM/PCL hybrid nanofibrous scaffold. *Mater. Des.* **2020**, *193*, 108773. [CrossRef]
31. Kim, T.H.; Jung, Y.; Kim, S.H. Nanofibrous Electrospun Heart Decellularized Extracellular Matrix-Based Hybrid Scaffold as Wound Dressing for Reducing Scarring in Wound Healing. *Tissue Eng. Part A* **2018**, *24*, 830–848. [CrossRef]

32. Kim, K.; Lee, J.Y.; Shin, J.; Yoo, Y.T. Fabrication of electropsun PLGA and small intestine submucosa-blended nanofibrous membranes and their biocompatibility for wound healing. *Fibers Polym.* **2017**, *18*, 231–239. [CrossRef]
33. Haider, A.; Haider, S.; Kang, I.-K. A comprehensive review summarizing the effect of electrospinning parameters and potential applications of nanofibers in biomedical and biotechnology. *Arab. J. Chem.* **2018**, *11*, 1165–1188. [CrossRef]
34. Coates, J. Interpretation of Infrared Spectra, A Practical Approach. In *Encyclopedia of Analytical Chemistry*; John Wiley & Sons Ltd.: Chichester, UK, 2006. [CrossRef]
35. Witt, J.; Mertsch, S.; Borrelli, M.; Dietrich, J.; Geerling, G.; Schrader, S.; Spaniol, K. Decellularised conjunctiva for ocular surface reconstruction. *Acta Biomater.* **2018**, *67*, 259–269. [CrossRef]
36. Grant, R.; Hallett, J.; Forbes, S.; Hay, D.; Callanan, A. Blended electrospinning with human liver extracellular matrix for engineering new hepatic microenvironments. *Sci. Rep.* **2019**, *9*, 1–12. [CrossRef]
37. Gao, S.; Guo, W.; Chen, M.; Yuan, Z.; Wang, M.; Zhang, Y.; Liu, S.; Xi, T.; Guo, Q. Fabrication and characterization of electrospun nanofibers composed of decellularized meniscus extracellular matrix and polycaprolactone for meniscus tissue engineering. *J. Mater. Chem. B* **2017**, *5*, 2273–2285. [CrossRef] [PubMed]
38. Wong, S.-C.; Baji, A.; Leng, S. Effect of fiber diameter on tensile properties of electrospun poly(ε-caprolactone). *Polymer* **2008**, *49*, 4713–4722. [CrossRef]
39. Postnikoff, C.K.; Pintwala, R.; Williams, S.; Wright, A.M.; Hileeto, D.; Gorbet, M.B. Development of a Curved, Stratified, In Vitro Model to Assess Ocular Biocompatibility. *PLoS ONE* **2014**, *9*, e96448. [CrossRef]
40. Bosworth, L.A.; Hu, W.; Shi, Y.; Cartmell, S.H. Enhancing Biocompatibility without Compromising Material Properties: An Optimised NaOH Treatment for Electrospun Polycaprolactone Fibres. *J. Nanomater.* **2019**, *2019*, 1–11. [CrossRef]
41. Ang, L.P.K.; Cheng, Z.Y.; Beuerman, R.W.; Teoh, S.H.; Zhu, X.; Tan, D.T.H. The Development of a Serum-Free Derived Bioengineered Conjunctival Epithelial Equivalent Using an Ultrathin Poly(ε-Caprolactone) Membrane Substrate. *Investig. Ophthalmol. Vis. Sci.* **2006**, *47*, 105–112. [CrossRef] [PubMed]
42. Drubin, D.G.; Nelson, W.J. Origins of Cell Polarity. *Cell* **1996**, *84*, 335–344. [CrossRef]
43. Koufakis, D.I.; Karabatsas, C.H.; Sakkas, L.I.; Alvanou, A.; Manthos, A.K.; Chatzoulis, D.Z. Conjunctival Surface Changes in Patients with Sjogren's Syndrome: A Transmission Electron Microscopy Study. *Investig. Ophthalmol. Vis. Sci.* **2006**, *47*, 541–544. [CrossRef]
44. Cennamo, G.L.; Del Prete, A.; Forte, R.; Cafiero, G.; Marasco, D. Impression cytology with scanning electron microscopy: A new method in the study of conjunctival microvilli. *Eye* **2008**, *22*, 138–143. [CrossRef] [PubMed]
45. Tatematsu, Y.; Ogawa, Y.; Shimmura, S.; Dogru, M.; Yaguchi, S.; Nagai, T.; Yamazaki, K.; Kameyama, K.; Okamoto, S.; Kawakami, Y.; et al. Mucosal microvilli in dry eye patients with chronic GVHD. *Bone Marrow Transplant.* **2012**, *47*, 416–425. [CrossRef] [PubMed]
46. Doughty, M.J.; Naase, T. Nucleus and cell size changes in human bulbar conjunctival cells after soft contact lens wear, as assessed by impression cytology. *Contact Lens Anterior Eye* **2008**, *31*, 131–140. [CrossRef] [PubMed]
47. Zorn-Kruppa, M.; Houdek, P.; Wladykowski, E.; Engelke, M.; Bartok, M.; Mewes, K.R.; Moll, I.; Brandner, J.M. Determining the Depth of Injury in Bioengineered Tissue Models of Cornea and Conjunctiva for the Prediction of All Three Ocular GHS Categories. *PLoS ONE* **2014**, *9*. [CrossRef] [PubMed]
48. Garcia-Posadas, L.; Soriano-Romaní, L.; López-García, A.; Diebold, Y. An engineered human conjunctival-like tissue to study ocular surface inflammatory diseases. *PLoS ONE* **2017**, *12*. [CrossRef] [PubMed]
49. Sekiguchi, R.; Yamada, K.M. Basement Membranes in Development and Disease. *Curr. Top. Dev. Biol.* **2018**, 143–191. [CrossRef]
50. Makuloluwa, A.K. Development of a Synthetic Substrate for Conjunctival Cell Transplantation. Ph.D. Thesis, University of Liverpool, Liverpool, UK, 2017. [CrossRef]
51. Schlötzer-Schrehardt, U.; Dietrich, T.; Saito, K.; Sorokin, L.; Sasaki, T.; Paulsson, M.; Kruse, F. Characterization of extracellular matrix components in the limbal epithelial stem cell compartment. *Exp. Eye Res.* **2007**, *85*, 845–860. [CrossRef]
52. Marçal, H.; Ahmed, T.; Badylak, S.F.; Tottey, S.; Foster, L.J.R. A comprehensive protein expression profile of extracellular matrix biomaterial derived from porcine urinary bladder. *Regen. Med.* **2012**, *7*, 159–166. [CrossRef] [PubMed]
53. Lindberg, K.; Badylak, S.F. Porcine small intestinal submucosa (SIS): A bioscaffold supporting in vitro primary human epidermal cell differentiation and synthesis of basement membrane proteins. *Burns* **2001**, *27*, 254–266. [CrossRef]

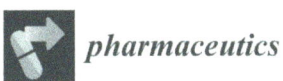

Article

Optimization of Collagen Chemical Crosslinking to Restore Biocompatibility of Tissue-Engineered Scaffolds

Mohammad Mirazul Islam [1], Dina B. AbuSamra [1], Alexandru Chivu [2], Pablo Argüeso [1], Claes H. Dohlman [1], Hirak K. Patra [2], James Chodosh [1] and Miguel González-Andrades [1,3,*]

[1] Department of Ophthalmology, Massachusetts Eye and Ear and Schepens Eye Research Institute, Harvard Medical School, Boston, MA 02114, USA; mohammad_islam@meei.harvard.edu (M.M.I.); dina_abusamra@meei.harvard.edu (D.B.A.); Pablo_Argueso@MEEI.HARVARD.EDU (P.A.); claes_dohlman@meei.harvard.edu (C.H.D.); james_chodosh@meei.harvard.edu (J.C.)
[2] Department of Surgical Biotechnology, University College London, London NW3 2PF, UK; a.chivu@ucl.ac.uk (A.C.); hirak.patra@ucl.ac.uk (H.K.P.)
[3] Maimonides Biomedical Research Institute of Cordoba (IMIBIC), Department of Ophthalmology, Reina Sofia University Hospital and University of Cordoba, 14004 Cordoba, Spain
* Correspondence: miguel.gonzalez@imibic.org

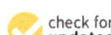

Citation: Islam, M.M.; AbuSamra, D.B.; Chivu, A.; Argüeso, P.; Dohlman, C.H.; Patra, H.K.; Chodosh, J.; González-Andrades, M. Optimization of Collagen Chemical Crosslinking to Restore Biocompatibility of Tissue-Engineered Scaffolds. *Pharmaceutics* 2021, *13*, 832. https://doi.org/10.3390/pharmaceutics13060832

Academic Editor: Charles M. Heard

Received: 23 April 2021
Accepted: 28 May 2021
Published: 3 June 2021

Publisher's Note: MDPI stays neutral with regard to jurisdictional claims in published maps and institutional affiliations.

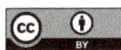

Copyright: © 2021 by the authors. Licensee MDPI, Basel, Switzerland. This article is an open access article distributed under the terms and conditions of the Creative Commons Attribution (CC BY) license (https://creativecommons.org/licenses/by/4.0/).

Abstract: Collagen scaffolds, one of the most used biomaterials in corneal tissue engineering, are frequently crosslinked to improve mechanical properties, enzyme tolerance, and thermal stability. Crosslinkers such as 1-ethyl-3-(3-dimethylaminopropyl) carbodiimide hydrochloride (EDC) are compatible with tissues but provide low crosslinking density and reduced mechanical properties. Conversely, crosslinkers such as glutaraldehyde (GTA) can generate mechanically more robust scaffolds; however, they can also induce greater toxicity. Herein, we evaluated the effectivity of double-crosslinking with both EDC and GTA together with the capability of sodium metabisulfite (SM) and sodium borohydride (SB) to neutralize the toxicity and restore biocompatibility after crosslinking. The EDC-crosslinked collagen scaffolds were treated with different concentrations of GTA. To neutralize the free unreacted aldehyde groups, scaffolds were treated with SM or SB. The chemistry involved in these reactions together with the mechanical and functional properties of the collagen scaffolds was evaluated. The viability of the cells grown on the scaffolds was studied using different corneal cell types. The effect of each type of scaffold treatment on human monocyte differentiation was evaluated. One-way ANOVA was used for statistical analysis. The addition of GTA as a double-crosslinking agent significantly improved the mechanical properties and enzymatic stability of the EDC crosslinked collagen scaffold. GTA decreased cell biocompatibility but this effect was reversed by treatment with SB or SM. These agents did not affect the mechanical properties, enzymatic stability, or transparency of the double-crosslinked scaffold. Contact of monocytes with the different scaffolds did not trigger their differentiation into activated macrophages. Our results demonstrate that GTA improves the mechanical properties of EDC crosslinked scaffolds in a dose-dependent manner, and that subsequent treatment with SB or SM partially restores biocompatibility. This novel manufacturing approach would facilitate the translation of collagen-based artificial corneas to the clinical setting.

Keywords: cornea; collagen; double-crosslinking; carbodiimide; glutaraldehyde; sodium metabisulfite; sodium borohydride; EDC/NHS

1. Introduction

Data from the World Health Organization (WHO) indicate that the current transplantation rate of 100,800 solid organs per year fulfills less than 10% of the global demand [1]. Therefore, any advancement in the development of new biomaterials holds tremendous potential to fill the gap between the supply and demand of donated organs. Engineered organ development is based on the selection of appropriate biomaterials, which usually requires polymerization processes to form apposite structure of the target organ. Natural biomaterials, such as collagen, show superior biocompatibility but lack optimal mechanical properties. Despite that, collagen-based biomaterials are widely used for tissue engineering because of their excellent properties for creating regenerative cell-free scaffolds for tissue engineering as seen in early clinical evaluations [2–4]. The clinical success of collagen scaffolds is based on their excellent biocompatibility. However, bioactivity is hindered mostly by poor mechanical behavior and a high vulnerability to enzymatic digestion [5]. These weaknesses make collagen scaffolds unsuitable for transplantation in patients with severe inflammatory disease conditions in which high levels of host proteolytic enzymes are present.

Crosslinkers are commonly used to produce collagen-based scaffolds with physicochemical properties similar to healthy tissues and organs, including mechanical properties, enzyme tolerance capacity, and thermal stability. Collagen can be crosslinked with different strategies that include chemical [6], physical [7], and enzymatic [8] crosslinking. One of the most commonly used is the zero-length chemical crosslinking using 1-ethyl-3-(3-dimethylaminopropyl) carbodiimide hydrochloride (EDC) and N-hydroxysuccinimide (NHS), which have been proven effective for crosslinking of collagen fibres [9]. This approach results in a lower crosslinking density than other chemical (e.g., GTA, formaldehyde) and physical crosslinking methods (e.g., ionizing irradiation or UV light, dehydrothermal, pressure), but has been shown to have promising biofunctional outcomes [3], unlike more hostile crosslinking techniques that are associated with inflammatory responses and worse biological outcomes [10]. Crosslinking using EDC involves the activation of carboxylic acid groups of collagen to give o-acylisourea groups, which form crosslinks after reaction with free amine groups of the collagen and finally formed amide bonds [11]. In this process, EDC does not incorporate into the crosslinked structure. Because of that, this type of crosslinking is called zero-length crosslinking; however, there are non-zero-length crosslinkers that get incorporated into the crosslinked structure with a series of chemical reactions [12]. Although EDC/NHS forms rigid zero-length crosslinking of the collagen, the collagen hydrogel still remain susceptible to collagenase degradation and the mechanical strength of crosslinked collagen is not satisfactory [5].

To address the lack of enzymatic stability and mechanical strength of EDC-crosslinked collagen scaffolds, several research groups have proposed other crosslinkers for collagen, such as glutaraldehyde (GTA) [13]. GTA is a non-zero-length crosslinker that generates a more rigid biomacromolecular network, associated with the incorporation of covalent bonds (Schiff bases) [14] between polypeptide chains of the collagen. GTA has been used for clinical applications, not only as a crosslinker but also as a sterilizing agent, including the fabrication of bioprostheses for human implantation [15]. However, other medical applications of GTA crosslinking are generally restricted as chemical modification of biomaterials by GTA may pose a significant risk for toxicity [16,17]. Thus, there is a need to optimize the GTA-based crosslinking in order to maximize the improvement of physicochemical properties of artificial tissues and organs while minimizing its toxic effect.

The balance between mechanical resistance, including enzymatic stability, and cytotoxicity can be achieved by two main approaches. On the one hand, as we have shown previously, different crosslinkers can be combined to crosslink collagen in order to acquire the beneficial effect of each crosslinker [18]. GTA has not been previously used in combination with other more biocompatible crosslinkers with the direct purpose of reducing the exposure to GTA in order to decrease GTA-induced cytotoxicity. However, as an evaluation of physical properties of collagen membranes, it was shown that GTA can increase the crosslinking density of a previously crosslinked matrix using dimethyl suberimidate as first crosslinker [19]. On the other hand, different research groups have shown that the aldehyde groups introduced in the crosslinked biopolymers with GTA can be masked with different chemical treatments (i.e., glycine) to reduce the cytotoxicity of glutaraldehyde [20].

Therefore, we aimed to optimize double-crosslinking of collagen scaffolds using EDC/NHS and GTA, including masking chemical treatments in order to manufacture mechanically and enzymatically strong implants while reducing the cytotoxic effect of the crosslinkers. We focused on the corneal application because of the high requirements in terms of mechanical and optical behavior, in addition to biocompatibility. Herein, we crosslinked collagen with EDC and post-treated with GTA, followed by different neutralizing chemical agents (i.e., sodium metabisulfite (SM) and sodium borohydride (SB)) to restore the biocompatibility of the implants. Our result demonstrated that GTA improves the mechanical properties of the EDC crosslinked implants in a dose-dependent manner, and a final masking of the free aldehyde group on the scaffold with SM or SB can restore biocompatibility.

2. Materials and Method

Type I porcine atelocollagen was purchased from Nippon Meat Packers Inc. (Tokyo, Japan). All reagents were of analytical grade and used as received. All the chemicals were purchased from Sigma-Aldrich (St. Louis, MO, USA) if not mentioned otherwise.

2.1. Fabrication of Collagen Hydrogel

Hydrogel encompassed 10% (wt/wt) collagen was made following previously described protocol [18]. Collagen solution was buffered with 150 µL of 0.63 M 2-(N-Morpholino)ethane-sulfonic acid, 4-Morpholineethanesulfonic acid monohydrate (MES) buffer in a syringe mixing system. Then, the collagen solution was adjusted to pH 5 with 2.0 M aqueous NaOH. Calculated volumes of aqueous solutions of 1-ethyl-3-(3-dimethylaminopropyl) carbodiimide (EDC) and its co-reagent N-hydroxysuccinimide (NHS), both at 10% (wt/vol), were added to the collagen solution (EDC: Collagen-NH_2 (mol:mol) = 0.7:1 and EDC:NHS (mol:mol) = 2:1). Every addition was followed by thorough mixing. The final mixed solution was immediately dispersed onto a glass plate to a thickness of 500 µm, similar to the human cornea. The hydrogels were cured at 100% humidity at room temperature for 16 h and then at 37 °C for 5 h. After demolding, hydrogels were washed thoroughly with phosphate-buffered saline (PBS).

2.2. Double-Crosslinking with GTA

Different molar concentrations of GTA were used to double-crosslink the collagen hydrogels. The molar ratio of GTA:Collagen-NH_2 was set at x:1, where x was gradually increased to 0.018, 0.18, 0.45, 0.9, and 2.7. Depending on x, hydrogels were named as 1, 2, 3, 4, and 5, respectively. Three 6 mm diameter hydrogels were placed in a glass vial with 1 mL PBS containing a specific amount of GTA and the vial was kept under continuous shaking at 150 rpm for 4 h. After GTA crosslinking, the hydrogels were washed rigorously with PBS overnight at room temperature. We used neutral pH conditions for GTA crosslinking. At acidic conditions, GTA crosslinking is usually slow and gives materials of lower thermal stability [21].

2.3. Masking Unreacted Aldehyde Groups

Double-crosslinked hydrogels were treated with different chemicals to mask the unreacted aldehyde group from the hydrogel to reduce cytotoxicity. Sodium metabisulfite 1% (wt/vol) (SM) and Sodium borohydride 1% (wt/vol) (SB) were independently used for 1 h and 10 min, respectively, to treat the hydrogels under constant shaking at room temperature. We also tested the efficacy of 200 mM glycine, 200 nM lysine, 10% citric acid, 200 mg/mL NaOH and 4 M NaCl for 1.5 h to mask unreacted aldehyde groups of the double-crosslinked hydrogel. However, due to their inability to prevent cytotoxicity, these groups were taken out from the further studies, continuing the evaluation of SM and SB.

2.4. Optical Transmission

The optical transmissions of the hydrogels were examined by a UV-Vis spectrometer (Molecular Devices SpectraMax 384 Plus Microplate Reader, Molecular Devices; San Jose, CA, USA). Six mm diameter trephined discs of the hydrogels were placed in individual wells of a 96-well quartz microplate, and their optical transmittance was recorded from 200–800 nm in quartz microplate at 1 nm wavelength increments. The transmittance of the samples was corrected with blank water media and the mean transmittance (%) for each group was calculated and plotted as a function of wavelength.

2.5. In Vitro Biodegradation

The resistance of the hydrogels against collagenase digestion was determined as we previously described [22]. In brief, hydrogels were placed in a vial containing 5 U/mL collagenase from *Clostridium histolyticum* (Sigma-Aldrich, St. Louis, MO, USA) in 0.1 M Tris-HCl (pH 7.4) and 5 mM $CaCl_2$ at 37 °C. The collagenase solution was replenished every 8 h and the percent residual mass of the sample was measured at different time points after removing the hydrogels from the solution and gently blotted on the filter paper to remove the surface water.

2.6. Mechanical Characterization

Mechanical characterization of the hydrogels was conducted using a mechanical tester (Mark-10 ESM 303, Copiague, NY, USA). To measure the compressive modulus, cylindrical samples (diameter = 6.0 mm, and thickness = 0.5 μm) were placed in the mechanical tester and measurement was performed with crosshead speed of 0.5 mm/min. The compressive stress was recorded as a function of the strain. Load displacement extracted data were translated to engineering stress–strain data by incorporating the cross-sectional areas and the original thickness of the hydrogels. The obtained stress/strain curve was used to extract the compressive modulus of each hydrogel.

2.7. Water Content Measurement

The water content of hydrogels was determined to ensure uniformity using previously published protocol [3] with modifications. In brief, hydrated hydrogels were removed from PBS; the surface was gently blotted dry and then immediately weighed on a microbalance to record the wet weight (W_0) of the hydrogels. Dry weight of the same hydrogels was obtained by drying the samples at 50 °C until constant mass was achieved (W).

The equilibrated water content of the hydrogels (W_t) was calculated according to the following equation: $W_t = (W_0 - W)/W_0 \times 100\%$.

2.8. Fourier-Transform Infrared Spectroscopy (FTIR)

FTIR was performed on a Jasco attenuated total reflectance FTIR 4200 spectrometer (ATR FT/IR-4200, Jasco, Tokyo, Japan), averaging 30 scans between 4000 cm^{-1} and 600 cm^{-1}, at a resolution of 2 cm^{-1}. The measurements were performed on the samples in hydrated form, as well as after drying in a vacuum desiccator for 24 h.

2.9. Contact Angle Measurement

The surface hydrophilicity of different hydrogel samples was studied by contact angle measurements. A drop of 3 μL dH_2O was deposited onto each hydrogel by a micro-syringe and images were taken with Dino-light digital microscope (AnMo Electronics Corporation, Hsinchu, Taiwan). The contact angle was measured with ImageJ (U.S. National Institutes of Health, Bethesda, MD, USA).

2.10. In Vitro Biocompatibility

Human corneal cells were used to evaluate the biomaterials as the proposed modification could be applied for the improvement of collagen based artificial cornea development. The cornea is a non-compartmented, solid, transparent organ that is comprised mainly of three distinct cell types. Each of these corneal cell populations behaves differently in response to the specific properties of the biomaterial. For that reason, we specifically checked all three principal cell types in conjugation with the modified double-crosslinked hydrogels.

2.10.1. Human Corneal Epithelial Cells (HCEC)

The biocompatibility of the hydrogels was tested using SV40-immortalized HCEC, kindly provided by Professor May Griffith, as previously reported [23]. The hydrogels were cut into 6 mm diameter segments and 5000 HCEC were seeded on top of each for culture with DMEM/Ham's F-12 media (Corning, Manassas, VA, USA) supplemented with 10% Newborn Calf Serum (NCS) (HyClone, Logan, UT, USA), 10 ng/mL epidermal growth factor (EGF) (Life Technologies, Frederick, MD, USA), 5 ug/mL Human Insulin (Sigma-Aldrich, St. Louis, MO, USA) and 1% penicillin/streptomycin (Gibco, Life Technologies Corporation, Grand Island, NY, USA), at 37 °C and 5% CO_2. Cells seeded on tissue culture plates (TCP) were used as control. AlamarBlue study was performed at day 1, day 4, and day 7 after cell seeding. At each time point, the tissue culture media was removed and replaced with fresh media (100 µL) containing resazurin sodium salt (0.004% w/v) and incubated for 4 h. Afterwards, the media (95 µL) were removed from each well and pipetted into a new 96-well plate and read on a BioTek plate reader (Synergy 2, BioTek Instruments; Winooski, VT, USA) at 530/25 nm for excitation and 600/25 nm for emission. At day 7, live/dead staining was performed with a staining kit (Life Technologies Corporation, Carlsbad, CA, USA), where cells were double-stained by calceinacetoxymethyl (Calcein AM) and ethidium homodimer-1 (EthD-1). Images were taken by using a fluorescence microscope (Zeiss Axio Observer Z1, Carl Zeiss Microimaging GmbH, Jena, Germany). The transcellular barrier function of stratified corneal epithelial cells was evaluated with the rose bengal anionic dye (Acros Organics; Morris Plains, NJ, USA) as described previously [24].

2.10.2. Human Corneal Fibroblasts (HCF)

Immortalized human corneal fibroblasts (HCF), kindly donated by Professor James V Jester, were used for evaluating the cellularization potential. Around 5000 HCF were cultured on the top of the hydrogels and cultured with DMEM/Ham's F-12 media supplemented with 10% fetal bovine serum (FBS) (Life Technologies Corporation, Carlsbad, CA, USA) for seven days at 37 °C in 5% CO_2. AlamarBlue assay was performed at day 1, 4, and 7 after cell seeding and live/dead staining was performed at day 7.

2.10.3. Human Corneal Endothelial Cells (CEC)

Telomerase immortalized human corneal endothelial cells (CEC), kindly provided by Professor Ula Jurkunas, were cultured on the top of hydrogels. Cells were cultured in Opti-MEM I with Glutamax-I media (Life Technologies Corporation, Carlsbad, CA, USA) supplemented with 8% (v/v) FBS, 5 ng/mL EGF (EMD Millipore Corporation, Temecula, CA, USA), 0.2 mg/mL calcium chloride (Fisher Scientific Company, Fair Lawn, NJ, USA), 0.8 mg/mL chondroitin sulfate-A (Sigma-Aldrich, St. Louis, MO, USA), 0.25 mg/mL Gentamycin (Life Technologies Corporation), 1% (v/v) Antibiotic-Antimycotic solution (Life Technologies Corporation), and 0.1 mg/mL bovine pituitary extract (Alfa Aesar, Ward Hill, MA, USA) for 7 days. Approximately 5000 CEC were seeded on the top of the hydrogels and incubated at 37 °C in 5% CO_2. Media was changed every other day. AlamarBlue assay was performed at day 1, 4, and 7 after cell seeding, and live/dead staining was performed at day 7.

2.11. Hydrogel Composition and Influence on Human Adaptive Immunity

Human monocytic THP-1 cells were used to determine the effect of the hydrogels on human adaptive immunity. THP-1 cells were cultured on the hydrogels in RPMI (Gibco) media supplemented with 10% FBS, 1% penicillin/streptomycin and 50 µM β-mercaptoethanol (Gibco) and culture for 6 days at 37 °C in 5% CO_2. THP-1 cells culture on TCP with or without Lipopolysaccharide (1× LPS, Invitrogen, Carlsbad, CA, USA) were used as controls. Morphological changes of the cells were evaluated by 20× phase contrast images taken at days 2 and 6 with Nikon Eclipse (TS100) microscope. LPS was used as a control to induce THP-1 cell differentiation into macrophage-like cells. The influence of hydrogels on pro-inflammatory macrophage differentiation was evaluated by labeling the cells after culture for 6 days with direct-conjugate antibody against CD86 (pro-inflammatory M1 marker) (Table 1). Data were acquired using a BD LSR II and analyzed using FlowJo software (Becton, Dickinson and Company, Franklin Lakes, NJ, USA).

Table 1. Antibodies for Flow Cytometry.

Target	Antibody	Supplier	Dilution Factor
CD86	APC Mouse Anti-Human CD86, Clone 2331 (FUN-1)	BD Bioscience, Odenton, MD, USA	1/20
Isotype Control for CD86	APC Mouse IgG1, κ, Clone MOPC-21	BD Bioscience	1/20

2.12. Statistical Analysis

One-way ANOVA with Tukey post hoc test was performed to compare mechanical and functional characteristic properties. A value of $p < 0.05$ was considered statistically significant. n.s., *, **, ***, and **** represent p greater than 0.05, $p < 0.05$, $p < 0.01$, $p < 0.001$, and $p < 0.0001$, respectively. For cell culture study, statistics were not denoted on the graph due to over crowdedness in the figure; however, result elaboration contains the specific statistics data. The GraphPad Prism Software (GraphPad Software, San Diego, CA, USA) was used to analyze the data.

3. Results

3.1. Collagen Hydrogel

The hydrogels were developed using collagen as base materials through EDC/NHS crosslinking. The treatments were performed on the base materials and untreated samples served as controls (Figure 1). Post-formulation treatments started with treating hydrogels with different concentrations of GTA solution for producing a mechanically and enzymatically reinforced material suitable for fabrication of the implants.

The compressive modulus was measured to evaluate the mechanical properties of the hydrogel; strong materials exhibit a higher compressive modulus. Post-formulation GTA-treatment (PFGT) significantly increased the mechanical property of EDC-treated hydrogels with respect to the untreated control (non-PFGT) in a dose-dependent manner, reaching a plateau at 1.5MPa. Significant improvement was achieved between 1 and 3 ($p = 0.0019$), 4 ($p = 0.0048$), and 5 ($p = 0.0055$) GTA hydrogels in PFGT groups (Figure 2A). Although GTA concentrations increased, there was no significant difference in mechanical property between 2, 3, 4, and 5 PFGT hydrogels groups.

The UV–Vis spectroscopy revealed that the final PFGT products were transparent (Figure 2B). Transparency to UVB (280–315 nm) was more prominent for control and 1 hydrogels (~70%). UVB transmission was ~30% for all other hydrogels. The PFGT 3 hydrogel formulation more effectively blocked UVA (315–400 nm). The optical evaluation of the hydrogels showed high levels of optical transmission (>80%) in the visible spectrum (between 400 and 800 nm) for the control and 1 hydrogel groups (Figure 2B). Higher doses of GTA led to a decrease of the transmission of visible violet (380–450 nm) and blue (450–485 nm) light. This resulted in color changes after GTA treatment, where yellowing of the hydrogel was observed. Transmission of other visible light (485–800 nm) was similar for all the hydrogels.

Solutions with excess collagenase were used to evaluate the enzymatic stability of the samples in comparison to control non-PFGT hydrogel. Control hydrogels completely degraded within 4 hours (Figure 2C). The lowest concentration of GTA (hydrogel 1) retained a mass of more than 15% after 10 h. All other PFGT groups were stable through 30 h. Approximately 30% residual mass was present for the 3 and 4 PFGT formulations after 30 h collagenase treatment. Like mechanical property, enzymatic stability did not increase further after 3 PFGT hydrogel formulation (Figure 2C).

3.2. Masking of Unreacted Aldehyde Groups of GTA

The aldehyde groups introduced in the PFGT hydrogels were quenched by sodium metabisulfite or sodium borohydride, separately, to compare the masking potential of these two chemicals. Based on the mechanical and enzymatic properties, only PFGT 3 hydrogels were used for the aldehyde masking study, in comparison to unmodified PFGT 3 hydrogels. Sodium metabisulfite treated and sodium borohydride treated hydrogels were abbreviated as 3-SM and 3-SB hydrogel, respectively.

Hydrogels were characterized similarly to evaluate the effect of post-chemical treatment with SM or SB on the PGTA 3 hydrogels. Compressive modulus studies showed that post-chemical treatment of the PGTA hydrogel does not mechanically alter the hydrogel (Figure 3A). The compressive modulus of the hydrogels was 1.5 MPa with non-significant ($p = 0.1989$) differences between hydrogels.

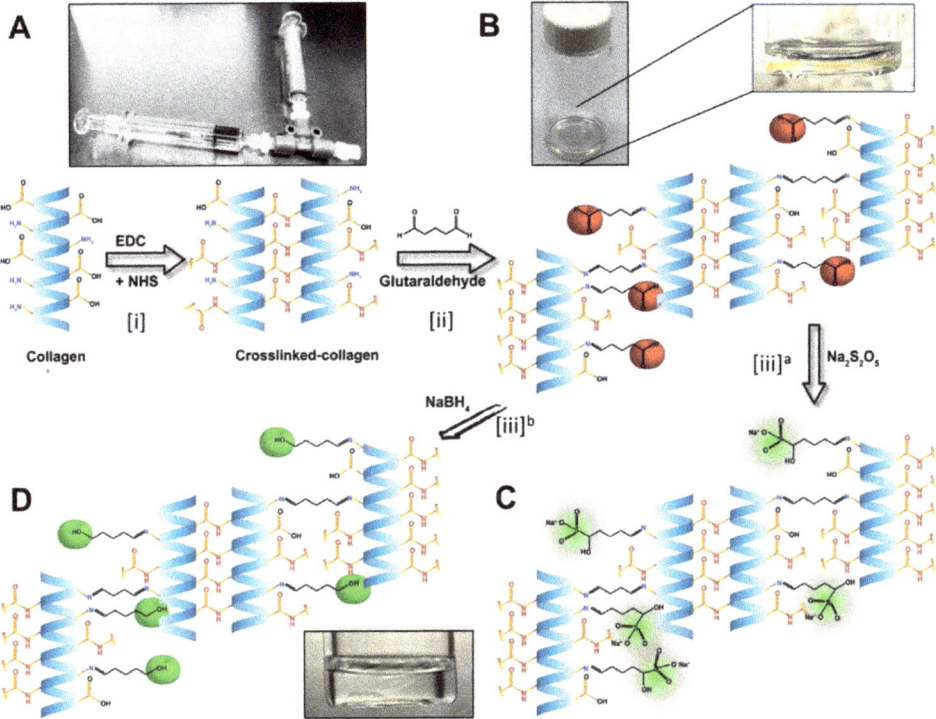

Figure 1. Stepwise illustration of the chemical reactions in the development of the biomaterials. (**A**) Illustration of the EDC/NHS crosslinking of the collagen. The T-piece syringe mixing system was used for making the hydrogels. (**B**) Hydrogels from the previous step crosslinked with GTA, leaving the unreacted aldehyde groups marked as red. Magnified image of a hydrogel in the GTA solution. (**C**) Neutralization of the free aldehyde groups with Sodium metabisulfite ($Na_2S_2O_5$; in green). Alternatively, (**D**) neutralization of the free aldehyde groups by Sodium borohydride ($NaBH_4$) and conversion of aldehyde group to alcohol groups (green).

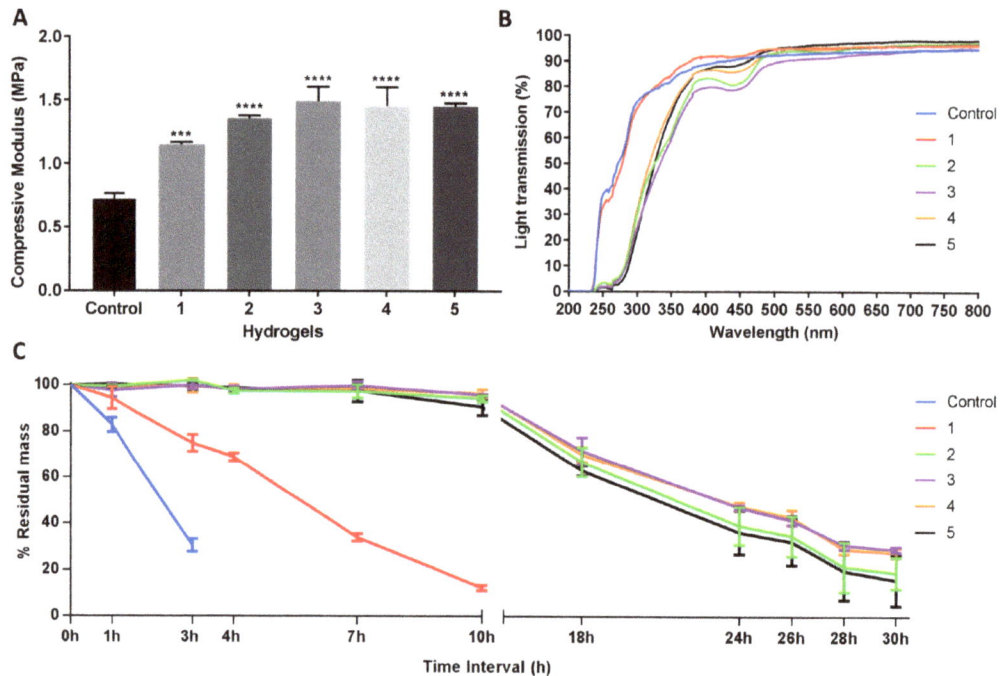

Figure 2. Mechanical and functional assessment of the collagen hydrogels, comparing the control (EDC/NHS crosslinked hydrogel) with double-crosslinked hydrogels with different concentrations of GTA (1, 2, 3, 4, and 5 PFGT hydrogels). (**A**) Compressive modulus was measured to evaluate the mechanical properties of the hydrogels. *** and **** represent $p < 0.001$ and $p < 0.0001$, respectively. (**B**) Optical evaluation of the hydrogels was carried out based on the analysis of light transmission through the different samples, from UV to visual wavelengths. (**C**) Treatment with collagenase was performed and residual mass (presented against time in hours (h)) of the hydrogels was calculated. For all panels, quantitative results were reported as the mean ± S.D. from three independent hydrogels and results were compared between groups.

Changes in light transmission were prominent between chemically treated and untreated PFGT 3 hydrogels. Post-crosslinked chemical treatment removes the yellow color (Figure 1) and rendered the hydrogel completely transparent at the visible, violet, and blue light spectrums (Figure 3B). UVA and UVB transmission were also increased but less so compared to the control hydrogel.

The effect of post-chemical treatment on enzymatic stability was also evaluated and examined for 7 h to determine the pattern of the enzymatic degradation, similar to Figure 2C. SB or SM-treated PGTA 3 hydrogels were equally stable to non-treated PFGT 3 hydrogels up to 7 h, and the residual mass was close to the initial weight at the end of each study (Figure 3C). The pattern of degradation was similar to the extended time study previously performed (Figure 2C).

Water content of the control hydrogel was similar to non-treated PFGT 3 hydrogel, although there were significant differences between control and 3-SB and 3-SM hydrogels. However, for all hydrogels, the water content was more than 80% (Figure 3D).

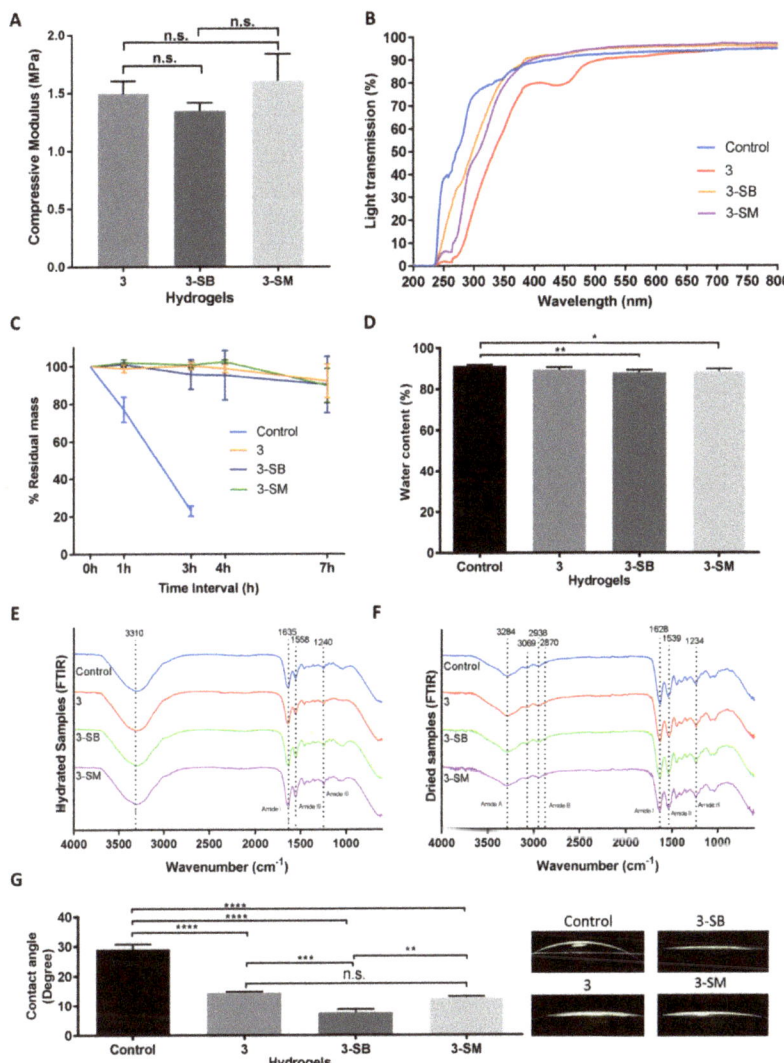

Figure 3. Mechanical and functional assessment of the collagen hydrogels, comparing the control (EDC/NHS) with post-formulation GTA-treatment (PFGT) 3 hydrogels before and after post-crosslinked chemical treatment. Sodium metabisulfite treated and Sodium borohydride treated hydrogels were abbreviated as 3-SM and 3-SB hydrogel, respectively. (**A**) Compressive modulus was measured to evaluate the mechanical properties of the 3 hydrogels. (**B**) Optical evaluation of the hydrogels was carried out based on the analysis of light transmission. (**C**) Collagenase study was performed and residual mass (presented against time in hours (h)) of the hydrogels were calculated. (**D**) Water content measurement (%) among the hydrogels compared with control hydrogels. FTIR spectra of hydrated (**E**) and dried (**F**) hydrogel samples. (**G**) Representative micrographs of water contact angles of different hydrogels with the corresponding contact angle measurement. For all panels, quantitative results were reported as the mean ± S.D. from three independent samples and results compared between groups. n.s., *, **, ***, and **** represent p greater than 0.05, $p < 0.05$, $p < 0.01$, $p < 0.001$, and $p < 0.0001$, respectively.

The FTIR spectra of the hydrated gel (Figure 3E) exhibited amide I bands at 1635 cm^{-1} attributed to stretching of C=O bonds of the polypeptide chains, as well as amide II and amide III bands at 1558 cm^{-1} and 1240 cm^{-1}, respectively, associated with in-plane N-H bending, C-N stretching, and C-H stretching. The potential amide A and amide B bands were obscured by the presence of a broad band centred at 3310 cm^{-1} characteristic of O-H stretching vibration mode of water. The dried hydrogel samples (Figure 3F) showed similar spectral features to the ones in the hydrated state, with slightly shifted band positions. The FTIR spectra showed amide A bands associated with N-H stretching at 3284 cm^{-1}, with shoulders at 3069 cm^{-1} corresponding to sp^2 C-H stretching of aromatic residues. The amide B double bands were observed at 2938 cm^{-1} and 2870 cm^{-1} corresponding to the two stretching modes of CH$_2$. Stretching of C=O bonds of the polypeptide backbone was indicated by the presence of the amide I band at 1628cm^{-1}. Amide II and amide III bands at 1539 cm^{-1} and 1234cm^{-1} respectively were indicative of N-H in plane bending vibrations coupled with C-N and C-H stretching. The remaining signals were assigned as follows: 1447 cm^{-1} O-H bending coupled with C-H scissoring, 1395 cm^{-1} carboxyl O-H bending, broad 1078 cm^{-1}–1030 cm^{-1} double-band C-O stretching.

Contact angle analysis was carried out to evaluate the wettability of the hydrogel surface (Figure 3G). Water placed on control hydrogels showed significantly greater contact angle (mean, 29.03 ± 1.72) than water placed on treated hydrogels. Only the contact angle on non-treated PGTA 3 hydrogel was comparable to 3-SM hydrogel. The lowest contact angle was found on 3-SB hydrogels (mean, 7.76 ± 1.06), and was significantly different from the control hydrogel ($p < 0.0001$).

3.3. In Vitro Biocompatibility

The three major corneal cell types, HCEC, HCF, and CEC, were used to evaluate the biocompatibility of the hydrogels. Post-chemical treated 3 hydrogels were used for this experiment and unmodified hydrogels and TCP were used as controls. AlamarBlue assay was performed to evaluate cell metabolic activity (Figure 4A) and a live-dead assay (Figure 4B) was done to evaluate cytotoxicity related to hydrogel treatments. AlamarBlue assay showed that non-chemical treated 3 hydrogels were not biocompatible for any of the 3 corneal cells types, and this was confirmed by cytotoxicity testing. Sodium metabisulfite and sodium borohydride both prominently improved biocompatibility of the PFGT 3 hydrogel and facilitated the growth of corneal cells. Cell growth was better on the control non-treated hydrogels and on TCP than on to PFGT 3 hydrogels.

The HCEC metabolic activity was superior on control hydrogels and the lowest cell growth was observed on PFGT 3 hydrogels at days 1 to 4. However, the metabolic activity of HCEC on all hydrogels became similar at day 7, showing non-significant differences ($p = 0.1855$). Live-dead staining data were similar. In the Rose Bengal assay, all the hydrogels showed a normal pattern of corneal epithelial cell stratification, with multiple non-stained areas where differentiated surface epithelial cells excluded the dye (Figure 4C).

HCF metabolic activity differences were prominent from day 4 of the cell culture. 3-SB hydrogels facilitated the growth of HCF and there was no significant difference in metabolic activity at day 7 between control hydrogels and 3-SB hydrogels ($p = 0.4273$). HCF metabolic activity was significantly lower at day 7 on 3-SM hydrogels compared to control hydrogels ($p = 0.0090$). Live-dead staining revealed that HCF became confluent at day 7 on 3-SB hydrogels, similar to control hydrogels and TCP.

CEC grew on hydrogels treated with both chemicals, whereas non-chemical treated hydrogels were not CEC compatible. There was no significant difference of cell growth between 3-SB and 3-SM hydrogels at day 7 ($p = 0.1175$). However, the cell number was higher on 3-SM hydrogels, and similar to control hydrogels and TCP ($p = 0.2682$ and 0.0646, respectively). Live-dead staining showed confluence of CEC by day 7 on all hydrogels and on TCP, except for non-chemical treated PGTA 3 hydrogels.

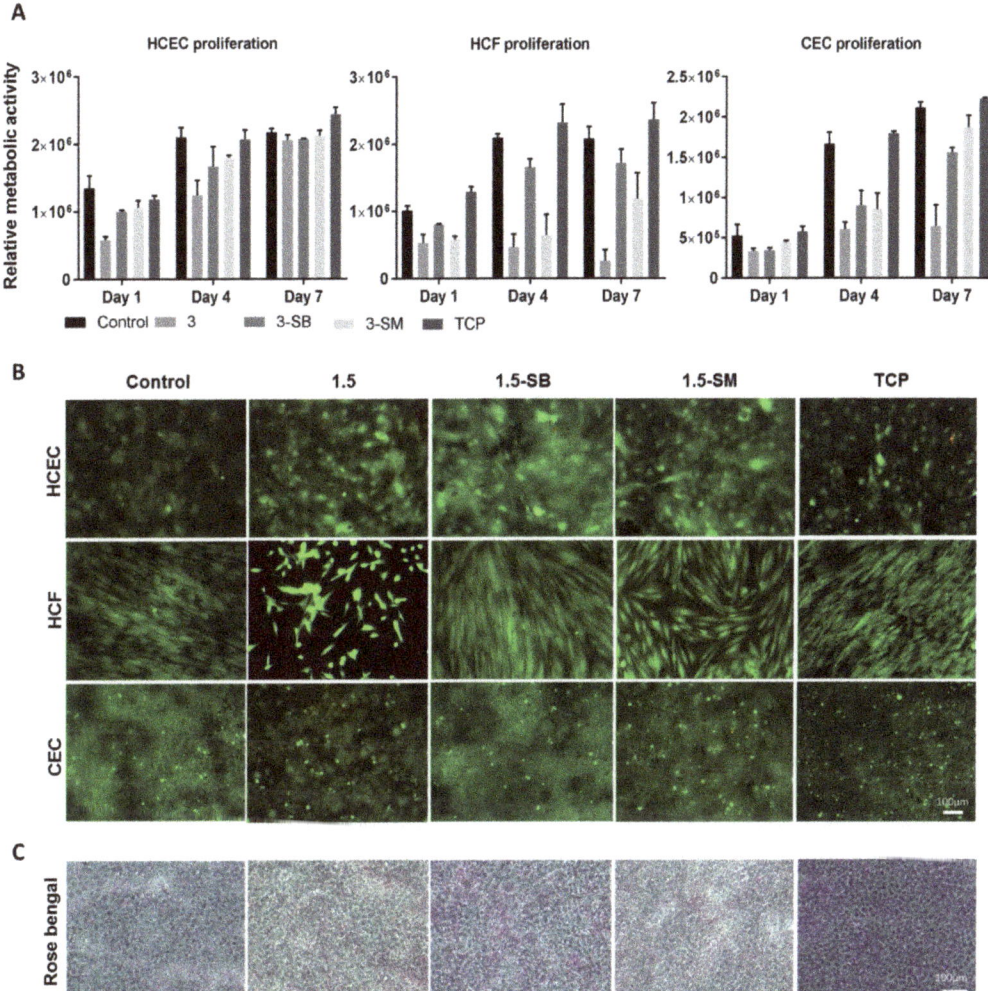

Figure 4. Biocompatibility studies of hydrogels 3 with three corneal cell types. (**A**) Metabolic activity study with individual cells at different time points, compared between hydrogels, with tissue culture plate (TCP) as a positive control. Quantitative results were reported as the mean ± S.D. (arbitrary unit) from three independent samples at each time points. (**B**) Live/dead staining of human corneal epithelial cells (HCEC), human corneal fibroblasts (HCF) and human corneal endothelial cells (CEC) on PFGT 3 hydrogels before and after post-crosslinked chemical treatment, compared with control hydrogel. All the images were taken at 7 days of cell culture. (**C**) Rose Bengal assay showed a normal pattern of stratification of the corneal epithelial cells, exhibiting multiple non-stained areas where the stratified epithelial barrier function excludes the dye. Scale bars are 100 μm.

3.4. In Vitro Evaluation of Human Adaptive Immunity in Presence of the Hydrogels

We wanted to determine whether the monocytic cell line (THP-1) when cultured for 5 days on different PFGT 3 hydrogels would differentiate towards a pro-inflammatory M1 (CD86) macrophage phenotype. When LPS was not added in the media, no morphological changes were visible; however, when LPS was used in the media, the change in cell size and morphology were observed on TCP, which proved the differentiation potential of the THP-1 cells (Figure 5A). Expression of CD86 was evaluated after 6 days of culture on different hydrogels and TCP with or without LPS. Significant overexpression of CD86 (polarization toward M1 inflammatory macrophage) was noticed only on non-PFGT 3 hydrogels compare to the control ($p = 0.0109$). CD86 expression did not differ significantly between 3-SB and 3-SM hydrogels and the control (Figure 5B).

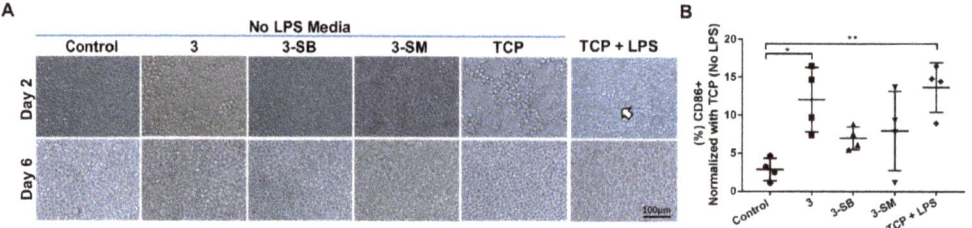

Figure 5. Human monocytic THP-1 cell polarization to M1 macrophage phenotypes in presence or absence of hydrogels and LPS. (**A**) THP-1 cells were cultured on different hydrogels and on TCP for 6 days. Morphological changes of cultured cells in presence of LPS are marked with arrow. (**B**) At day 6, the expression of CD86 (pro-inflammatory M1 marker) was evaluated and compared between the hydrogel groups, and percentage expression data was normalized to TCP (No LPS). Quantitative results were reported as the mean ± S.D. from four independent samples. * and ** represent $p < 0.05$, and $p < 0.01$, respectively.

4. Discussion

The present study compared the effects of crosslinking collagen with two robust crosslinking agents, EDC and GTA. The results support a novel strategy to reduce the cytotoxic effect of the crosslinkers while strengthening the mechanical properties of the biomaterial, all without compromising the optical properties and enzymatic stability of the implant. Although EDC crosslinking did not show direct cytotoxic effects, GTA crosslinking of EDC crosslinked hydrogels induced cytotoxic effects. To address this concern, we restored cell biocompatibility by treating the double EDC/GTA crosslinked hydrogel with different chemicals (SB or SM).

There is a shortage of donor corneas to treat visual impairment due to corneal diseases, resulting in 10 million untreated patients with 1.5 million additional patients needing a transplant every year [25,26]. Only 1 donor cornea is available for 70 needed [27]. Hence, developing alternatives to human corneal donation is an urgent need. Crosslinked artificial corneas have been considered as a potential alternative to human donor corneas for transplantation, and have been shown in clinical trials to restore vision [3,28]. For the most part, collagen in these artificial corneas has been crosslinked with EDC and NHS. The EDC/NHS crosslinked hydrogel is mechanically weak and susceptible to enzymatic degradation. Therefore, there is an unmet need to generate stable collagen-based biomaterials. We have previously shown that double-crosslinking of collagen can be achieved by using EDC together with a bi-functional epoxy-based cross-linker, 1,4-butanediol diglycidyl ether [18]. We also demonstrated that this improves the elasticity and tensile strength of the collagen implants. In the current report, we have used two crosslinkers, EDC and GTA, to take advantage of the beneficial effects of each but at minimal concentrations. We show that this strategy reduces toxicity, and at the same time increases the mechanical and enzymatic stability of the hydrogels. The base hydrogel was made with collagen crosslinked with EDC/NHS, where the molar ratio EDC:Collagen-NH$_2$ (mol:mol) = 0.7:1. EDC:Collagen-NH$_2$ = 0.5–0.7 : 1 have been studied extensively as artificial corneas, and some formulations that have been transplanted into human patients [28,29]. Variation in the molar ratio of EDC:Collagen-NH$_2$ was based on the type of collagen, its source, and the purpose of the study. Increased ratio of EDC can be used but will produce nonhomogenous hydrogels as the EDC becomes gelatinous very quickly and will not allow formation of particular organ structures such as the cornea. In our work, the hydrogels were treated with different concentrations of GTA for 4 h. In vitro biocompatibility studies of biomaterials with only GTA have shown that crosslinking with GTA for 24 h is not well-tolerated by human corneal epithelial cells [30]. In our study, we only used one time point, and we are aware that incubation for different time points could have produced different outcomes; it was shown that longer reaction times or higher GTA concentrations results in a decrease in free amine groups in the reaction [31].

We also found that the lowest concentration (PFGT 1 hydrogels) of GTA significantly increased the mechanical properties and enzymatic stability of the hydrogel. This is predictable as GTA crosslinking of collagen takes place through a reaction of the aldehyde groups of GTA with the amine groups of lysine or hydroxylysine residues [31]. While calculating the EDC concentration to make the hydrogel, we left unreacted lysine residues to react with GTA for secondary crosslinking. These conditions were gradually increased with increased concentrations of GTA, but at some point, increasing the GTA concentration (PFGT 5 hydrogels) did not alter the properties of the hydrogels, possibly due to saturation of the lysine group on the hydrogel. Cheung et al. proposed another explanation. They showed that lower concentrations of GTA were more effective in tissue crosslinking compared to higher concentrations, as high concentrations of GTA promote rapid surface crosslinking of the tissue, generating a barrier that prevents the diffusion of GTA into the tissue [32]. It was also shown that with high concentrations of GTA, the arrangement of collagen fibrils became very compact. Therefore, although the GTA dosage was increased, there was only a relatively small improvement in thermal stability and resistance to collagenase [13]. This was confirmed by our collagenase study in which PFGT 3 hydrogels exhibited maximum stability against collagenase, and that addition of more GTA (PFGT 5 hydrogels) did not render the hydrogel more stable. Our results parallel the previously published report that GTA-treated amniotic membrane is resistant to enzymatic digestion. Results from this latter study showed that the crosslinked membrane was preserved for up to 90 days without any signs of dissolution and maintained good transparency [33]. In our study, collagen gels crosslinked with GTA showed a yellowish color, which might be attributed to the self-polymerization of GTA molecules [13,34].

The challenging part of this project was to make the hydrogel biocompatible. For better GTA crosslinking, the reactions were carried out at neutral pH which induced the formation of reactive polymers. It has been suggested that the cytotoxicity and calcification arise from the propensity of GTA to form reactive polymers [35]. When human endothelial cells were seeded on untreated GTA-fixed aortic wall pieces, only limited adhesion (24%) was seen and no viable cells were found after 1 week [36]. On GTA-fixed heart valves, cell attachment was poor and no viable cells were observed [37]. Moreover, exposure time is also important. In vitro biocompatibility studies showed that the amniotic membranes (AM) crosslinked with GTA for 24 h do not support human corneal epithelial cell cultures, while AM treated with GTA for 6 h facilitated the expansion and transplantation of limbal epithelial progenitor cells [30]. Other research groups have showed that aldehyde groups introduced in the crosslinked biopolymers treated with GTA can be quenched with citric acid [36,37] and glycine [30,38] to reduce cytotoxicity. However, in our work we treated PFGT 3 hydrogels with citric acid, glycine, or lysine with no success as the toxicity of the hydrogels was not eliminated (data not shown). In contrast, the toxicity of GTA was reduced by reaction with sodium bisulfite via formation of a proposed GTA-bisulfite complex [39]. To our knowledge, neither SB nor SM has been used previously on GTA crosslinked biomaterials to improve biocompatibility. Another quenching agent we used was sodium borohydride. SB has been used as an aldehyde blocking reagent for electron microscope histochemistry [40] and for quenching of GTA-induced fluorescence in immunofluorescence on tissue sections [41].

Treatment with SB and SM had no adverse effect on the mechanical properties of double-crosslinked hydrogels. Enzymatic stability was similar before and after SB or SM treatment. Moreover, our studies confirmed that post-chemical treatment with SB or SM on double-crosslinked hydrogels rendered them optically clear and biocompatible. SB treated-hydrogels were similar to the control hydrogel in regard to transparency. The treatment with SB and SM will reduce aldehyde group and introduce the more hydrophilic hydroxyl or sulphate group and hence the product becomes more transparent. As the cornea is the main refractive element of the eye and serves as the main ocular diopter to transmit light for vision, high optical clarity is a key property that needs to be replicated in any artificial replacement [42]. The water content of human cornea is 80% and that of the collagen hydrogels was around 90% [18]. By FTIR spectra analysis of hydrated samples, we observed the typical collagen bands such as amide A at ~3310 cm^{-1}, amide I at 1600–1700 cm^{-1}, amide II at 1500–1550 cm^{-1}, and amide III at 1200–1300 cm^{-1} [43]; however, amide B at ~3063 cm^{-1} corresponding to the collagen was missing. When dried sample was analyzed, amide B was observed and all bands shifted to the same degree across all the hydrogels. Shifting of bands is correlated with the degree of crosslinking [43] and in our case the modification of functional groups was similar for control and PFGT hydrogels. When GTA reacts with the lysine residues of proteins, the aldimine linkage (CH=N) forms, which has the characteristic absorption at 1450 cm^{-1} [44]. This band was missing even for non-PFGT hydrogels, which may be because of the minute modification of the lysine groups after double-crosslinking, although this slight modification contributed significantly to change the properties of the hydrogels. The contact angle significantly decreased after GTA crosslinking, resulting in more hydrophilic surfaces. This type of surface facilitates cell adherence and migration, which could lead to a rapid cellularization of the scaffold.

Immune cells, particularly monocytes and macrophages, play a critical role in determining success or failure of implant acceptance by the recipient [45]. Therefore, controlling macrophage polarity is one approach to control inflammation and prevent failure of implanted biomaterials [46]. Human monocytic THP-1 cells have been previously used to evaluate M1 macrophage differentiation in response to biomaterials [46,47]. We used THP-1 cells and monitored the expression of CD86 to determine the response to differently treated hydrogels. As macrophages are classically activated in vitro by bacterial cell wall components [48], we also used LPS as control for the differentiation of these cells on TCP. In general, reduced biocompatibility is associated with increased CD86 (M1 macrophage marker) expression [47]. We found that CD86 expression increased after GTA crosslinking in PFGT 3 hydrogels. However, treatment of hydrogels with SB or SM mitigated the overexpression of CD86.

5. Conclusions

Our results demonstrate that double-crosslinking improves the mechanical properties of the scaffolds, and the treatment with SB or SM improves biocompatibility. This unique developmental approach should facilitate the use of collagen-based implants in regenerative medicine.

Author Contributions: Conceptualization, M.M.I. and M.G.-A.; methodology, M.M.I., D.B.A., and A.C.; formal analysis, M.M.I., D.B.A., P.A., H.K.P., and M.G.-A.; investigation, M.M.I. and M.G.-A.; writing—original draft preparation, M.M.I.; writing—review and editing, P.A., C.H.D., H.K.P., J.C. and M.G.-A.; supervision, M.G.-A. All authors have read and agreed to the published version of the manuscript.

Funding: This research was funded by Boston Keratoprosthesis fund (Boston, MA, USA).

Institutional Review Board Statement: Not applicable.

Informed Consent Statement: Not applicable.

Data Availability Statement: The datasets generated during and/or analysed during the current study are available from the corresponding author on reasonable request.

Conflicts of Interest: The authors do not have any conflict of interest to declare.

References

1. World Health Organization (WHO). Transplantation. Available online: www.who.int/transplantation/gkt/statistics/en/ (accessed on 10 May 2021).
2. Edin, E.; Simpson, F.; Griffith, M. Synthesis and Application of Collagens for Assembling a Corneal Implant. *Methods Mol. Biol.* **2020**, *2145*, 169–183.
3. Islam, M.M.; Buznyk, O.; Reddy, J.C.; Pasyechnikova, N.; Alarcon, E.I.; Hayes, S.; Lewis, P.; Fagerholm, P.; He, C.; Iakymenko, S.; et al. Biomaterials-enabled cornea regeneration in patients at high risk for rejection of donor tissue transplantation. *NPJ Regen. Med.* **2018**, *3*, 2. [CrossRef]
4. Buznyk, O.; Pasyechnikova, N.; Islam, M.M.; Iakymenko, S.; Fagerholm, P.; Griffith, M. Bioengineered Corneas Grafted as Alternatives to Human Donor Corneas in Three High-Risk Patients. *Clin. Transl. Sci.* **2015**, *8*, 558–562. [CrossRef] [PubMed]
5. Ahn, J.-I.; Kuffova, L.; Merrett, K.; Mitra, D.; Forrester, J.V.; Li, F.; Griffith, M. Crosslinked collagen hydrogels as corneal implants: Effects of sterically bulky vs. non-bulky carbodiimides as crosslinkers. *Acta Biomater.* **2013**, *9*, 7796–7805. [CrossRef]
6. Zeugolis, D.I.; Paul, R.G.; Attenburrow, G. Post-self-assembly experimentation on extruded collagen fibres for tissue engineering applications. *Acta Biomater.* **2008**, *4*, 1646–1656. [CrossRef]
7. Haugh, M.G.; Jaasma, M.J.; O'Brien, F.J. The effect of dehydrothermal treatment on the mechanical and structural properties of collagen-GAG scaffolds. *J. Biomed. Mater. Res. A* **2009**, *89*, 363–369. [CrossRef]
8. Chau, D.Y.; Collighan, R.J.; Verderio, E.A.; Addy, V.L.; Griffin, M. The cellular response to transglutaminase-cross-linked collagen. *Biomaterials* **2005**, *26*, 6518–6529. [CrossRef]
9. Islam, M.M.; Griffith, M.; Merrett, K. Fabrication of a human recombinant collagen-based corneal substitute using carbodiimide chemistry. *Methods Mol. Biol.* **2013**, *1014*, 157–164. [PubMed]
10. Chvapil, M.; Speer, D.; Mora, W.; Eskelson, C. Effect of tanning agent on tissue reaction to tissue implanted collagen sponge. *J. Surg. Res.* **1983**, *35*, 402–409. [CrossRef]
11. Damink, L.H.O.; Dijkstra, P.J.; van Luyn, M.J.; van Wachem, P.B.; Nieuwenhuis, P.; Feijen, J. Cross-linking of dermal sheep collagen using a water-soluble carbodiimide. *Biomaterials* **1996**, *17*, 765–773. [CrossRef]
12. Hwang, Y.J.; Granelli, J.; Lyubovitsky, J. Effects of zero-length and non-zero-length cross-linking reagents on the optical spectral properties and structures of collagen hydrogels. *ACS Appl. Mater. Interfaces* **2012**, *4*, 261–267. [CrossRef]
13. Tian, Z.; Liu, W.; Li, G. The microstructure and stability of collagen hydrogel cross-linked by glutaraldehyde. *Polym. Degrad. Stab.* **2016**, *130*, 264–270. [CrossRef]
14. Jayakrishnan, A.; Jameela, S.R. Glutaraldehyde as a fixative in bioprostheses and drug delivery matrices. *Biomaterials* **1996**, *17*, 471–484. [CrossRef]
15. Bigi, A.; Cojazzi, G.; Panzavolta, S.; Rubini, K.; Roveri, N. Mechanical and thermal properties of gelatin films at different degrees of glutaraldehyde crosslinking. *Biomaterials* **2001**, *22*, 763–768. [CrossRef]
16. Lai, J.Y.; Ma, D.H.; Cheng, H.Y.; Sun, C.C.; Huang, S.J.; Li, Y.T.; Hsiue, G.H. Ocular biocompatibility of carbodiimide cross-linked hyaluronic acid hydrogels for cell sheet delivery carriers. *J. Biomater. Sci. Polym. Ed.* **2010**, *21*, 359–376. [CrossRef]
17. Lai, J.Y. Biocompatibility of chemically cross-linked gelatin hydrogels for ophthalmic use. *J. Mater. Sci. Mater. Med.* **2010**, *21*, 1899–1911. [CrossRef]
18. Koh, L.B.; Islam, M.M.; Mitra, D.; Noel, C.W.; Merrett, K.; Odorcic, S.; Fagerholm, P.; Jackson, W.B.; Liedberg, B.; Phopase, J.; et al. Epoxy cross-linked collagen and collagen-laminin Peptide hydrogels as corneal substitutes. *J. Funct. Biomater.* **2013**, *4*, 162–177. [CrossRef]
19. Charulatha, V.; Rajaram, A. Influence of different crosslinking treatments on the physical properties of collagen membranes. *Biomaterials* **2003**, *24*, 759–767. [CrossRef]
20. Matsuda, S.; Iwata, H.; Se, N.; Ikada, Y. Bioadhesion of gelatin films crosslinked with glutaraldehyde. *J. Biomed. Mater. Res.* **1999**, *45*, 20–27. [CrossRef]
21. Peng, Y.Y.; Glattauer, V.; Ramshaw, J.A.M. Stabilisation of Collagen Sponges by Glutaraldehyde Vapour Crosslinking. *Int. J. Biomater.* **2017**, *2017*, 8947823. [CrossRef] [PubMed]
22. Islam, M.M.; Ravichandran, R.; Olsen, D.; Ljunggren, M.K.; Fagerholm, P.; Lee, C.J.; Griffith, M.; Phopase, J. Self-assembled collagen-like-peptide implants as alternatives to human donor corneal transplantation. *RSC Adv.* **2016**, *6*, 55745–55749. [CrossRef]
23. Islam, M.M.; Sharifi, R.; Mamodaly, S.; Islam, R.; Nahra, D.; Abusamra, D.B.; Hui, P.C.; Adibnia, Y.; Goulamaly, M.; Paschalis, E.I.; et al. Effects of gamma radiation sterilization on the structural and biological properties of decellularized corneal xenografts. *Acta Biomater.* **2019**, *96*, 330–344. [CrossRef]
24. Gonzalez-Andrades, M.; Sharifi, R.; Islam, M.M.; Divoux, T.; Haist, M.; Paschalis, E.I.; Gelfand, L.; Mamodaly, S.; di Cecilia, L.; Cruzat, A.; et al. Improving the practicality and safety of artificial corneas: Pre-assembly and gamma-rays sterilization of the Boston Keratoprosthesis. *Ocul. Surf.* **2018**, *16*, 322–330. [CrossRef]
25. Whitcher, J.P.; Srinivasan, M.; Upadhyay, M.P. Corneal blindness: A global perspective. *Bull. World Health Organ.* **2001**, *79*, 214–221. [PubMed]
26. World Health Organization (WHO). Prevention of Blindness and Visual Impairment. Available online: www.who.int/blindness/publications/globaldata/en/#:~{}:text=Globally%20the%20number%20of%20people,blindness%20is%20cataract%20(51%25) (accessed on 10 May 2021).
27. Gain, P.; Jullienne, R.; He, Z.; Aldossary, M.; Acquart, S.; Cognasse, F.; Thuret, G. Global survey of corneal transplantation and eye banking. *JAMA Ophthalmol.* **2016**, *134*, 167–173. [CrossRef] [PubMed]

28. Fagerholm, P.; Lagali, N.S.; Merrett, K.; Jackson, W.B.; Munger, R.; Liu, Y.; Polarek, J.W.; Soderqvist, M.; Griffith, M. A biosynthetic alternative to human donor tissue for inducing corneal regeneration: 24-month follow-up of a phase 1 clinical study. *Sci. Transl. Med.* **2010**, *2*, 46–61. [CrossRef] [PubMed]
29. Islam, M.M.; Cėpla, V.; He, C.; Edin, J.; Rakickas, T.; Kobuch, K.; Ruželė, Ž.; Jackson, W.B.; Rafat, M.; Lohmann, C.P.; et al. Functional fabrication of recombinant human collagen–phosphorylcholine hydrogels for regenerative medicine applications. *Acta Biomater.* **2015**, *12*, 70–80. [CrossRef]
30. Lai, J.Y.; Ma, D.H. Glutaraldehyde cross-linking of amniotic membranes affects their nanofibrous structures and limbal epithelial cell culture characteristics. *Int. J. Nanomed.* **2013**, *8*, 4157–4168. [CrossRef]
31. Damink, L.H.H.O.; Dijkstra, P.J.; van Luyn, M.J.A.; van Wachem, P.B.; Nieuwenhuis, P.; Feijen, J. Glutaraldehyde as a crosslinking agent for collagen-based biomaterials. *J. Mater. Sci. Mater. Med.* **1995**, *6*, 460–472. [CrossRef]
32. Cheung, D.T.; Perelman, N.; Ko, E.C.; Nimni, M.E. Mechanism of crosslinking of proteins by glutaraldehyde III. Reaction with collagen in tissues. *Connect. Tissue Res.* **1985**, *13*, 109–115. [CrossRef]
33. Spoerl, E.; Wollensak, G.; Reber, F.; Pillunat, L. Cross-linking of human amniotic membrane by glutaraldehyde. *Ophthalmic Res.* **2004**, *36*, 71–77. [CrossRef]
34. Chandran, P.L.; Paik, D.C.; Holmes, J.W. Structural mechanism for alteration of collagen gel mechanics by glutaraldehyde crosslinking. *Connect. Tissue Res.* **2012**, *53*, 285–297. [CrossRef]
35. Rasmussen, K.E.; Albrechtsen, J. Glutaraldehyd. The influence of pH, temperature, and buffering on the polymerization rate. *Histochemistry* **1974**, *38*, 19–26. [CrossRef]
36. Gulbins, H.; Goldemund, A.; Anderson, I.; Haas, U.; Uhlig, A.; Meiser, B.; Reichart, B. Preseeding with autologous fibroblasts improves endothelialization of glutaraldehyde-fixed porcine aortic valves. *J. Thorac. Cardiovasc. Surg.* **2003**, *125*, 592–601. [CrossRef]
37. Kim, S.S.; Lim, S.H.; Cho, S.W.; Gwak, S.J.; Hong, Y.S.; Chang, B.C.; Park, M.H.; Song, K.W.; Choi, C.Y.; Kim, B.S. Tissue engineering of heart valves by recellularization of glutaraldehyde-fixed porcine valves using bone marrow-derived cells. *Exp. Mol. Med.* **2006**, *38*, 273–283. [CrossRef]
38. Lai, J.-Y.; Li, Y.-T. Evaluation of cross-linked gelatin membranes as delivery carriers for retinal sheets. *Mater. Sci. Eng. C* **2010**, *30*, 677–685. [CrossRef]
39. Jordan, S.L.; Russo, M.R.; Blessing, R.L.; Theis, A.B. Inactivation of glutaraldehyde by reaction with sodium bisulfite. *J. Toxicol. Environ. Health* **1996**, *47*, 299–309. [CrossRef]
40. Craig, A.S. Sodium borohydride as an aldehyde blocking reagent for electron microscope histochemistry. *Histochemistry* **1974**, *42*, 141–144. [CrossRef] [PubMed]
41. Tagliaferro, P.; Tandler, C.J.; Ramos, A.J.; Saavedra, J.P.; Brusco, A. Immunofluorescence and glutaraldehyde fixation. A new procedure based on the Schiff-quenching method. *J. Neurosci. Methods* **1997**, *77*, 191–197. [CrossRef]
42. Merrett, K.; Fagerholm, P.; McLaughlin, C.R.; Dravida, S.; Lagali, N.; Shinozaki, N.; Watsky, M.A.; Munger, R.; Kato, Y.; Li, F.; et al. Tissue-Engineered Recombinant Human Collagen-Based Corneal Substitutes for Implantation: Performance of Type I versus Type III Collagen. *Investig. Ophthalmol. Vis. Sci.* **2008**, *49*, 3887–3894. [CrossRef] [PubMed]
43. Chang, M.C.; Tanaka, J. FT-IR study for hydroxyapatite/collagen nanocomposite cross-linked by glutaraldehyde. *Biomaterials* **2002**, *23*, 4811–4818. [CrossRef]
44. Nguyen, T.; Lee, B. Fabrication and characterization of cross-linked gelatin electro-spun nano-fibers. *J. Biomed. Sci. Eng.* **2010**, *3*, 1117–1124. [CrossRef]
45. Anderson, J.M.; Rodriguez, A.; Chang, D.T. Foreign body reaction to biomaterials. *Semin. Immunol.* **2008**, *20*, 86–100. [CrossRef] [PubMed]
46. Cha, B.H.; Shin, S.R.; Leijten, J.; Li, Y.C.; Singh, S.; Liu, J.C.; Annabi, N.; Abdi, R.; Dokmeci, M.R.; Vrana, N.E.; et al. Integrin-Mediated Interactions Control Macrophage Polarization in 3D Hydrogels. *Adv. Healthc. Mater.* **2017**, *6*, 1700289. [CrossRef]
47. McTiernan, C.D.; Simpson, F.C.; Haagdorens, M.; Samarawickrama, C.; Hunter, D.; Buznyk, O.; Fagerholm, P.; Ljunggren, M.K.; Lewis, P.; Pintelon, I.; et al. LiQD Cornea: Pro-regeneration collagen mimetics as patches and alternatives to corneal transplantation. *Sci. Adv.* **2020**, *6*, eaba2187. [CrossRef] [PubMed]
48. Genin, M.; Clement, F.; Fattaccioli, A.; Raes, M.; Michiels, C. M1 and M2 macrophages derived from THP-1 cells differentially modulate the response of cancer cells to etoposide. *BMC Cancer* **2015**, *15*, 577. [CrossRef] [PubMed]

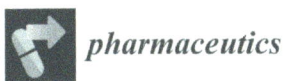

Article

Generation of a Biomimetic Substitute of the Corneal Limbus Using Decellularized Scaffolds

David Sánchez-Porras [1], Manuel Caro-Magdaleno [2], Carmen González-Gallardo [3], Óscar Darío García-García [1,4], Ingrid Garzón [1], Víctor Carriel [1], Fernando Campos [1,*] and Miguel Alaminos [1,*]

[1] Department of Histology and Tissue Engineering Group, Faculty of Medicine, Universidad de Granada and Instituto de Investigación Biosanitaria ibs.GRANADA, E18016 Granada, Spain; david.s.p.94@gmail.com (D.S.-P.); garciagarciaoscar2b@gmail.com (Ó.D.G.-G.); igarzon@ugr.es (I.G.); vcarriel@ugr.es (V.C.)

[2] Division of Ophthalmology, University Hospital Virgen Macarena, Universidad de Sevilla, E41009 Seville, Spain; drmanuelcaro@gmail.com

[3] Division of Ophthalmology, University Hospital San Cecilio, E18016 Granada, Spain; carmengonzalez23283@hotmail.com

[4] Doctoral Programme in Biomedicine, Escuela Internacional de Posgrado, Universidad de Granada, E18071 Granada, Spain

* Correspondence: fcampos@ugr.es (F.C.); malaminos@ugr.es (M.A.); Tel.: +34-958-243-515 (M.A.)

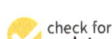

Citation: Sánchez-Porras, D.; Caro-Magdaleno, M.; González-Gallardo, C.; García-García, Ó.D.; Garzón, I.; Carriel, V.; Campos, F.; Alaminos, M. Generation of a Biomimetic Substitute of the Corneal Limbus Using Decellularized Scaffolds. *Pharmaceutics* 2021, *13*, 1718. https://doi.org/10.3390/pharmaceutics13101718

Academic Editors: Yolanda Diebold and Laura García-Posadas

Received: 24 August 2021
Accepted: 13 October 2021
Published: 17 October 2021

Publisher's Note: MDPI stays neutral with regard to jurisdictional claims in published maps and institutional affiliations.

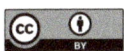

Copyright: © 2021 by the authors. Licensee MDPI, Basel, Switzerland. This article is an open access article distributed under the terms and conditions of the Creative Commons Attribution (CC BY) license (https://creativecommons.org/licenses/by/4.0/).

Abstract: Patients with severe limbal damage and limbal stem cell deficiency are a therapeutic challenge. We evaluated four decellularization protocols applied to the full-thickness and half-thickness porcine limbus, and we used two cell types to recellularize the decellularized limbi. The results demonstrated that all protocols achieved efficient decellularization. However, the method that best preserved the transparency and composition of the limbus extracellular matrix was the use of 0.1% SDS applied to the half-thickness limbus. Recellularization with the limbal epithelial cell line SIRC and human adipose-derived mesenchymal stem cells (hADSCs) was able to generate a stratified epithelium able to express the limbal markers p63, pancytokeratin, and crystallin Z from day 7 in the case of SIRC and after 14–21 days of induction when hADSCs were used. Laminin and collagen IV expression was detected at the basal lamina of both cell types at days 14 and 21 of follow-up. Compared with control native limbi, tissues recellularized with SIRC showed adequate picrosirius red and alcian blue staining intensity, whereas limbi containing hADSCs showed normal collagen staining intensity. These preliminary results suggested that the limbal substitutes generated in this work share important similarities with the native limbus and could be potentially useful in the future.

Keywords: corneal limbus; decellularized xenograft; recellularization; mesenchymal stem cells

1. Introduction

Numerous diseases, including trauma, infections, congenital malformations, degeneration, and other conditions, may affect the transparency of the human cornea and cause blindness [1]. Cornea transplantation or keratoplasty is the gold-standard treatment for severe corneal diseases. However, keratoplasty is subjected to donor shortage [2], and is contraindicated in patients with severe limbal damage and limbal stem cell deficiency (LSCD) [3]. Patients affected by severe LSCD typically show corneal conjunctivalization and neovascularization, and the management of this condition is challenging [4].

In cases with unilateral disease, LSCD can be treated by transplanting autologous limbal tissue from a healthy eye to a damaged eye [5]. Autologous grafts are free from the risk of immune rejection, but are not available in bilateral cases and can potentially compromise the healthy donor eye, resulting in LSCD [6]. If an autologous transplant is not available, patients can be treated with allogeneic limbal grafts obtained from cadaveric or living donors [5,6]. Allogeneic grafts are also subjected to important concerns, such as the risk of immune rejection [5] and graft survival [7]. The lack of a fully safe and efficient treatment makes necessary the search of therapeutic alternatives.

In this regard, the development of cell culture methods allowing cell isolation and expansion is a major advance in the treatment of LSCD [6]. Using small limbal tissue biopsies, current technology allows the generation of limbal stem cell populations that can be implanted in patients with LSCD [8]. Cultured limbal stem cells can be grafted as isolated cells or by using different types of carriers and biomaterials such as the human amniotic membrane, fibrin, collagen, or synthetic biopolymers [9–11]. Alternative approaches such as the use of cultured oral mucosa keratinocytes have also been proposed for LSCD treatment [12]. Although promising, the clinical usefulness of most of these treatments should still be demonstrated.

Development of novel tissue engineering technologies allowed the design and construction of human organs that could replace damaged tissues [13]. Bioartificial tissues and organs can be generated using different methods and techniques. Two of the most promising methods are organ bioprinting [14,15] and scaffolds seeded with living cells [16,17]. On the one hand, bioprinting offers the possibility of fabricating complex constructs in which cells and biomaterials can be precisely deposited in a specific 3D structure. However, the fine structure of the human cornea and corneal limbus is very complex, and alternative approaches including the development of transparent bio-inks and complex design protocols are in need to generate efficient limbal substitutes using bioprinting [14,15]. On the other hand, cell-seeded scaffolds have been extensively used in cornea tissue engineering. In general, these methods make use of different types of biomaterials that can be prepared in the laboratory and subsequently seeded with living cells to generate a tissue substitute [16,17]. In the case of the cornea, several models of bioartificial corneas have been developed [18,19], and some of these models have been clinically evaluated [20–22]. Again, these techniques need to be significantly improved to allow the efficient reproduction of the delicate histoarchitecture of these tissues.

One of the possible biofabrication alternatives used in cornea tissue engineering is xenograft decellularization. Decellularized natural tissues have the advantage of faithfully reproducing the native extracellular matrix (ECM) [23]. Although a number of works have focused on the development of decellularization protocols applied to the native cornea, a fully efficient protocol able to preserve all ECM components is in need. In general, cornea xenografts can be decellularized by using chemical, physical, and biological methods [24]. Chemical protocols typically use different types of detergents such as sodium dodecyl sulfate (SDS) and Triton X-100, although ethylenediaminetetraacetic acid (EDTA) and hypertonic salts have also been used [25,26]. Physical methods are mostly based on freeze-thawing, osmotic pressure, and lyophilization, whereas biological protocols make use of enzymes such as trypsin, DNAse, and RNAse [24,27]. Although little clinical experience is available for the use of decellularized corneal xenografts, some preliminary clinical trials have pointed out the biosafety and functionality of decellularized porcine corneas in patients subjected to lamellar keratoplasty [26–29].

Regarding the corneal limbus, very few works focused on the optimization of decellularization protocols specifically applied to this structure [30]. Allocated at the transition between the cornea and the sclera, the corneal limbus plays a key role in maintaining corneal physiology, and its integrity and function are crucial for a normal corneal homeostasis [31]. The three-dimensional structure of the limbus is very complex. The crypts of the limbus form specific pocket-like structures containing fibrovascular Vogt palisades that make up a fundamental micro-niche that houses and supports the limbal stem cells [32].

Unfortunately, the complex structure of the limbus is very difficult to reproduce in the laboratory using standard tissue engineering protocols. However, the use of decellularization methods applied to the native limbi provides the specific morphology, structure, and protein composition of the corneal limbus [30], and offers the opportunity of obtaining adequate limbal scaffolds for use in tissue engineering. In fact, some preliminary reports using SDS and NaCl decellularization protocols have described the efficient generation of limbal substitutes for use in regenerative medicine [11,28,30].

On the other hand, the search for alternative sources of extraocular cells free from the drawbacks and limitations associated with autologous limbal cells used in the treatment of LSCD is in need [33]. In this sense, a possible alternative is the use of human adipose-derived mesenchymal stem cells (hADSCs), which have previously been shown to have differentiation potential to several types of corneal cells both ex vivo and in vivo [34].

In the present preliminary work, we evaluated several decellularization methods applied to the corneal limbus, and we generated recellularized limbal xenografts for future use in patients with limbal damage using two different cell sources.

2. Materials and Methods

2.1. Obtaining Decellularized Xenografts from Native Limbi

The study protocol is schematically summarized in Figure 1.

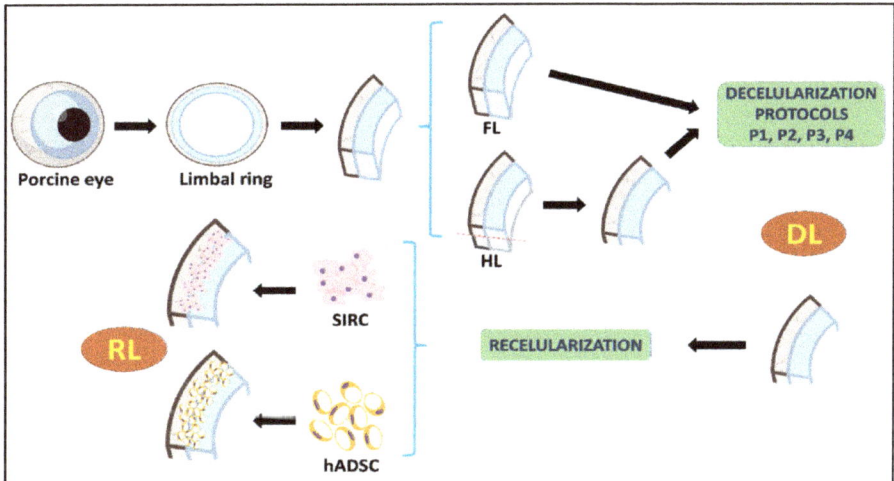

Figure 1. Schematic representation of the study protocol used in the present work. Fl: full-thickness limbus; HL: half-thickness limbus; DL: decellularized limbus; RL: recellularized limbus.

Fresh porcine eyes were obtained from a local slaughterhouse. On arrival to the laboratory, eyes were washed in PBS and the corneal limbus was carefully dissected using sterile scissors. Limbi contained 2–3 mm of sclera and 3–4 mm of cornea. Limbal rings were washed thoroughly in PBS with a mixture of antibiotics and antimycotics containing penicillin (1000 U/mL), streptomycin (1000 µg/mL), and amphotericin B (2.5 µg/mL) (Merck, Darmstadt, Germany), and the rest of the uvea, retina, iris, and ciliary body were removed with forceps. The rings were then sectioned into fragments approximately 1 cm in length consisting of the full-thickness limbus (FL). Parts of these fragments were then sectioned in two halves using a surgical blade to separate the anterior part of the limbus (the most superficial) from the posterior part (the most profound). Only the anterior half of the limbal fragments, corresponding to the half-thickness limbus (HL), was used.

Both the FL and HL were subjected to four decellularization protocols combining several types of detergents (to dissolve cell membranes), distilled water (to induce osmotic cell lysis), NaCl (to promote cell swelling), and enzymes (to remove nucleic acids) (all these components were purchased from Merck):

- Protocol P1: Double-distilled water (ddH_2O) for 24 h; 0.1% sodium dodecyl sulphate (SDS) (3 incubations of 24 h each).

- Protocol P2: ddH$_2$O for 24 h; 0.1% SDS for 24 h; wash in PBS; 1.5 M of NaCl (2 incubations of 24 h each).
- Protocol P3: ddH$_2$O for 24 h; 0.1% SDS for 24 h; wash in PBS; 1% sodium deoxycholate (SDC) for 24 h; wash in PBS; 0.6% triton X-100 for 24 h; wash in PBS; 100 mg/L of DNAse and 20 mg/L of RNAse for 45 min.
- Protocol P4: ddH$_2$O for 24 h; 0.1% SDS for 24 h; wash in PBS; 1% sodium deoxycholate (SDC) for 24 h; wash in PBS; 0.6% triton X-100 for 24 h; wash in PBS; 100 mg/L of DNAse and 20 mg/L of RNAse for 45 min; wash in PBS; 0.05% Trypsin for 1 h.

All detergents were dissolved in ddH$_2$O. DNAse, RNAse, and trypsin were used at 37 °C. All incubations were performed with agitation. After decellularization, decellularized limbi (DLs) were washed 5 times in cold PBS (15 min each time) and stored at 4 °C.

To assess transparency, DLs were placed on a black background and photographed.

2.2. Evaluation of Decellularization Efficiency in DL

To determine the efficiency of the four decellularization protocols applied to the corneal limbus, DLs were analyzed using DNA quantification and 4′,6-diamidino2-phenylindole (DAPI) staining. To quantify residual DNA in DLs, tissues were trimmed and processed using the QIAamp DNA Mini Kit (Qiagen, Hilden, Germany). Isolated DNA was dissolved in water and quantified using a NanoDrop 2000 spectrophotometer (Thermo Fisher Scientific, Waltham, MA, USA). Results were then normalized with respect to the weight of dry tissue as previously reported [35,36], and 10 measurements were made per sample. To identify the presence of nuclei or nuclei remnants in DLs, each tissue was fixed in formalin and embedded in paraffin as described below, and tissue sections were obtained using a microtome. Sections were dewaxed, rehydrated, stained with DAPI, coverslipped, and examined with a Nikon Eclipse i90 fluorescent microscope.

2.3. Generation of Recellularized Limbal Substitutes by Tissue Engineering

The DLs showing the best results were further recellularized with two types of cells: the limbal epithelial cell line SIRC (Statens Seruminstitut Rabbit Cornea) and primary cell cultures of mesenchymal stem cells (MSCs) derived from the adipose tissue (hADSCs). SIRC was purchased from ATCC (ref: CCL-60), whereas hADSCs were obtained by the enzymatic digestion of small human adipose tissue biopsies, as previously reported [37]. Both cell types were cultured in Dulbecco's modified Eagle's medium (DMEM) supplemented with 10% fetal bovine serum and 1% antibiotics/antimycotics (all from Merck) using standard cell culture conditions.

To obtain recellularized limbi (RLs), DLs were first functionalized to increase the adhesiveness of the decellularized scaffold and promote cell attachment by incubating the tissues in fetal bovine serum for 24 h with slight agitation.

After functionalization, SIRC and hADSCs were trypsinized and carefully seeded on the surface of the DL (170,000 cells per cm^2 of sample). To promote attachment, cells were resuspended in a minimal amount of medium (50 µL) and DLs were immobilized using agarose casts, as previously reported [38]. In order to induce epithelial differentiation of both cell types seeded on the RL, these tissues were cultured for 21 days in EM epithelial differentiation medium containing epithelial growth and differentiation factors, as previously described [39]. The EM medium consisted of a mixture of 150 mL of HAM-F12, 300 mL of DMEM, 50 mL of fetal bovine serum, 1% antibiotics/antimycotics, 24 µg/mL of adenine, 5 µg/mL of insulin, 1.3 ng/mL of triiodothyronine, 0.4 µg/mL of hydrocortisone, and 10 ng/mL of EGF (epidermal growth factor) (all of them, from Merck).

Preliminary transmittance analysis was carried out on RLs and controls using a SmartSpec 3000 spectrophotometer (Bio-Rad, Hercules, CA, USA). Each sample was analyzed at three wavelengths (400, 550, and 700 nm) using three replicates, and average values were obtained.

2.4. Histological Analyses of DL and RL

Control porcine and human native limbi, and DLs and RLs were fixed in 4% neutral buffered formaldehyde, dehydrated in increasing concentrations of ethanol, cleared in xylene, and embedded in paraffin following routine protocols. In addition, 5 µm sections were obtained with a microtome, mounted on glass slides, dewaxed, and rehydrated with an ethanol series.

To evaluate tissue morphology and structure, sections were stained with hematoxylin-eosin (HE) (Panreac AppliChem, Barcelona, Spain). The structure and composition of the tissue extracellular matrix (ECM) were evaluated by identifying collagen fibers and proteoglycans using picrosirius red (PSR) and alcian blue (AB) histochemistry, as previously reported [36,40] (reagents from Panreac AppliChem).

In order to identify specific components of the epithelial and basement membrane layers of RLs, controls and RLs were subjected to immunohistochemistry for p63, pancytokeratin, crystallin Z (CRY-Z), laminin, and collagen IV. In brief, tissue sections were subjected to antigen retrieval with pH 8 EDTA buffer (25 min at 95 °C) for p63, pancytokeratin, and collagen IV or with pH 6 citrate buffer (25 min at 95 °C) for CRY-Z and laminin, and endogenous peroxidase was quenched with H_2O_2. Then, samples were preincubated in a blocking solution containing horse serum and incubated with the following primary antibodies: anti-p63 (Master Diagnostica, Granada, Spain, prediluted), anti-pancytokeratin (Master Diagnostica, prediluted), anti-CRY-Z (Abcam, Cambridge, UK, dilution 1:250), anti-laminin (Abcam, dilution 1:200), and anti-collagen IV (Master Diagnostica, prediluted). After washing in PBS, tissues were incubated in secondary anti-mouse or anti-rabbit antibodies labeled with peroxidase (ImmPRESS reagent kit, Vector Laboratories; Burlingame, CA, USA, prediluted), washed in PBS, and incubated with diaminobenzidine (DAB) (Vector Laboratories). In all cases, positive and negative control tissues were used, with negative controls corresponding to tissue sections subjected to the same protocol, except that the primary antibody was replaced by PBS to show the negative staining signal. Samples were then counterstained with Harry's hematoxylin and coverslipped.

2.5. Quantitative Analysis and Statistics

Stained tissues were analyzed with an Eclipse 90i microscope (Nikon, Tokyo, Japan), and images were obtained using the same conditions (magnification, exposure time, contrast, etc.) for all samples stained with the same method to allow signal quantification. White light was used to analyze all samples, and polarized light microscopy was used to evaluate DL tissues stained with PSR.

For PSR and AB histochemistry, the staining signal intensity and area fraction were quantified using the ImageJ software (National Institutes of Health, Bethesda, MD, USA), as previously reported [41]. Briefly, each histological image was analyzed by randomly selecting 10 points (for intensity) and 10 square areas (for area fraction), and both the signal intensity and the area occupied by the positive staining signal were calculated by the program, the background signal was subtracted, and averages were obtained for each type of sample. Results obtained for each sample were statistically compared with controls using the Mann–Whitney tests with the RealStatistics software (Dr. Charles Zaiontz, Purdue University, West Lafayette, IN, USA).

For the immunohistochemical analyses, results were semiquantitatively categorized as strongly positive signal (+++), positive signal (++), slightly positive signal (+), or negative signal (−), as previously reported [39].

3. Results

3.1. Decellularization Efficiency of the Different Protocols Applied to the Porcine Limbus

Analysis of the different decellularization protocols studied in this work revealed that the four protocols were able to efficiently decellularize the porcine corneal limbus. First, the efficiency of the decellularization process was evaluated by quantification of the residual DNA present in each type of sample. Results showed very high DNA content in control limbi (1742.58 ± 62.06 ng of DNA per mg of dry weight of tissue), whereas DL tissues subjected to decellularization had very low amounts of DNA, with all protocols showing less than 50 ng of DNA per mg of dry weight of tissue for both the FL and HL, thus fulfilling the requirements for decellularized tissues [35] (Figure 2). Differences with control FL and HL were statistically significant for all groups, but comparisons among the different types of decellularized tissues showed nonsignificant differences.

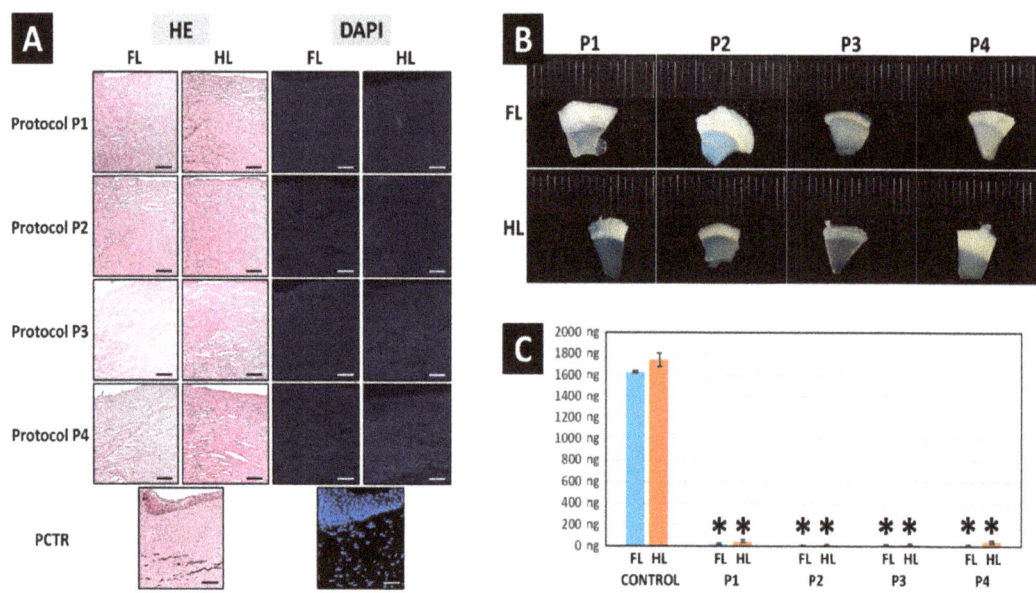

Figure 2. Analysis of native porcine limbus (PCTR) and decellularized limbi using four different decellularization methods (P1 to P4). Each decellularization protocol was applied to the full-thickness limbus (FL) and the half-thickness limbus (HL). (A) Histological analysis using hematoxylin-eosin (HE) and DAPI. (B) Macroscopical images showing transparency levels of each DL on a black scale in millimeters. (C) Quantification of residual DNA (in ng of DNA per mg of dry weight of tissue) in controls and DL. Asterisks (*) represent statistically significant differences with both the FL and the HL controls ($p < 0.05$). Nonsignificant differences were found among the different samples decellularized with P1, P2, P3, and P4. Scale bars: 50 µm.

In order to evaluate the decellularization efficiency at the histological level (Figure 2), controls and DLs decellularized with each protocol were analyzed histologically using HE staining. As shown in Figure 1, native control limbi showed abundant cells at the epithelial and stromal layers of the tissue. However, the use of the four decellularization methods evaluated here resulted in a complete absence of detectable cells or cell debris in all DLs, for both the HE and DAPI staining methods, with no differences among samples, suggesting that the four methods described here were fully efficient, although the typical pocket-like structures found in the limbal area were not detected in DLs.

Strikingly, we found that tissues decellularized with protocols P1, followed by P2, showed the most appropriate results in terms of transparency, especially when HLs were used. In contrast, P3 and P4 resulted in an important alteration of corneal transparency (Figure 2).

3.2. Histochemical Analysis of ECM Components Preservation in Decellularized Limbi

The effects of each decellularization protocol on the structure and composition of the tissue ECM were evaluated using PSR and AB (Figures 3 and 4). As expected, we first found that native control limbi showed high PSR staining intensity and area fraction, suggesting that a high number of collagen fibers were present in these tissues. Then, the analysis of DLs revealed a significant decrease in PSR intensity and area fraction in all samples ($p < 0.05$), except for HLs treated with the P1 protocol, which were comparable to controls for PSR staining intensity but were significantly lower than controls for the area fraction occupied by collagen fibers.

When polarized light was applied, we found that control corneas showed several types of properly oriented collagen fibers, with a mixture of red, orange, yellow, and green fibers. However, DLs tended to show a decrease in red and orange colors, especially in FLs and in HLs treated with protocol P3, suggesting a decrease in thick, mature fibers and an alteration of fiber alignment and orientation in these samples, as previously suggested [42].

Analysis of tissue proteoglycans using AB staining showed a significant decrease in the staining signal intensity in all samples, as compared to control native tissues ($p < 0.05$). However, when the area fraction corresponding to an AB-positive signal was analyzed, we found a significant decrease in FLs decellularized with P1 and in HLs treated with P2 and P3, with the rest of samples being comparable to controls ($p > 0.05$).

On the other hand, our preliminary analysis of the transparency of RLs showed that the average transmittance of these tissues ranged between 31.49 ± 9.14% of the transmittance of HCTR found in RLs recellularized with hADSCs at 21 days of follow-up and 102.44 ± 32.06% for limbi recellularized with SIRC at day 21 (Supplementary Table S1).

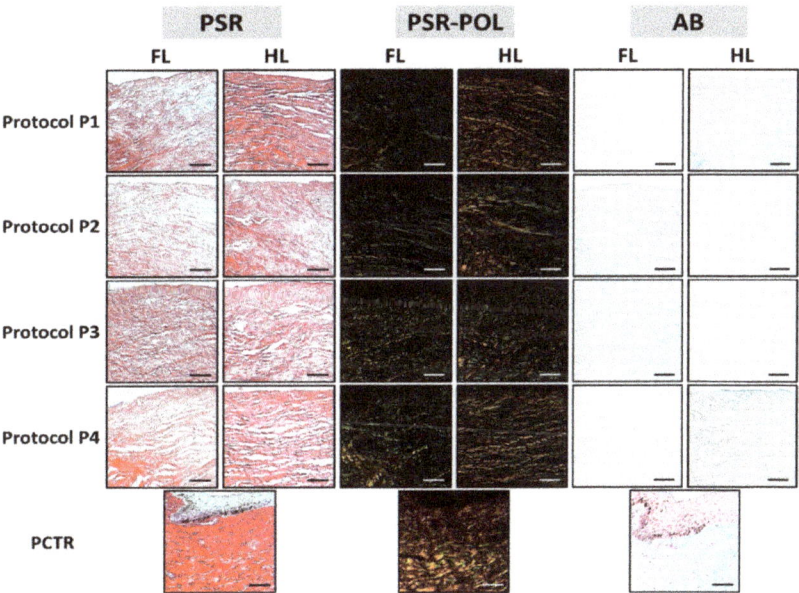

Figure 3. Histochemical analysis of native porcine limbus (PCTR) and decellularized limbi using four different decellularization methods (P1 to P4). Each decellularization protocol was applied to the full-thickness limbus (FL) and the half-thickness limbus (HL). PSR: picrosirius red, PSR-POL: polarized-light picrosirius red, AB: alcian blue. Scale bars: 50 μm.

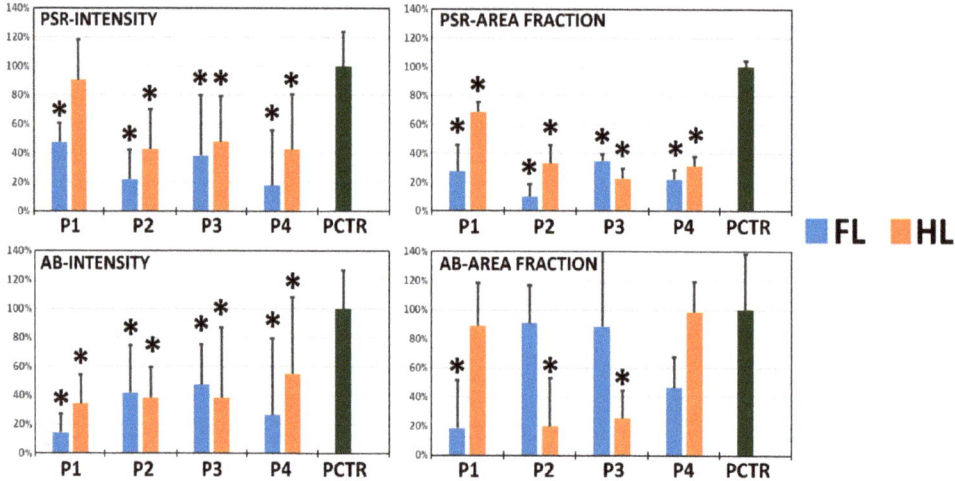

Figure 4. Quantitative analysis of the picrosirius red (PSR) and alcian blue (AB) staining intensity and area fraction of decellularized limbi (DLs). Four decellularization protocols (P1 to P4) were applied to the full-thickness limbus (FL, blue bars) and the half-thickness limbus (HL, orange bars). Results are shown as average values normalized with respect to the native porcine limbus used as control (PCTR, green bars), which is considered as 100%, with error bars corresponding to standard deviations. Asterisks (*) represent statistically significant differences with the native porcine limbus used as control ($p < 0.05$).

3.3. Histological Analysis of Recellularized Limbi

In the present work, we used DLs decellularized with protocol P1 applied to HLs, as this method allowed an efficient decellularization with the best results in terms of ECM preservation. When these tissues were recellularized with SIRC rabbit cornea epithelial cells, we found that cells tended to attach to the DL surface, forming a multilayered cell stratum, and tended to allocate in the pocket-like structures found in DLs (Figure 5). In addition, we found that the number of cells in each RL was high from the first analysis time at day 7, with very few changes at days 14 and 21. Cells showed several intercellular spaces at days 7 and 14, but not at day 21, when cells became more densely packed, although the well-organized structure of the native cornea epithelium was not reached.

Analysis of RLs containing hADSCs revealed that this type of cell was also able to attach to the tissue surface, but the number of cells was low at day 7, with few cell layers, and increased at day 14, with several cell layers. Interestingly, some of the cells became detached from the decellularized scaffold at day 21. As for the SIRC cells, abundant intercellular spaces were found among hADSCs, and differed from the fine structure of the control tissues. Interestingly, the morphology of the hADSCs grown on the surface of the RL was elongated and spindle-shaped, whereas SIRC displayed a more rounded or polygonal shape.

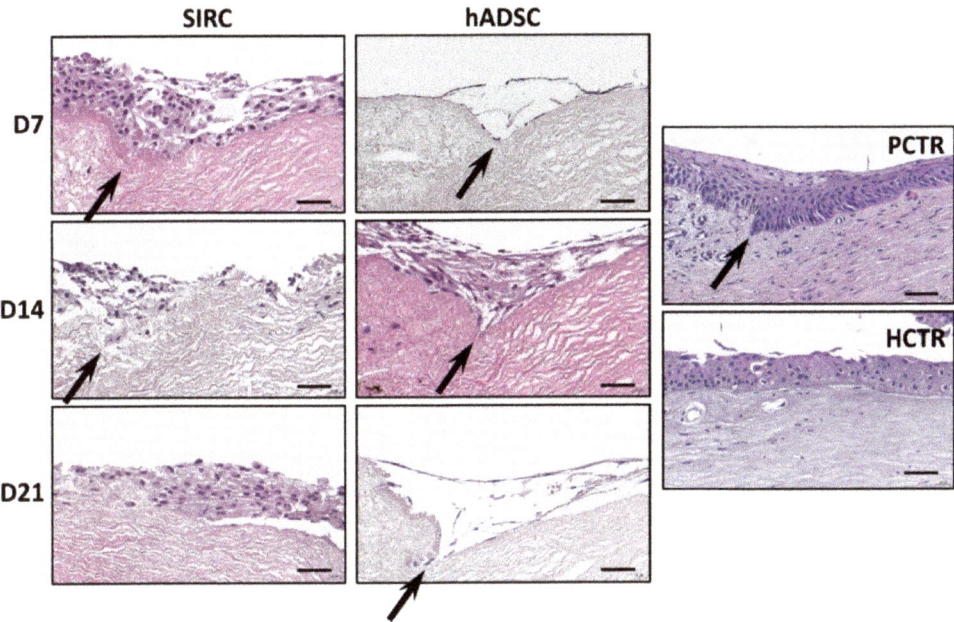

Figure 5. Histological analysis of native controls and RLs recellularized with SIRC epithelial cells and hADSCs, at days 7 (D7), 14 (D14), and 21 (D21) of follow-up using hematoxylin-eosin staining (HE). PCTR: Native porcine limbus used as control. HCTR: Native human limbus used as control. Pocket-like structures found in some of the images have been highlighted with arrows. Scale bars: 50 μm.

3.4. Evaluation of Limbal Cell Markers in Recellularized Limbi

In the first place, we analyzed the expression of the limbal stem cell marker p63 in controls and RLs (Figure 6). As expected, epithelial cells found in control limbi were strongly positive (+++), especially in the human limbus and in the basal layer of the porcine limbus. When the RLs were analyzed, we found that tissues recellularized with SIRC epithelial cells showed positive p63 expression (++) from day 7 to day 21, although at a lower level than controls. However, hADSCs showed negative p63 expression (−) at days 7 and 14, and became positive (++) at day 21. Then, we assessed the expression of pancytokeratin in each type of sample, and we found a strongly positive signal (+++) in human and porcine control limbi, and a positive expression in RLs containing SIRC cells at 7, 14, and 21 days of follow-up. In addition, the expression was negative (−) in RLs recellularized with hADSCs kept ex vivo for 7 days, slightly positive at day 14, and became positive at day 21. Finally, our analysis of CRY-Z proteins revealed that human epithelial cells were strongly positive, although porcine cornea cells were negative for this marker. RLs containing SIRC were positive at the three time periods analyzed here, whereas RLs containing hADSCs were negative at day 7, and slightly positive at days 14 and 21 of follow-up ex vivo.

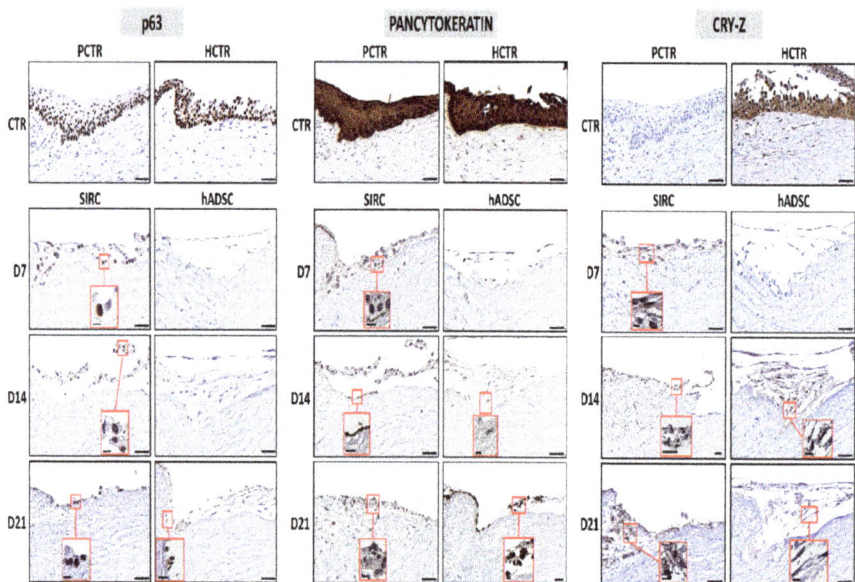

Figure 6. Immunohistochemical analysis of the corneal epithelial cell markers p63, pancytokeratin, and crystallin Z (CRY-Z) in RLs recellularized with SIRC cells and hADSCs at days 7 (D7), 14 (D14), and 21 (D21) of follow-up, porcine native limbus (PCTR), and human native limbus (HCTR). Insets correspond to higher-magnification images of cells showing the expression of each analyzed marker in the RL tissues. Scale bars: 50 μm for large images and 10 μm for the insets.

3.5. Immunohistochemical Analysis of Basement Membrane Components in Recellularized Limbi

Two of the main components of the basement membrane—laminin and collagen IV—were analyzed by immunohistochemistry (Figure 7). In this regard, our results demonstrated that the human native cornea expressed both proteins at the basement membrane of the epithelial cells, although the porcine cornea was negative for the two markers analyzed here. RLs containing SIRC cells were negative for laminin at all follow-up times, but were positive for collagen IV at days 14 and 21, being negative at day 7. However, RLs generated with hADSCs were negative for laminin and collagen IV at day 7 and became positive at days 14 and 21 for both markers. As expected, blood vessels found at the limbal tissue showed a positive staining signal for both laminin and collagen IV.

3.6. Histochemical Analysis of ECM Components in Recellularized Limbi

Once recellularized, two major ECM components were analyzed in RL samples using PSR and AB (Figures 8 and 9). When the staining intensity was analyzed in samples stained with PSR, we found that the highest intensity corresponded to the native limbus controls. However, differences between controls and all types of RLs were nonsignificant at 7, 14, and 21 days ($p > 0.05$). However, we found that all RLs had lower PSR area fractions than native controls did at the three times, with significant differences between the native limbi and all types of RLs.

Analysis of ECM proteoglycans using AB histochemistry first revealed that the lowest staining intensity corresponded to RLs containing hADSCs, with statistically significant differences with native limbi for the three time periods analyzed here. In contrast, RLs generated with SIRC showed nonsignificant differences with controls at all times. Finally, we found that the area occupied by AB-positive staining was significantly lower in all types of RLs than in native controls at all times, with very few differences among RL samples and times.

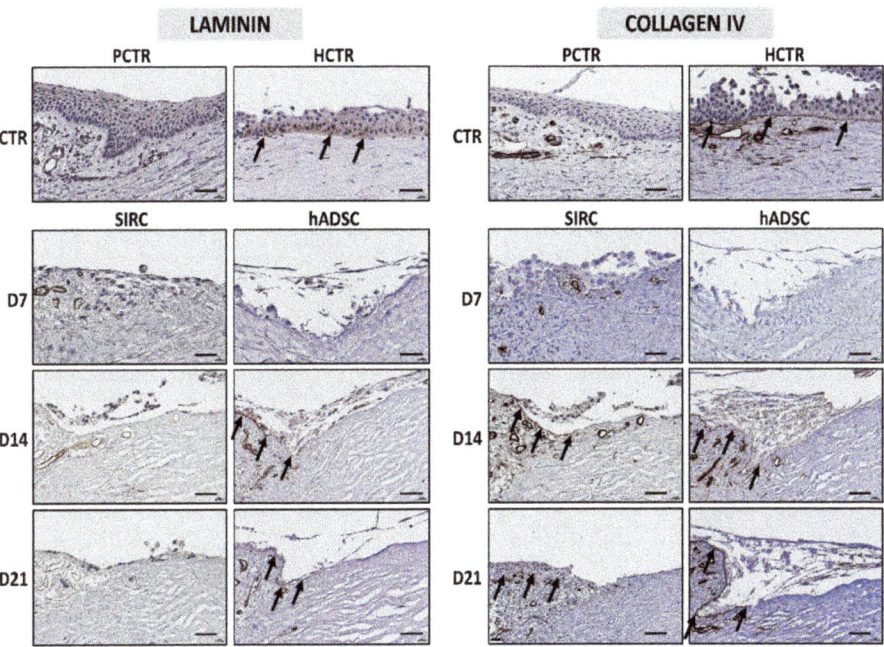

Figure 7. Immunohistochemical analysis of the basement membrane markers laminin and collagen IV in RLs recellularized with SIRC cells and hADSCs at days 7 (D7), 14 (D14), and 21 (D21) of follow-up, porcine native limbus (PCTR), and human native limbus (HCTR). Illustrative areas of the basement membrane stained by the immunohistochemical procedure are highlighted with arrows. Scale bars: 50 μm.

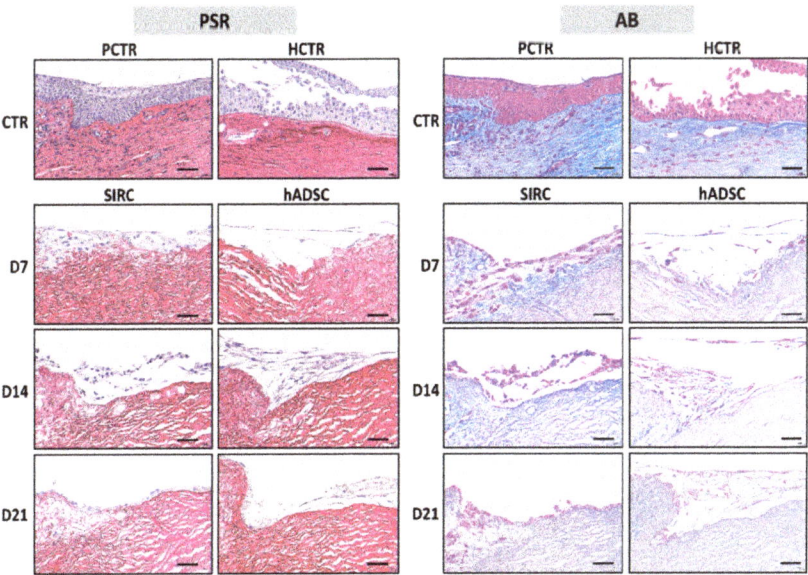

Figure 8. Histochemical analysis of native porcine limbus (PCTR), native human limbus (HCTR), and limbi recellularized with SIRC cells and hADSCs evaluated at days 7 (D7), 14 (D14), and 21 (D21) of follow-up. PSR: picrosirius red, AB: alcian blue. Scale bars: 50 μm.

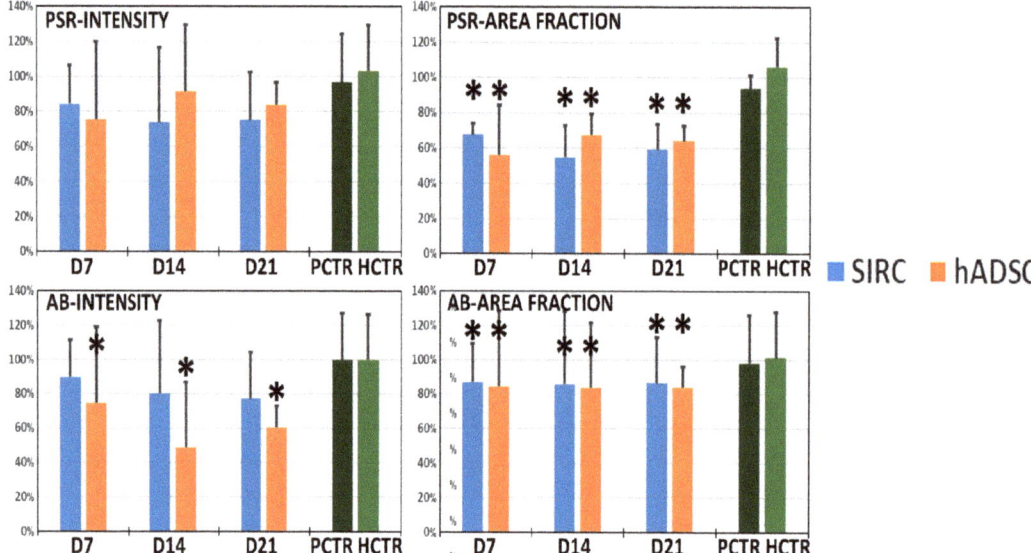

Figure 9. Quantitative analysis of the picrosirius red (PSR) and alcian blue (AB) staining intensity and area fraction of recellularized limbi (RLs). Results are shown as average values normalized with respect to the native limbi used as controls and shown in green (PCTR and HCTR), whose mean is considered as 100%, with error bars corresponding to standard deviations. Asterisks (*) represent statistically significant differences with both controls (PCTR and HCTR) ($p < 0.05$).

4. Discussion

LSCD is a severe condition causing cornea opacification, conjunctival pannus, and blindness that can be secondary to chemical or thermal injuries, autoimmune diseases such as the Stevens–Johnson syndrome, mucous membrane pemphigoid, and hereditary diseases such as aniridia [43]. Current treatments are challenging, especially in cases with structural damage of the limbal area, which is not a candidate to cell therapy. In fact, maintenance of the crypt-like structures in which limbal stem cells reside is fundamental for these cells to survive and exert their function in the limbus, and structural alterations of this niche would lead to stem cell death [6].

In the present preliminary work, we generated several types of limbal substitutes that could be used in the future to replace the damaged limbus using both a corneal and an extracorneal cell source. Although the present report is a preliminary work, our results suggest that these bioartificial limbi display several similarities with the native limbus and, thus, could be potentially useful for the treatment of LSCD.

In the first place, we evaluated several decellularization protocols applied to the native porcine limbus. Decellularization of native organs allows the obtaining of biological scaffolds composed of natural extracellular matrix (ECM) that can be used in regenerative medicine for tissue and organ replacement [35]. Compared with strategies based on scaffolds generated de novo such as fibrin, collagen, or agarose applied to cornea tissue engineering [20,44], decellularization offers the possibility of obtaining a scaffold containing the Vogt palisades and crypt-like structures that are required for a proper limbal function [30]. In addition, previous works have demonstrated that the porcine limbus is structurally similar to the human limbus [45].

Xenografts obtained by the decellularization of animal tissues can be used to reproduce human tissues and organs in the laboratory [46]. Compared with human tissues, xenografts are easily available and accessible, and can be obtained with very few ethical concerns. However, xenogeneic scaffolds may not be able to fully reproduce the structure and biochemical composition of the human tissues, and the expression of relevant antigenic components should be controlled before clinical use, as antigenicity could hinder the use of xenografts in regenerative medicine [47].

Numerous protocols have been described to date for the decellularization of different types of corneal xenografts [24]. However, very little information is available on decellularization of the corneal limbus. In a preliminary work, we demonstrated previously that the porcine cornea can be decellularized in toto, including the limbus, using SDS detergents [25]. Then, Huang et al. used a combined protocol using a mixture of salts, enzymes, and SDC and demonstrated that the porcine limbus could be decellularized and then recellularized with cultured cells [48]. Very recently, Isidan et al. compared several methods applied to the whole porcine cornea and confirmed our preliminary results suggesting that SDS is the most effective decellularization agent for the whole cornea [28]. Based on the protocols described in all these previous reports, we selected four decellularization methods that were evaluated in the present work. In general, these methods were based on the use of the anionic detergents SDS and SDC, the nonionic surfactant Triton X-100, hypertonic NaCl, and trypsin digestion.

Previous reports have suggested that decellularization of the whole cornea is challenging, and the efficiency of the decellularization protocols may be reduced when the whole tissue is subjected to decellularization [28]. For this reason, we evaluated each decellularization protocol on both the full-thickness limbus and the half-thickness limbus. Our results showed that all protocols were efficient on both the FL and the HL tissues, suggesting that the four protocols evaluated here were fully successful and are appropriate for decellularization of the porcine limbus. However, protocol P1, which is based on the use of SDS detergent, was able to preserve the limbus ECM components and transparency more efficiently than other protocols could, especially when HLs were used. Although differences were found with control native corneas, and the crypt-like structures were not detectable, probably due to tissue swelling, the collagen staining intensity and the proteoglycans area fraction were comparable with controls. For these reasons, and due to the fact that protocol P1 is one of the simplest decellularization protocols, we could recommend this protocol applied to HLs for porcine limbus decellularization. This is in agreement with previous results obtained by our group [25] and by other research groups [28]. However, additional analyses based on biochemical characterization of the decellularized limbi should be performed to confirm these findings. In addition, our analysis of transparency was very preliminary, and in-depth analyses able to quantify the transmittance of each DL with higher accuracy should be performed before and after glycerol treatment—to reduce swelling—as suggested [49].

An important issue related to decellularized tissues is biomechanical behavior. In general, it is well known that the biomechanical properties of tissues are important variables affecting tissue function and cell mechanotransduction [50]. However, the decellularization process may significantly alter the structure of the tissue ECM and, thus, the biomechanical properties of the decellularized scaffolds, which could alter the phenotype, proliferation capability, and differentiation potential of the cells cultured on this scaffold and modify cell behavior and tissue regeneration [51]. In fact, it has been demonstrated that decellularized corneal xenografts vary their biomechanical properties after decellularization [52]. Therefore, a thorough analysis of the biomechanical properties of the DL generated in the present work is in need.

Once decellularized, DLs should be repopulated with limbal stem cells for clinical use. Recellularization is also challenging, as not all cell types are able to grow and differentiate on decellularized scaffolds. In the present work, we assessed two different types of cells for limbal recellularization: corneal epithelial cells and extracorneal cells with differentiation potential (hADSCs). The use of alternative cell sources was previously suggested by several researchers, who demonstrated that hADSCs have intrinsic potential to differentiate into several cornea cell phenotypes both ex vivo and in vivo [33,34,53]. First, different types of MSCs were differentiated into stromal keratocytes using conditioning media [34], suggesting that these cells could be used to support epithelial cell growth and differentiation.

However, these cells were also demonstrated to have a differentiation potential into cornea epithelial cells [33,34,53], which supports their use as alternative cell sources in cornea and limbus recellularization. In general, our results suggest that both types of cells were able to attach to this scaffold and showed several markers of cell differentiation on the decellularized biomaterials. Interestingly, the morphology of each cell type was different, and hADSCs showed the typical structure of MSCs, and abundant intercellular spaces, at day 21. In general, these findings support the preferential use of SIRC over hADSCs, as SIRC cells are specifically committed to the limbal epithelial cell lineage, whereas hADSCs correspond to the undifferentiated phenotype that is typical of MSCs [54].

Although further research should determine the role of serum functionalization, the fact that cells were able to adhere to the decellularized scaffold could be related to the functionalization step applied to the DL. Previous reports have shown that most biomaterials lack specific signals that are necessary for cell differentiation and function, and surface functionalization with serum proteins could contribute to mimic the in vivo scenario and improve biomaterial functionality [55]. A possible concern of tissue functionalization with serum is the possibility of inducing cells to differentiate to noncorneal cell lineages, such as the vascular phenotype. Future studies should determine if functionalization is necessary and if alternative methods can be applied to DLs.

To determine the feasibility of the scaffolds generated in this work to support limbal cell differentiation, we analyzed the expression of several markers of epithelial differentiation. In general, our results obtained ex vivo suggest that none of the cell types were able to fully differentiate and mature on the scaffold, although partial signs of epithelial differentiation were found. Concretely, SIRC cells were able to express the epithelial markers p63, pancytokeratin, and CRY-Z from the beginning, with no time-dependent differences. This is in agreement with the limbal epithelial stem cell nature of these cells and their intrinsic differentiation status [56]. However, hADSCs were initially negative for these three markers, as is the case of all types of human MSCs, but became positive or slightly positive for the three epithelial markers after 21 days of ex vivo differentiation induction using conditioning media. These results confirm the differentiation capability of hADSCs to the epithelial cell lineage under certain circumstances, as previously suggested [57,58]. Previous results published by our group demonstrated that these cells, which can be harvested autologously, can be differentiated ex vivo using conditioning media, although differentiation is not complete ex vivo and the in vivo environment is required for terminal differentiation [58]. Interestingly, hADSCs were already used to efficiently recellularize acellular scaffolds obtained from human corneas [59]. Future studies should be carried out on animal models to determine if these cells are able to fully differentiate into epithelial cells upon in vivo induction, as demonstrated for the skin and oral mucosa [58,60]. Moreover, additional research is in need to fully characterize the cells grown on the decellularized scaffolds to determine their exact phenotype. Specifically, immunostaining with the Ki-67 proliferation marker and labeling with BrdU should determine the proliferation potential of these cells, whereas co-staining with limbal stem cell markers such as ABCG2, p63, and cytokeratin 15 should demonstrate their stem cell identity [61].

One of the main factors influencing epithelial cell attachment is the basement membrane. Evaluation of this structure showed that two of its major components—laminin and collagen IV—were detectable in RLs from day 14 onward, suggesting that an incipient basement membrane was formed between the scaffold and the cells seeded on top. The fact that RLs containing SIRC were negative for laminin could be explained by the fact that the anti-laminin antibody used in this work was specific anti-human.

In addition, the quantification of two key components of the limbus ECM revealed that RLs containing SIRC cells had adequate collagen fibers and proteoglycans—in terms of staining intensity—although the area fraction was not comparable to controls. The fact that SIRC cells are already committed to the limbal phenotype, whereas hADSCs are much more undifferentiated, may explain these findings. Despite its effect on collagen and proteoglycans quantification likely being very low or negligible, it is also possible that ECM components found in RLs may be affected by tissue functionalization with serum.

The present work has several limitations. The first one is the need of carrying out additional analyses, such as a biochemical analysis, to confirm the histological, histochemical, and immunohistochemical results showed here, as well as extensive analysis of tissue transparency after decellularization and recellularization. Furthermore, DLs should be analyzed using transmission electron microscopy techniques to determine if the limbal crypts are intact after the decellularization process. In addition, DLs should be recellularized with human primary limbal stem cells, and the expression of relevant stem cell markers should be assessed in these cells such as specific limbal stem cell markers and cell proliferation markers, to determine the real potential of the decellularized scaffolds. Future analyses should address all these issues.

In summary, the preliminary results obtained in the present work demonstrated that the porcine cornea limbus can be efficiently decellularized using the protocols described here, and that recellularization with epithelial or mesenchymal cells allows the successful generation of RLs with potential clinical usefulness. Future experiments in animal models should determine the in vivo usefulness of these limbal substitutes. Among their possible clinical applications, the limbal substitutes described here could be used as advanced therapies and medicinal products in patients with severe structural alteration of the limbus and loss of the micro-niche of the limbal stem cells.

5. Patents

MCM and MA are coauthors of patent application number PCT/ES2020/070168, "decellularized limbus".

Supplementary Materials: The following are available online at https://www.mdpi.com/article/10.3390/pharmaceutics13101718/s1, Table S1: Preliminary analysis of light transmittance at three different wavelengths (400, 550 and 700 nm) as determined by spectrophotometric analysis of human native limbus (HCTR) and RL decellularized with SIRC and hADSC cells at days 7, 14 and 21 of follow-up. Values correspond to percentages of transmittance using the values obtained in HCTR as reference (100% transmittance).

Author Contributions: Conceptualization, D.S.-P., M.A., C.G.-G. and M.C.-M.; methodology, V.C., F.C. and I.G.; formal analysis, M.A. and D.S.-P.; investigation, D.S.-P. and M.C.-M.; resources, Ó.D.G.-G.; writing—original draft preparation, D.S.-P.; writing—review and editing, M.A., I.G., V.C. and M.C.-M. All authors have read and agreed to the published version of the manuscript.

Funding: This work was supported by the Spanish Plan Nacional de Investigación Científica, Desarrollo e Innovación Tecnológica (I+D+i) of the Spanish Ministry of Economy and Competitiveness (Instituto de Salud Carlos III), Grants FIS PI20/0317 and ICI21-00010, cofinanced by FEDER funds (European Union). This work was also supported by grant PI-0086-2020 from Consejería de Salud y Familias, Junta de Andalucía, Spain, and grant B-CTS-504-UGR20 (Proyectos de I+D+i en el marco del Programa Operativo FEDER Andalucía 2014–2020) from the University of Granada, Consejería de Transformación Económica, Industria, Conocimiento y Universidades, Junta de Andalucía, and European Union (cofinanced by FEDER funds).

Institutional Review Board Statement: The study was conducted according to the guidelines of the Declaration of Helsinki and approved by the Institutional Ethics Committee of the Province of Granada (Comité Ético de Investigación, CEIM/CEI), refs. [10,20], date of approval 9 December 2020.

Informed Consent Statement: Informed consent was obtained from all subjects involved in the study.

Data Availability Statement: The data presented in this study are available on request from the corresponding authors.

Acknowledgments: Authors are thankful for the technical assistance provided by Fabiola Bermejo-Casares and Paloma de la Cueva Batanero. Results of this work could be part of the PhD dissertation of Óscar-Darío García-García.

Conflicts of Interest: The authors declare no conflict of interest. The funders had no role in the design of the study; in the collection, analyses, or interpretation of data; in the writing of the manuscript, or in the decision to publish the results.

References

1. Jhanji, V.; Billig, I.; Yam, G.H.-F. Cell-Free Biological Approach for Corneal Stromal Wound Healing. *Front. Pharmacol.* **2021**, *12*, 671405. [CrossRef]
2. Gain, P.; Jullienne, R.; He, Z.; Aldossary, M.; Acquart, S.; Cognasse, F.; Thuret, G. Global Survey of Corneal Transplantation and Eye Banking. *JAMA Ophthalmol.* **2016**, *134*, 167–173. [CrossRef]
3. Bremond-Gignac, D.; Copin, H.; Benkhalifa, M. Corneal epithelial stem cells for corneal injury. *Expert Opin. Biol. Ther.* **2018**, *18*, 997–1003. [CrossRef] [PubMed]
4. Singh, A.; Sangwan, V.S. Mini-Review: Regenerating the Corneal Epithelium With Simple Limbal Epithelial Transplantation. *Front. Med.* **2021**, *8*, 673330. [CrossRef] [PubMed]
5. Figueiredo, F.; Glanville, J.; Arber, M.; Carr, E.; Rydevik, G.; Hogg, J.; Okonkwo, A.; Figueiredo, G.; Lako, M.; Whiter, F.; et al. A systematic review of cellular therapies for the treatment of limbal stem cell deficiency affecting one or both eyes. *Ocul. Surf.* **2021**, *20*, 48–61. [CrossRef] [PubMed]
6. Adil, M.T.; Henry, J.J. Understanding cornea epithelial stem cells and stem cell deficiency: Lessons learned using vertebrate model systems. *Genesis* **2021**, *59*, e23411. [CrossRef] [PubMed]
7. Miri, A.; Al-Deiri, B.; Dua, H.S. Long-term Outcomes of Autolimbal and Allolimbal Transplants. *Ophthalmology* **2010**, *117*, 1207–1213. [CrossRef] [PubMed]
8. Rama, P.; Matuska, S.; Paganoni, G.; Spinelli, A.; De Luca, M.; Pellegrini, G. Limbal Stem-Cell Therapy and Long-Term Corneal Regeneration. *N. Engl. J. Med.* **2010**, *363*, 147–155. [CrossRef] [PubMed]
9. Galindo, S.; de la Mata, A.; López-Paniagua, M.; Herreras, J.M.; Pérez, I.; Calonge, M.; Nieto-Miguel, T. Subconjunctival injection of mesenchymal stem cells for corneal failure due to limbal stem cell deficiency: State of the art. *Stem Cell Res. Ther.* **2021**, *12*, 60. [CrossRef]
10. Deng, S.X.; Kruse, F.; Gomes, J.A.P.; Chan, C.C.; Daya, S.; Dana, R.; Figueiredo, F.C.; Kinoshita, S.; Rama, P.; Sangwan, V.; et al. Global Consensus on the Management of Limbal Stem Cell Deficiency. *Cornea* **2020**, *39*, 1291–1302. [CrossRef]
11. Shafiq, M.A.; Milani, B.Y.; Djalilian, A.R. In Vivo Evaluation of a Decellularized Limbal Graft for Limbal Reconstruction. *Int. J. Tissue Eng.* **2014**, *2014*, e754245. [CrossRef]
12. Nishida, K.; Yamato, M.; Hayashida, Y.; Watanabe, K.; Yamamoto, K.; Adachi, E.; Nagai, S.; Kikuchi, A.; Maeda, N.; Watanabe, H.; et al. Corneal Reconstruction with Tissue-Engineered Cell Sheets Composed of Autologous Oral Mucosal Epithelium. *N. Engl. J. Med.* **2004**, *351*, 1187–1196. [CrossRef]
13. Arenas-Herrera, J.E.; Ko, I.K.; Atala, A.; Yoo, J.J. Decellularization for whole organ bioengineering. *Biomed. Mater.* **2013**, *8*, 014106. [CrossRef]
14. Ng, W.L.; Chua, C.K.; Shen, Y.-F. Print Me an Organ! Why We Are Not There Yet. *Prog. Polym. Sci.* **2019**, *97*, 101145. [CrossRef]
15. Lee, J.M.; Ng, W.L.; Yeong, W.Y. Resolution and shape in bioprinting: Strategizing towards complex tissue and organ printing. *Appl. Phys. Rev.* **2019**, *6*, 011307. [CrossRef]
16. Melchels, F.; Barradas, A.; van Blitterswijk, C.; de Boer, J.; Feijen, J.; Grijpma, D.W. Effects of the architecture of tissue engineering scaffolds on cell seeding and culturing. *Acta Biomater.* **2010**, *6*, 4208–4217. [CrossRef] [PubMed]
17. Melchels, F.; Tonnarelli, B.; Olivares, A.L.; Martin, I.; Lacroix, D.; Feijen, J.; Wendt, D.J.; Grijpma, D.W. The influence of the scaffold design on the distribution of adhering cells after perfusion cell seeding. *Biomaterials* **2011**, *32*, 2878–2884. [CrossRef]
18. Khosravimelal, S.; Mobaraki, M.; Eftekhari, S.; Ahearne, M.; Seifalian, A.M.; Gholipourmalekabadi, M. Hydrogels as Emerging Materials for Cornea Wound Healing. *Small* **2021**, *17*, e2006335. [CrossRef]
19. Guérin, L.-P.; Le-Bel, G.; Desjardins, P.; Couture, C.; Gillard, E.; Boisselier, E.; Bazin, R.; Germain, L.; Guérin, S. The Human Tissue-Engineered Cornea (hTEC): Recent Progress. *Int. J. Mol. Sci.* **2021**, *22*, 1291. [CrossRef]
20. Rico-Sánchez, L.; Garzón, I.; González-Andrades, M.; Ruíz-García, A.; Punzano, M.; Lizana-Moreno, A.; Muñoz-Ávila, J.I.; Sánchez-Quevedo, M.D.C.; Martínez-Atienza, J.; Lopez-Navas, L.; et al. Successful development and clinical translation of a novel anterior lamellar artificial cornea. *J. Tissue Eng. Regen. Med.* **2019**, *13*, 2142–2154. [CrossRef]
21. Andrades, M.G.; Mata, R.; González-Gallardo, M.D.C.; Medialdea, S.; Arias-Santiago, S.; Martinez-Atienza, J.; Ruiz-García, A.; Pérez-Fajardo, L.; Lizana-Moreno, A.; Garzón, I.; et al. A study protocol for a multicentre randomised clinical trial evaluating the safety and feasibility of a bioengineered human allogeneic nanostructured anterior cornea in patients with advanced corneal trophic ulcers refractory to conventional treatment. *BMJ Open* **2017**, *7*, e016487. [CrossRef]
22. Buznyk, O.; Pasyechnikova, N.; Islam, M.M.; Iakymenko, S.; Fagerholm, P.; Griffith, M. Bioengineered Corneas Grafted as Alternatives to Human Donor Corneas in Three High-Risk Patients. *Clin. Transl. Sci.* **2015**, *8*, 558–562. [CrossRef]
23. Saldin, L.T.; Cramer, M.C.; Velankar, S.S.; White, L.J.; Badylak, S.F. Extracellular matrix hydrogels from decellularized tissues: Structure and function. *Acta Biomater.* **2017**, *49*, 1–15. [CrossRef]
24. Yoon, C.H.; Choi, H.J.; Kim, M.K. Corneal xenotransplantation: Where are we standing? *Prog. Retin. Eye Res.* **2021**, *80*, 100876. [CrossRef] [PubMed]

25. Andrades, M.G.; Carriel, V.; Rivera-Izquierdo, M.; Garzón, I.; González-Andrades, E.; Medialdea, S.; Alaminos, M.; Campos, A. Effects of Detergent-Based Protocols on Decellularization of Corneas with Sclerocorneal Limbus. Evaluation of Regional Differences. *Transl. Vis. Sci. Technol.* **2015**, *4*, 13. [CrossRef] [PubMed]
26. Pang, K.; Du, L.; Wu, X. A rabbit anterior cornea replacement derived from acellular porcine cornea matrix, epithelial cells and keratocytes. *Biomaterials* **2010**, *31*, 7257–7265. [CrossRef] [PubMed]
27. Li, Q.; Wang, H.; Dai, Z.; Cao, Y.; Jin, C. Preparation and Biomechanical Properties of an Acellular Porcine Corneal Stroma. *Cornea* **2017**, *36*, 1343–1351. [CrossRef]
28. Isidan, A.; Liu, S.; Chen, A.M.; Zhang, W.; Li, P.; Smith, L.J.; Hara, H.; Cooper, D.K.C.; Ekser, B. Comparison of porcine corneal decellularization methods and importance of preserving corneal limbus through decellularization. *PLoS ONE* **2021**, *16*, e0243682. [CrossRef] [PubMed]
29. Zhang, M.-C.; Liu, X.; Jin, Y.; Jiang, D.-L.; Wei, X.-S.; Xie, H.-T. Lamellar Keratoplasty Treatment of Fungal Corneal Ulcers with Acellular Porcine Corneal Stroma. *Arab. Archaeol. Epigr.* **2015**, *15*, 1068–1075. [CrossRef]
30. Spaniol, K.; Witt, J.; Mertsch, S.; Borrelli, M.; Geerling, G.; Schrader, S. Generation and characterisation of decellularised human corneal limbus. *Graefe's Arch. Clin. Exp. Ophthalmol.* **2018**, *256*, 547–557. [CrossRef]
31. Seyed-Safi, A.G.; Daniels, J.T. The limbus: Structure and function. *Exp. Eye Res.* **2020**, *197*, 108074. [CrossRef]
32. Shortt, A.J.; Secker, G.A.; Munro, P.M.; Khaw, P.T.; Tuft, S.J.; Daniels, J.T. Characterization of the Limbal Epithelial Stem Cell Niche: Novel Imaging Techniques Permit In Vivo Observation and Targeted Biopsy of Limbal Epithelial Stem Cells. *Stem Cells* **2007**, *25*, 1402–1409. [CrossRef]
33. Galindo, S.; Herreras, J.M.; López-Paniagua, M.; Rey, E.; De La Mata, A.; Plata-Cordero, M.; Calonge, M.; Nieto-Miguel, T. Therapeutic Effect of Human Adipose Tissue-Derived Mesenchymal Stem Cells in Experimental Corneal Failure Due to Limbal Stem Cell Niche Damage. *Stem Cells* **2017**, *35*, 2160–2174. [CrossRef] [PubMed]
34. Zhang, L.; Coulson-Thomas, V.J.; Ferreira, T.G.; Kao, W.W.Y. Mesenchymal stem cells for treating ocular surface diseases. *BMC Ophthalmol.* **2015**, *15*, 155. [CrossRef] [PubMed]
35. Crapo, P.M.; Gilbert, T.; Badylak, S.F. An overview of tissue and whole organ decellularization processes. *Biomaterials* **2011**, *32*, 3233–3243. [CrossRef] [PubMed]
36. Philips, C.; Cornelissen, M.; Carriel, V. Evaluation methods as quality control in the generation of decellularized peripheral nerve allografts. *J. Neural Eng.* **2018**, *15*, 021003. [CrossRef]
37. Mailey, B.; Hosseini, A.; Baker, J.; Young, A.; Alfonso, Z.; Hicok, K.; Wallace, A.M.; Cohen, S.R. Adipose-Derived Stem Cells: Methods for Isolation and Applications for Clinical Use. *Methods Mol. Biol.* **2014**, *1210*, 161–181. [CrossRef]
38. El Soury, M.; García-García, D.; Moretti, M.; Perroteau, I.; Raimondo, S.; Lovati, A.; Carriel, V. Comparison of Decellularization Protocols to Generate Peripheral Nerve Grafts: A Study on Rat Sciatic Nerves. *Int. J. Mol. Sci.* **2021**, *22*, 2389. [CrossRef]
39. Garzón, I.; Jaimes-Parra, B.; Pascual-Geler, M.; Cózar, J.; Sánchez-Quevedo, M.; Mosquera-Pacheco, M.; Sánchez-Montesinos, I.; Fernández-Valadés, R.; Campos, F.; Alaminos, M. Biofabrication of a Tubular Model of Human Urothelial Mucosa Using Human Wharton Jelly Mesenchymal Stromal Cells. *Polymers* **2021**, *13*, 1568. [CrossRef]
40. Carriel, V.; Campos, A.; Alaminos, M.; Raimondo, S.; Geuna, S. Staining Methods for Normal and Regenerative Myelin in the Nervous System. *Methods Mol. Biol.* **2017**, *1560*, 207–218. [CrossRef]
41. Chato-Astrain, J.; Philips, C.; Campos, F.; Durand-Herrera, D.; García-García, O.D.; Roosens, A.; Alaminos, M.; Campos, A.; Carriel, V. Detergent-based decellularized peripheral nerve allografts: An in vivo preclinical study in the rat sciatic nerve injury model. *J. Tissue Eng. Regen. Med.* **2020**, *14*, 789–806. [CrossRef] [PubMed]
42. Drifka, C.R.; Loeffler, A.G.; Mathewson, K.; Mehta, G.; Keikhosravi, A.; Liu, Y.; Lemancik, S.; Ricke, W.; Weber, S.M.; Kao, W.J.; et al. Comparison of Picrosirius Red Staining With Second Harmonic Generation Imaging for the Quantification of Clinically Relevant Collagen Fiber Features in Histopathology Samples. *J. Histochem. Cytochem.* **2016**, *64*, 519–529. [CrossRef] [PubMed]
43. Oie, Y.; Komoto, S.; Kawasaki, R. Systematic review of clinical research on regenerative medicine for the cornea. *Jpn. J. Ophthalmol.* **2021**, *65*, 169–183. [CrossRef] [PubMed]
44. Tidu, A.; Schanne-Klein, M.-C.; Borderie, V.M. Development, structure, and bioengineering of the human corneal stroma: A review of collagen-based implants. *Exp. Eye Res.* **2020**, *200*, 108256. [CrossRef] [PubMed]
45. Notara, M.; Schrader, S.; Daniels, J.T. The Porcine Limbal Epithelial Stem Cell Niche as a New Model for the Study of Transplanted Tissue-Engineered Human Limbal Epithelial Cells. *Tissue Eng. Part A* **2011**, *17*, 741–750. [CrossRef]
46. Wong, M.L.; Griffiths, L.G. Immunogenicity in xenogeneic scaffold generation: Antigen removal vs. decellularization. *Acta Biomater.* **2014**, *10*, 1806–1816. [CrossRef] [PubMed]
47. Platt, J.; Disesa, V.; Gail, D.; Massicot-Fisher, J.; National Heart, Lung, and Blood Institute Heart and Lung Xenotransplantation Working Group. Recommendations of the National Heart, Lung, and Blood Institute Heart and Lung Xenotransplantation Working Group. *Circulation* **2002**, *106*, 1043–1047. [CrossRef]
48. Huang, M.; Li, N.; Wu, Z.; Wan, P.; Liang, X.; Zhang, W.; Wang, X.; Li, C.; Xiao, J.; Zhou, Q.; et al. Using acellular porcine limbal stroma for rabbit limbal stem cell microenvironment reconstruction. *Biomaterials* **2011**, *32*, 7812–7821. [CrossRef]
49. Murab, S.; Ghosh, S. Impact of osmoregulatory agents on the recovery of collagen conformation in decellularized corneas. *Biomed. Mater.* **2016**, *11*, 065005. [CrossRef]

50. Wang, M.; Cui, C.; Ibrahim, M.M.; Han, B.; Li, Q.; Pacifici, M.; Lawrence, J.T.R.; Han, L.; Han, L.-H. Regulating Mechanotransduction in Three Dimensions using Sub-Cellular Scale, Crosslinkable Fibers of Controlled Diameter, Stiffness, and Alignment. *Adv. Funct. Mater.* **2019**, *29*, 1808967. [CrossRef]
51. Jiang, Y.; Li, R.; Han, C.; Huang, L. Extracellular matrix grafts: From preparation to application (Review). *Int. J. Mol. Med.* **2021**, *47*, 463–474. [CrossRef] [PubMed]
52. Marin-Tapia, H.A.; Romero-Salazar, L.; Arteaga-Arcos, J.C.; Rosales-Ibáñez, R.; Mayorga-Rojas, M. Micro-mechanical properties of corneal scaffolds from two different bio-models obtained by an efficient chemical decellularization. *J. Mech. Behav. Biomed. Mater.* **2021**, *119*, 104510. [CrossRef] [PubMed]
53. Nieto-Miguel, T.; Galindo, S.; Reinoso, R.; Corell, A.; Martino, M.; Pérez-Simón, J.A.; Calonge, M. In VitroSimulation of Corneal Epithelium Microenvironment Induces a Corneal Epithelial-like Cell Phenotype from Human Adipose Tissue Mesenchymal Stem Cells. *Curr. Eye Res.* **2013**, *38*, 933–944. [CrossRef] [PubMed]
54. Garzon, I.; Chato-Astrain, J.; Campos, F.; Fernandez-Valades, R.; Sanchez-Montesinos, I.; Campos, A.; Alaminos, M.; D'Souza, R.N.; Martin-Piedra, M.A. Expanded Differentiation Capability of Human Wharton's Jelly Stem Cells Toward Pluripotency: A Systematic Review. *Tissue Eng. Part B Rev.* **2020**, *26*, 301–312. [CrossRef] [PubMed]
55. Mateos-Timoneda, M.A.; Levato, R.; Puñet, X.; Cano, I.; Castano, O.; Engel, E. Biofunctionalization of Polymeric Surfaces. In Proceedings of the 2015 37th Annual International Conference of the IEEE Engineering in Medicine and Biology Society (EMBC), Milan, Italy, 25–29 August 2015; pp. 1745–1748.
56. Olivieri, M.; Cristaldi, M.; Pezzino, S.; Rusciano, D.; Tomasello, B.; Anfuso, C.D.; Lupo, G. Phenotypic characterization of the SIRC (Statens Seruminstitut Rabbit Cornea) cell line reveals a mixed epithelial and fibroblastic nature. *Exp. Eye Res.* **2018**, *172*, 123–127. [CrossRef] [PubMed]
57. Bandeira, F.; Goh, T.-W.; Setiawan, M.; Yam, G.H.-F.; Mehta, J.S. Cellular therapy of corneal epithelial defect by adipose mesenchymal stem cell-derived epithelial progenitors. *Stem Cell Res. Ther.* **2020**, *11*, 14. [CrossRef]
58. Martin-Piedra, M.; Alfonso-Rodriguez, C.; Zapater, A.; Durand-Herrera, D.; Chato-Astrain, J.; Campos, F.; Sanchez-Quevedo, M.; Alamino, M.; Garzon, I. Effective use of mesenchymal stem cells in human skin substitutes generated by tissue engineering. *Eur. Cells Mater.* **2019**, *37*, 233–249. [CrossRef]
59. del Barrio, J.L.A.; Chiesa, M.; Garagorri, N.; Garcia-Urquia, N.; Fernandez-Delgado, J.; Bataille, L.; Rodriguez, A.; Arnalich-Montiel, F.; Zarnowski, T.; de Toledo, J.P.; et al. Acellular human corneal matrix sheets seeded with human adipose-derived mesenchymal stem cells integrate functionally in an experimental animal model. *Exp. Eye Res.* **2015**, *132*, 91–100. [CrossRef]
60. Garzón, I.; Miyake, J.; González-Andrades, M.; Carmona, R.; Carda, C.; Sánchez-Quevedo, M.D.C.; Campos, A.; Alaminos, M. Wharton's Jelly Stem Cells: A Novel Cell Source for Oral Mucosa and Skin Epithelia Regeneration. *Stem Cells Transl. Med.* **2013**, *2*, 625–632. [CrossRef]
61. Tsai, R.J.-F.; Tsai, R.Y.-N. Ex Vivo Expansion of Corneal Stem Cells on Amniotic Membrane and Their Outcome. *Eye Contact Lens* **2010**, *36*, 305–309. [CrossRef]

MDPI
St. Alban-Anlage 66
4052 Basel
Switzerland
Tel. +41 61 683 77 34
Fax +41 61 302 89 18
www.mdpi.com

Pharmaceutics Editorial Office
E-mail: pharmaceutics@mdpi.com
www.mdpi.com/journal/pharmaceutics

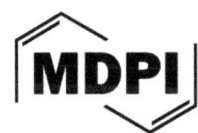

www.ingramcontent.com/pod-product-compliance
Lightning Source LLC
LaVergne TN
LVHW070409100526
838202LV00014B/1424